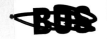

Natural Medicine
First Aid Remedies

Natural Medicine First Aid Remedies

SELF-CARE TREATMENTS FOR 100+ COMMON CONDITIONS

STEPHANIE MAROHN

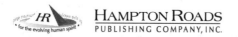

HAMPTON ROADS
PUBLISHING COMPANY, INC.

Cover design by Steve Amarillo
Cover art by Corbis Images
Illustrations by Anne L. Dunn

Hampton Roads Publishing Company, Inc.
1125 Stoney Ridge Road
Charlottesville, VA 22902

434-296-2772
fax: 434-296-5096
e-mail: hrpc@hrpub.com
www.hrpub.com

If you are unable to order this book from your local
bookseller, you may order directly from the publisher.
Call 1-800-766-8009, toll-free.

Library of Congress Catalog Card Number: 2001091197
ISBN 1-57174-218-2
10 9 8 7 6 5 4 3 2 1
Printed on acid-free paper in Canada

Disclaimer

The information in this book is not intended to replace the medical advice of the reader's own healthcare practitioner or to contradict the medical or surgical decisions regarding any ailment of the reader by his or her physician of choice. Herbs, supplements, and other therapies included in this book produce varying effects depending on the person, which reflects the inherent individualized property of natural medicine. The author and publisher disclaim responsibility for how you choose to employ the information in this book and the results or consequences of any of the treatments covered.

Acknowledgments

My deep gratitude to all the practitioners who contributed protocols to this book. I am so admiring of the fine work you are doing in the world. Thank you all for the time and energy you generously gave to this project, and for your willingness to share your expertise. It was a pleasure meeting you, whether by phone, e-mail, or in person.

Special thanks to Patricia Kaminski, who contributed all the flower essence protocols in the book, based on the vast clinical research she and Richard Katz have conducted through the Flower Essence Society. Thank you, too, Patricia, for your feedback along the way and the whiffs of mountain air in your e-mails.

Special thanks also to Katrina Raphaell, who contributed the majority of the stone/crystal protocols. You are a true gem, Katrina, in the most magical and powerful sense of the word.

My appreciation to Robyn Klein for putting me in touch with a network of truly inspired herbalists.

Great thanks and mea culpa salaams to my friends for their understanding of my unavailability and forgetfulness of important occasions during the white heat of writing this book.

Thank you to Nancy Gallenson, whose fabulous ballet classes provide a body and soul antidote to long hours at the computer.

My gratitude to Hampton Roads for their vision and mission in publishing. I am honored to be part of the family.

And the final thanks go to my brilliant friend and editor Richard Leviton, who never fails to inspire me in multiple realms.

Contents

Part III: About the Therapies

Introduction

Natural medicine first aid may be the first or the last natural therapy people use, depending on whether they arrive at its use in an inductive or deductive fashion. Some people find their way to alternative medicine through the safe and effective remedies it has to offer for minor, everyday health ailments. Struck by how well it works, these people often begin to investigate the use of alternative therapies for more serious health conditions. Teething is a good example of this process. It has brought more people to homeopathy than any other condition, as a homeopathic physician who contributed to this book states. Because homeopathic remedies work to ease the process of teething, highly pleased parents then take a closer look at the therapy that produced this minor miracle. Homeopathy is just one of the therapies included in this book that wins converts by the efficacy of its simple remedies.

Conversely, other people find their way to alternative medicine through a serious illness, in many cases, unfortunately, using it as the last resort. Even for patients who seek natural therapy only when their conditions are advanced or entrenched, the results are frequently impressive. People who have this experience often come to rely on alternative medicine for most of their health problems. But natural first aid may be the last bastion of care. People are used to popping an antacid when they have heartburn or spraying a synthetic antibacterial spray on a child's cut. While they will avoid the big guns of conventional medicine, they consider the minor remedies harmless, if they consider the matter at all.

There are two problems with this approach. One is that conventional over-the-counter remedies for minor health ailments are, for the most part, chemical based or contain chemical additives. We all ingest, inhale, or are exposed to hundreds of chemicals simply by living our lives in today's world—chemicals in our food, air, and water, in cleaning and other household products, in office equipment, even in furnishings at home and at work. Chemical toxins accumulate in our bodies over our lifetime, and our immune and other systems struggle to cope with the toxic load. In the interests of our health, it behooves us to try to cut down the load wherever we can. There is no need for any of us to be using chemical medicines when natural medicines work so well. First aid is one area where you can avoid the chemicals.

The second problem with relying on conventional medicine for minor ailments is that conventional remedies work by suppressing symptoms and have few if any healing effects. While antibacterial spray might keep your cut from getting infected, it won't do anything to help it heal. Why not use an essential oil or herbal preparation that does both (and contains no chemicals)?

The suppression of symptoms has a more serious impact when it comes to noninjury ailments. Alternative medicine is based on a holistic view of the body, meaning that the body is regarded as a whole, as a unit of interrelated parts and systems, and treatment addresses the whole body rather than focusing on symptoms. According to alternative medicine (and clinical evidence supports this view), suppression of symptoms (as with the use of antibiotics, for example) drives the illness deeper into the body, where it may produce a more serious condition. So instead of suppressing symptoms, natural medicine relieves discomfort while aiding the body in correcting the underlying imbalance that produced the symptoms in the first place. As an example, one remedy for hemorrhoids is the herb red root, which has long been used to clear lymphatic congestion. The connection? A stagnant lymph system is often a factor in the development of hemorrhoids.

If you are in the category of those who use alternative medicine for the big stuff, but reach for the ibuprofen when you have a muscle ache, you might want to reconsider, based on the above points. If you are someone who has never used natural medicine, first aid is a great introduction. After all, the stakes are low—what do you really have to lose?

The term "first aid" as I am employing it goes far beyond first aid as most people think of it—emergency medicine for accidents or injuries. Obviously, when you look at the table of contents for this book, you see that most of the ailments listed don't fall into the category of accident or injury. The conditions I include are common ailments that can benefit from self-care as the first line of treatment. The remedies offered here can be the first aid you turn to, if you will. Perhaps that was the original meaning of the term. This is not to say the remedies should be regarded as a replacement for medical care. Some of the conditions in this book require consultation with a qualified health practitioner.

In some instances, the remedies can provide relief until you can get to the doctor for more comprehensive treatment. In other instances, they may be all you need to resolve your ailment. Even with conditions such as psoriasis or edema, which tend to indicate a deeper problem, the remedies may be sufficient, since they have healing as well as symptom-relieving properties. In still other instances, you might discover that your health problem requires further treatment. You have a flu that you just can't shake or a urinary tract infection that won't go away. Or your psoriasis recurs every time you stop using the remedies. If that is the case, you need to seek medical help to determine the causes behind the intractability of your ailment and pursue deeper treatment.

You may want to consider consulting a practitioner of one or more of the therapies covered in this book. While these therapies can be quite effective when used for first aid, this is kindergarten activity compared to what they are capable of. As one practitioner I interviewed put it, "Asking a homeopath for first aid remedies is like asking a physicist to do a division problem for you." As holistic therapies, they can effect profound healing on all levels—physical, emotional, psychological, and spiritual. You may notice results in these areas from the remedies offered here.

Here are a few points on using this book:

Part I covers the basic items to stock in your natural medicine chest or first aid kit. They are the natural remedies that leading alternative medicine practitioners consider most important to include. Consider this simply a template. As you use the remedies throughout the book, you will discover which ones you use most often and which work best for you.

Part II is the A-to-Z of common ailments, with protocols in eight different therapies for treatment to choose from: essential oils, flower essences, food therapy, herbal medicine, homeopathy, nutritional supplements, reflexology, and stone/crystal therapy. You can use one or combine several to treat a given ailment. The therapies complement each other. In some cases, practitioners offer combination protocols. Many alternative medicine practitioners contributed protocols to this book. The protocols that are not footnoted are based on personal interviews with these doctors and other healers.

Unless otherwise specified, the dosage amounts cited throughout part 2 are calculated for the average 150-pound adult. To convert the dosages for children, reduce the amount of the individual dose in proportion to their weight. The frequency of dosage stays the same, unless noted otherwise. A child weighing seventy-five pounds, for example, would take 250 milligrams of vitamin C three times daily if the amount listed for an adult is 500 milligrams three times daily.

If full instructions for a therapy protocol do not appear under a given condition, consult the section on that therapy in part 3 of the book, where the therapies and directions for their use are explained in detail. For example, the reflexology entry for each condition in part 2 simply indicates what point to stimulate on the foot. Turn to the reflexology section in part 3 for instructions on how to do that.

A final word:

May you not have to use this book often, and when you do, may the remedies heal you quickly.

Part I
The Top Natural
First Aid Remedies

The Top Ten Natural Medicine First Aid Remedies

Based on a survey of natural medicine literature and the practitioners who contributed protocols to this book, here are the top ten remedies, runners-up, and honorable mentions for a natural medicine chest or first aid kit. These remedies are the basics for safe, effective, natural treatment of common ailments at home, at work, and during travel. As you use protocols in the eight different therapies presented throughout this book, you will likely discover many other remedies that you want to include in your natural medicine apothecary.

1. Arnica

Arnica (*Arnica montana*) reduces swelling, stiffness, pain, and bruising. Stock both oral homeopathic Arnica (30c pellets) and topical ointment (arnica gel or homeopathic arnica ointment) to treat sore muscles, back pain, joint pain, sprains and strains, torn ligaments, and bruises.

2. Five Flower Formula (Rescue Remedy)

A flower essence formula indicated for physical and/or emotional trauma or shock, it brings immediate calm and emotional neutralizing. The five flower essences in this formula are Rock Rose, Clematis, Impatiens, Cherry Plum, and Star of Bethlehem.

3. Echinacea Tincture

An all-purpose internal and external antibiotic, echinacea (*Echinacea angustifolia, E. purpurea, E. spp.* [several species]) tincture can be used to clean wounds, support immunity, prevent a cold from coming on when taken at the first sign of symptoms, and treat flu and other infections, rashes, and fever blisters. You can also use echinacea internally and externally to treat snakebite; it has a long tradition of use for this purpose in Native American herbal medicine.

4. Healing Herbal Salve

A salve containing some combination of the herbs calendula (*Calendula officinalis*), comfrey (*Symphytum officinale*), and/or St. John's wort (*Hypericum perforatum*) can be applied to sores, cuts, scrapes, burns, or other skin injury as a disinfectant, to soothe the area, and to speed tissue repair. Calendula is antimicrobial, and comfrey has a remarkable ability to promote cell growth and close over a wound (for this reason, you shouldn't use comfrey on a puncture wound). Some salves include Lavender essential oil in the mix.

5. Lavender Essential Oil

An antiseptic, bactericidal, decongestant, analgesic (pain reliever), and sedative, Lavender essential oil has broad application. It can be used topically to treat burns, sunburn, insect bites and stings, and muscle aches and pains. Inhaled or applied topically, Lavender can relieve headaches (combine with Peppermint essential oil for extra headache-relieving benefits), reduce stress and jet lag, and promote relaxation. It is also an insect repellant.

6. Tea Tree Essential Oil

A powerful antiseptic and broad-spectrum antimicrobial, Tea Tree (*Melaleuca alternifolia*) essential oil (also known as Ti-Tree) can be used as a topical treatment for cuts, scrapes, burns, cold sores, acne, and fungal or bacterial infections. Equal parts of Tea Tree and Lavender essential oils make an excellent topical antiseptic and antibacterial solution.

7. Peppermint

You may want to stock both peppermint (*Mentha piperata*) tincture and essential oil. The tincture can be taken orally, while the essential oil can be inhaled, as treatment for headaches and digestive complaints such as indigestion, gas, nausea, and motion sickness. Peppermint also has antimicrobial and antiviral properties. Peppermint essential oil is a good insect repellent. Lavender and Peppermint essential oils work well in combination, enhancing each other's effects.

8. Aloe Vera Gel

Aloe vera gel is highly soothing and healing for burns, sunburn, rashes, and insect bites and stings. It can also be used for chapped lips and to soften rough skin. The gel fresh from the plant is best, so for your natural medicine chest at home you can keep the houseplant on hand. Buy a high-quality gel for your travel first aid kit.

9. Activated Charcoal

Activated charcoal binds with toxins and bacteria and escorts them out of the body, which makes it an excellent remedy for food poisoning and diarrhea. In fact, charcoal has a long history of use not only for food poisoning, but for poisoning by deadly substances as well. It is not, however, a replacement for medical care when poison has been ingested. Activated charcoal is the pharmaceutical equivalent of the scrapings from burnt toast, and is widely available in drugstores and health food stores.

10. Homeopathic Belladonna

While there are many homeopathic remedies for fever, depending on the characteristics of the individual case, Belladonna is a common one. It is indicated for a fever with a sudden onset, flushed face, restlessness, and a pounding pulse. The fever may be accompanied by sore throat, cough, headache, or earache. Stock Belladonna 30c pellets.

Natural Medicine Runners-Up

The following five remedies were not cited as often as the ten listed above, but came in close behind.

11. *Cayenne Capsules*

Cayenne (*Capsicum minimum*) powder can be used to stop bleeding, improve digestion, stimulate the appetite, relieve gas, and help sweat out a cold or bronchitis. Cayenne also has pain-relieving properties, due to its active constituent capsaicin. You can mix the powder into a lotion or oil and massage into sore muscles or joints to ease aches and pains.

12. *Ginger*

Stock ginger capsules for motion sickness, nausea, stomachaches or other digestive problems, and sore throats. Ginger can also help sweat out a fever. The capsules can be swallowed as is or broken open to make a tea. You may want to keep some candied ginger on hand as well, as nibbling on a piece while traveling in a car or other moving vehicle can help prevent motion sickness.

13. Homeopathic Apis

This remedy is indicated for bee stings or other insect bites charactized by red swelling and stinging pain, and for conditions with hot, red swelling, such as hives and skin irritations. Stock Apis 30c pellets.

14. Eucalyptus Essential Oil

This essential oil (*Eucalyptus radiata*) is an antiseptic, decongestant, expectorant (loosens phlegm), anti-inflammatory, antiviral, and antibacterial agent. It can be used as an inhalant to clear sinus congestion, colds, coughs, and other respiratory ailments. Added to a lotion and applied topically, it can ease muscle and joint aches and pains.

15. *St. John's Wort Tincture*

St. John's wort (*Hypericum perforatum*) is another herb that has a wide range of uses. Although it is perhaps most commonly known for its antidepressant qualities, it is equally effective as an antiviral and anti-inflammatory and in speeding tissue repair. It is useful for sprains, bruises, swelling, cuts and other wounds, and insect bites and stings. The tincture or the oral homeopathic remedy Hypericum can also alleviate neuralgic (nerve) pain, and is indicated for shooting pain, such as that experienced when you shut your fingers in a door or drop something heavy on your toes.

Honorable Mentions

Witch hazel and hydrogen peroxide (3 percent H_2O_2) are good additions to a home medicine chest or first aid kit. They make excellent disinfectants for cuts, sores, and wounds, and have healing properties as well. Use them rather than rubbing alcohol, which should be avoided as it contains toxic denaturants (substances added to alter the alcohol) that only contribute to the body's toxic load.

Witch hazel is a distilled extract of the bark of the bush or small tree witch hazel (*Hamamelis virginiana*). Alcohol is used to preserve the extract, but you can get alcohol-free witch hazel. Witch hazel has been a home remedy for over a hundred years, and is widely available in drugstores and supermarkets. As a healing agent, it is an astringent, which means it tightens tissue, reduces secretions, and checks inflammation. Witch hazel can be used to stop bleeding, reduce the inflammation of bruises and other injuries, and heal burns and rashes.

Hydrogen peroxide provides a form of oxygen therapy, flooding tissues with healing oxygen and killing bacteria in the process. The foaming you see when you pour hydrogen peroxide on a cut is the oxygen at work. Due to its lack of toxicity, it can be used directly on mucous membranes, such as the lining of the mouth. Diluted and used as a mouthwash, it can help heal mouth and gum tissues.

Part II
Natural Medicine
First Aid Remedies for
102 Common Conditions

Abscess

 See Also   Bacterial Infection
Boil
Dental Abscess, for an abscess in the gums

An abscess is a collection or pocket of pus in a cavity formed by disintegrating tissue and surrounded by inflamed tissue. Pus itself is a product of inflammation, accumulating where infection is present. Abscesses can arise in any part of the body, but occur most often in the skin. Bacteria are frequently the source of the infection, but other microorganisms or an injury can also cause abscesses. Recurrent abscesses can be an indication of weakened immunity or toxicity in the system.

Symptoms include swelling, heat, redness, and throbbing of the affected area. The abscess increases in size as it fills with pus, and decreases when the pus is drained. If untreated, the abscess can spread, resulting in the formation of other abscesses, or the tissue can become fibrous, leaving a lump. A red line extending from the abscess is a sign of blood poisoning; seek medical care immediately.

Essential Oils

Chamomile, Lavender, and Tea Tree (*Melaleuca alternifolia*) are "the most effective oils for treating an abscess," says Patricia Davis, founder of the London School of Aromatherapy. They can be used singly or in combination. Put a few drops on a hot compress and place it over the abscess to draw out the infection and reduce the pain and inflammation. Leave the compress on until it cools. Repeat as needed.[1]

Flower Essences

Patricia Kaminski, an herbalist and flower essence therapist from Nevada City, California, recommends Self-Heal, used both topically and internally. For topical treatment, apply the flower essence and/or flower essence cream directly on the abscess 2–4 times daily. To speed healing, take 4 drops of the flower essence under the tongue 2–4 times daily. Continue treatment until the abscess is resolved.

Food Therapy

Eat:

Garlic, kelp, yogurt/kefir, pineapple (eat it by itself), foods high in vitamin A and beta-carotene. (For a list of foods containing these nutrients, see part 3, "Food Therapy," p. 374.)

Avoid:

Sugar (including fruit and fruit juice), simple carbohydrates such as white flour and white rice, and fried foods.

Herbal Medicine

Antibacterial herbs can be effective in resolving bacterial abscesses, including those caused by staph (*Staphylococcus* bacteria), says David Winston, A.H.G., a clinical herbalist and consultant from Washington, New Jersey. He suggests the following applications, which can also be used for boils.

Poultices: To open and drain an abscess that is red, hot, and inflamed, use one of the following poultices.

• Flaxseed: Put 2 tablespoons of flaxseed in a piece of cheesecloth and pour boiled water over/through it. The flaxseed will become gelatinous. When it is cool enough to apply to the skin without burning, spread it on the abscess and leave it on until it is cold. Do this twice daily for as long as necessary.

• Burdock (*Arctium lappa*) leaf: Put fresh burdock leaves in a blender with enough water to make a paste. Apply to the abscess and reapply when it dries out. Do this twice daily for as long as needed.

Topical antibacterial: You can use one or a combination of the following for as long as needed.

• Oregon grape (*Berberis aquifolium*) root: Make a decoction by putting 2 teaspoons of the herb in 1 cup of boiling water. Cover, simmer for 15–20 minutes, and steep for another 20 minutes. Soak a cloth with the decoction and lay it on the abscess. Wrap gauze around it and leave it on all day. Alternatively, you can use a tincture of Oregon grape root, but it can be painful to put that on an open abscess because of the alcohol in tinctures. Note: Oregon grape root will stain clothing yellow.

• Echinacea (*E. spp.*): Crush up the fresh root and add water to make a paste that resembles applesauce in consistency. Put it on the abscess, with a bandage on top of that so you can leave it on all day.

• St. John's wort (*Hypericum perforatum*) infused oil: This is known as hypericum oil, but the product label may read St. John's wort olive oil extract. Note that an infused oil is distinct from an essential oil or herbal tincture. It is the herb in a carrier oil such as olive oil, rather than an extract or an essential oil preserved in alcohol or glycerin. Dab the infused oil on the abscess 2–4 times daily, and cover with an adhesive bandage.

Homeopathy

Homeopathic physician Michael G. Carlston, M.D., of Santa Rosa, California, recommends the following remedies:

If the skin abscess is lingering, feels better with warmth, but does not produce much pain, use Silica *(Silicea)* 6c, 12c, or 30c. During the acute stage, take 2 or 3 pellets, or a couple of drops if taking in drop form, 2 to 3 times per day. You may need to take it for a week, but let your symptoms guide you. As they lessen, reduce the frequency of dosage. Don't keep taking the remedy when the abscess is gone.

If the abscess feels better with warmth but is painful, take Hepar sulphuris calcareum 6c, 12c, or 30c. It is likely that you'll need to take it 4 times a day. Again, let your symptoms be your guide. Reduce the frequency as your symptoms abate, and stop taking the remedy when the condition is resolved.

Nutritional Supplements

In addition to taking a multivitamin/mineral as a general practice, taking zinc, vitamin C, and vitamin A can help prevent the abscess from becoming a systemic infection, says Kathi Head, N.D., a naturopathic physician from Sandpoint, Idaho. Take 30 mg of zinc twice daily and 1,000 mg of vitamin C 3 times daily for a week or so. The dosage for vitamin A is 25,000 IU twice daily, but take it only for a week, and do not take it if you have any liver problems.

Reflexology

Treat the area of the foot corresponding to the part of the body where the abscess is located.

Stone/Crystal Therapy

For an abscess, use petrified palm, states Melody, author of the crystal reference series *Love Is in the Earth*. With hypoallergenic tape, secure the stone on or near the abscess, and leave it on for 2–3 days, until the condition is resolved.

Other Remedies

Applying warm compresses can ease the pain and swelling of a skin abscess, and speed drainage.

Putting a charcoal poultice on the abscess to draw out the infection works really well, says Dr. Head. Use activated charcoal powder or crush tablets and mix with hot water to make a paste. Put it on the abscess and cover with gauze. Alternate the charcoal poultice with a poultice made from the powder of Oregon grape or other berberine-containing herb (barberry, *Berberis vulgaris*, or goldenseal, *Hydrastis canadensis*) mixed with hot water. Berberine has antibiotic effects. By alternating the charcoal and the herb poultice, you both draw out and fight infection. Apply a new poultice 2–3 times daily. Continue the applications for a few days.

Acne

Acne is an inflammatory disease of the skin in which the sebaceous (oil-secreting) glands and hair follicles become infected, manifesting as blackheads, papules (red bumps), and/or pustules (pus- or lymph-filled bumps, or whiteheads). Common areas of acne eruption are the face, chest, back, and shoulders. Severe cases of acne can lead to scarring.

Acne is most associated with the increased hormonal activity of puberty, which increases the size and activity of the sebaceous glands. The elevated production of sebum (the fatty secretion that lubricates the skin) can cause the glands and follicles to become clogged, leading to inflammation and the eruption of acne. Similarly, the hormonal changes of pregnancy, menstruation, and menopause can produce brief flare-ups of acne, as can stress. Toxic buildup in the intestines can also be a factor.[1]

Essential Oils

Dab Lavender or Tea Tree (*Melaleuca alternifolia*) essential oil on pimples, says Mindy Green, A.H.G., M.S., an herbalist from Boulder, Colorado. Both are antibacterial and can help resolve a blemish quickly.

Flower Essences

For acne, take Crab Apple and Pretty Face essences, says Richard Katz, founder of the Flower Essence Society. Take 4 drops of each 2–4 times daily, or more often during acute episodes. You can also add the two essences to a base of Self-Heal cream (6–10 drops of each essence per 1 ounce of cream), and apply them topically, as needed. In extreme cases, induced by pronounced psychological stress, add Glassy Hyacinth and Star of Bethlehem to the protocol, in the same amounts as the other essences.

Food Therapy

Eat:

Fiber, raw and steamed vegetables, leafy greens, whole grains, yogurt, foods high in beta-carotene and zinc. (For a list of foods containing most of these nutrients, see part 3, "Food Therapy," p. 374.)

Nutritionist Ann Louise Gittleman, N.D., C.N.S., M.S., of Bozeman, Montana, points to the importance of: one, eating a good breakfast to start the day with stable blood sugar levels rather than with the wild fluctuations that go with a breakfast of coffee and/or pastry; and two, drinking plenty of water throughout the day to keep your system moving and help prevent the toxic buildup that can create skin problems.

Avoid:

Sugar (and limit fruit intake), soft drinks, alcohol, caffeine, white rice, white flour, iodized salt, fried and processed foods, dairy, animal fats, additives and preservatives, nightshade vegetables, food allergens.

"Sugar feeds the bacteria that can spur an acne breakout," says Dr. Gittleman. "Watch your zits melt when you cut out sugar." Although chocolate is not an acne trigger for everyone, she notes, it's best to avoid it because it's high in saturated fats, which are not good for anyone.

Herbal Medicine

Mindy Green recommends calendula (*Calendula officinalis*) flower and burdock (*Arctium lappa*) root, taken internally as a tea and used externally as a rinse or steam. Use one teaspoon of each per cup of boiled water. Steep for fifteen minutes, then strain. Drink a cup 1–4 times daily for 1–6 months. Use the tea as a rinse on the affected area as needed. As a steam bath for facial acne, heat the tea until it's steaming, put in a bowl, sit with your face in the steam rising from the bowl, and cover your head and the bowl to hold the steam in. Again, you can use this as needed.

Homeopathy

While acne is best treated by a constitutional remedy (consult a homeopath), the following may be helpful in the meantime, states Maesimund B. Panos, M.D.:[2]

Kali brom: often used for acne, especially if it is itchy and accompanied by restless sleep and unpleasant dreams.
Sulphur: for chronic acne with hard, rough skin, worsened by washing; especially indicated when sufferer is warm-blooded, sweats freely, and is often constipated.

Ant tart: for stubborn acne with many pustules.

Hepar sulph: for painful pustules; helps prevent them or bring them to a head.

Take the appropriate remedy in a 6x potency 3–4 times daily. As symptoms improve, decrease the frequency. Stop taking the remedy when the improvement is well established.

Nutritional Supplements

Dr. Gittleman recommends the following regimen for acne. Take the supplements at the dosages below until your acne clears up, then gradually reduce the dosages to one-half and continue at that level for maintenance.

Zinc: Take 30–45 mg daily (split into two doses). It is best to take zinc with food, as it causes nausea in some people. Taking zinc picolinate or another chelated form of zinc[3] reduces the likelihood of nausea. (Sufficient zinc in the body can also help reduce split ends in your hair and prevent stretch marks, which sometimes occur with the growth spurts of adolescence.)

Essential fatty acids:

Males—1 tablespoon of flaxseed oil (rich in omega-3 essential fatty acids) daily or 1,000 mg capsule 3 times daily.

Females—500 mg capsule containing a combination of flaxseed oil/evening primrose oil, 2 to 4 daily, or 1 to 2 tablespoons of the liquid combination daily. Dr. Gittleman suggests that women take flaxseed oil in combination with evening primrose oil (high in omega-6 essential fatty acids) because evening primrose has benefits for the menstrual cycle (specifically, cramps and menstrual-related migraines) as well as for acne.

Vitamin A: Take up to 25,000 IU daily. As vitamin A can be toxic in high doses, you should only take more than that if you are under the care of a qualified health practitioner. "Vitamin A is absolutely outstanding for acne," states Dr. Gittleman.

You can add chromium (200 mcg daily) and vitamin C (500–2,000 mg daily, divided over the day) to this program, if you like, says Dr. Gittleman. You can take these two supplements at these dosages indefinitely. Chromium helps to control blood sugar levels and therefore helps reduce the cravings for the sweets that should be avoided by someone prone to acne. Vitamin C helps maintain strong capillaries and is an important nutrient for the skin.

Reflexology

Endocrine system, intestines

Stone/Crystal Therapy

Use larimar, cuprite, or rose quartz, says Katrina Raphaell, crystal healing therapist and founder of the Crystal Academy of Advanced Healing Arts in Kapaa, Hawaii. Place the stone directly on the acne. Keep it in place for 5 minutes while visualizing your health goal (face free of blemishes, for example). Do this 3 times daily. You may also want to wear the stone, hold it, or carry it in your pocket for ongoing healing effects.

Allergic Reaction

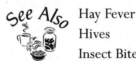
See Also
Hay Fever
Hives
Insect Bites and Stings
Poison Ivy/Oak Rash
Rash

An allergic reaction is an abnormal immune response to a substance (known as an allergen) that produces no reaction in a healthy immune system. An allergen can be anything you ingest, smell, touch, or inhale, from the common ragweed pollen to cat dander to a chemical in a cosmetic.

The body mobilizes the immune system to destroy what it perceives as a foreign invader, and releases histamine in the process. Histamine produces the inflammatory symptoms you experience during an allergic reaction. Such symptoms may include a runny nose and eyes, sinus congestion, sneezing, coughing, wheezing, headache, swelling, the outbreak of a rash, heat, and/or redness. The degree of reaction ranges from mild (as in runny eyes) to life-threatening (as when the body goes into anaphylactic shock and the level of inflammation can close off respiration), depending on how hypersensitive you are to the allergen.

If you are exposed to an allergen to which you know you are deathly allergic, seek emergency medical care immediately. The treatments discussed here are to ease the symptoms of non-life-threatening allergic reactions. Keep in mind, however, that these are merely first aid remedies. If you suffer from chronic allergies, it means you have an underlying immune imbalance and need to address it with deeper treatment in order to restore your health.

Essential Oils

For the eye symptoms of an allergic reaction (watering, itching, red eyes), Green Myrtle hydrosol can be effective, states Kurt Schnaubelt, Ph.D., scientific director of the Pacific Institute of Aromatherapy in San Rafael, California. While you cannot use essential oil in the eyes, you can use a hydrosol—aromatic water that is a coproduct of the essential oil distillation process. Spray the Green Myrtle hydrosol directly into the eyes up to 6 times per day to relieve allergic symptoms, says Dr. Schnaubelt.

Flower Essences

Yarrow Special Formula taken before exposure to known allergens can help prevent a reaction, notes flower essence therapist Patricia Kaminski of Nevada City, California. Take 4 drops 2–4 times daily. During exposure, take Yarrow Special Formula and Walnut, 4 drops of each 2–4 times daily or more often, as needed. If you have chronic allergies, you can take Yarrow Special Formula for several months to rebalance the system gradually.

Food Therapy

Eat:

Watercress, foods high in vitamins C and E. (For a list of foods containing these nutrients, see part 3, "Food Therapy," p. 374.) Drink plenty of water.

Avoid:

Additives, preservatives, cooked fats and oils, and common food allergens (see part 3, "Food Therapy," p. 374).

Herbal Medicine

. Ephedra (Ma-Huang, *Ephedra spp.*) tincture can be effective in relieving an allergic reaction, according to Amanda McQuade Crawford, M.N.I.M.H., Dip.Phyto., medical herbalist and director of the Ojai Center of Phytotherapy in Ojai, California. Take 10–15 drops of ephedra every 20–60 minutes as needed, up to 60 drops total in 24 hours. Do for 1–3 days, until you get symptomatic relief. If your symptoms continue unabated, you need to turn to other therapy. Ephedra should only be used on a short-term basis. It is best taken in combination with tinctures of bayberry (*Myrica cerifera*), yerba santa (*Eriodictyon californicum*), and/or licorice (*Glycrrhiza glabra*) root, according to Crawford, but you should consult an herbalist to have the blend formulated for you.

Nettle (*Urtica dioica*) leaf tincture can also be used for an allergic reaction, says Crawford, and it is safe to take for longer periods; follow the manufacturer's instructions.

Homeopathy

Naturopathic physicians Robert Ullmann, N.D., and Judyth Reichenberg-Ullmann, N.D., cite the following homeopathic remedies for allergic reaction:[1]

Allium cepa: if the nose is running like a faucet and the eyes are streaming.

Apis: if swelling and stinging pain that is better with cold application are the predominant symptoms.

Arsenicum: if the eyes are burning, there is a thin, burning nasal discharge, and you feel restless and anxious.

Urtica: if the allergic reaction is from eating shellfish or it feels like a burn or stinging nettles.

(For more homeopathic remedies for skin reactions, see "Rash.")

Take the appropriate remedy in a 30c potency every 2 hours until your symptoms improve. Stop taking the remedy, repeat if the symptoms return. If there is no improvement with 3 doses, you probably are not using the correct remedy.

Nutritional Supplements

Take 500 mg of vitamin C every 2 hours until the allergic reaction subsides, says Susan Roberts, N.D., a naturopathic physician from Portland, Oregon. She also advises drinking lots of water to help flush the toxins out of the body.

Reflexology

Treat the adrenal glands and the areas of the foot corresponding to the parts of the body where symptoms are the most pronounced.

Stone/Crystal Therapy

Bloodstone and hematite are the stones to use for an allergic reaction, states crystal healing therapist Katrina Raphaell of Kapaa, Hawaii. Place the stone directly on the body at the place of distress; for example, on a rash, or on your closed eyelids or against your nose if you are having eye and nose symptoms. Keep the stone in place for 5 minutes while visualizing your health goal. Do this 3 times daily. You can also wear the stone, hold it, or carry it in your pocket as continual healing.

Other Remedies

To ease an allergic reaction, stir 1/2 teaspoon of cream of tartar into 1/2 cup of warmed water (not microwaved), recommends Sue Reynolds, M.S.W., L.M.T., a certified herbalist and aromatherapist from Goleta, California. Continue to stir as you drink. Alkalinizing the body neutralizes the allergic mechanisms. As cream of tartar is strongly alkalinizing and will throw off your sodium-potassium balance, drink some water or juice with 1/2 teaspoon of salt dissolved in it half an hour after taking the cream of tartar. Sea salt is preferable and vegetable juice masks the salt taste best. You can take this two-phased remedy 2–3 times in several hours if necessary.

To produce the same effect, Drs. Ullmann and Reichenberg-Ullmann suggest a glass of water with 1–2 Alka-Seltzer Gold tablets or 1 teaspoon baking soda dissolved in it.[2]

Anxiety

The feeling variously described as dread, worry, uneasiness, apprehension, or brooding fear is familiar to everyone. We all experience anxiety to one degree or another in our lives. A certain amount of anxiety is part of being human, but if it reaches an uncomfortable level or begins to affect your functioning, you may want to try some of the following remedies. For serious anxiety disorders, seek medical attention.

Physical symptoms that can accompany anxiety include sweating, trembling, dry mouth, headache, muscle tension, rapid breathing, a racing pulse, stomach upset or tension, and nausea.

Essential Oils

To ease anxiety, herbalist Colleen K. Dodt recommends sprinkling 3–5 drops of Lavender essential oil on a tissue or handkerchief, carrying it with you, and inhaling the aroma, as needed.[1]

Herbalist Kathi Keville offers an anti-anxiety formula: Combine essential oils of Lavender (10 drops), Orange (10 drops), Marjoram (2 drops), and Cedarwood (2 drops) in 4 ounces of sweet almond oil. Use in any method of inhalation or topical delivery you like. For a bath oil, use 2 ounces of sweet almond oil rather than 4 ounces.[2]

Flower Essences

"Anxiety is a huge area of treatment in flower essence therapy because this therapy specializes in emotional disorders," states Patricia Kaminski, a flower essence therapist and educator from Nevada City, California. "Just as the Eskimos are intimately familiar with snow and have twenty-four words to describe it, we have many descriptions of anxiety. Each of these requires a different flower essence." Here are some common protocols:

St. John's Wort flower essence and St. John's Shield flower oil: for over-all symptoms of anxiety, especially when related to seasonal affective disorder (SAD; mood disturbance related to the reduced sunlight of winter months) or other life events that have altered the spiritual makeup of the individual.

Borage: when anxiety is accompanied by symptoms of heavyheartedness, such as grief.

Bleeding Heart: when anxiety stems from extreme attachment or loss of attachment to another.

Mimulus: when anxiety arises over small daily events, accompanied by irrational fears and phobias.

Mustard: for anxiety accompanied by intense mood swings.

Zinnia: as an antidote to moodiness and anxiety, and to bring a sense of humor and self-detachment.

Gentian: for anxiety that arises from a setback in life.

Larch: for anxiety over public performance.

Yarrow: for anxiety and a sense of unease produced by being overly sensitive to others.

Take 4 drops of the appropriate flower essence for your anxiety, 2–4 times daily, or more often during acute episodes. You can continue taking the remedy as needed.

Food Therapy

Eat:

Fresh vegetables, protein, parsley, sage, ginger, garlic, small frequent meals/snacks for stable blood sugar, foods high in magnesium, calcium, and vitamins B and C. (For a list of foods containing these nutrients, see part 3, "Food Therapy," p. 378.)

Avoid:

Caffeine, sugar, alcohol, refined and preserved foods

Herbal Medicine

Clinical herbalist and consultant David Winston, A.H.G., of Washington, New Jersey, suggests the following anti-anxiety herbal formula. Use tinctures of all in the proportions noted, and take 3–4 ml (roughly 3/5 to 4/5 of a teaspoon) of the combined tincture 3 times daily for as long as needed:

Motherwort (*Leonurus cardiaca*): 2 parts; tranquilizing, and helpful in slowing heart palpitations due to anxiety.

Blue vervain (*Verbena hastata*): 1 part; anxiolytic (anxiety-reducing) herb; if you experience nausea after taking the formula, try lowering the percentage of vervain in the mixture.

Kava-kava (*Piper methysticum*): 1 part; good for anxiety with muscle tension, more effective when used in a mix than when used alone.

Ashwagandha (*Withania somnifera*): 1 part; a calming, adaptogenic (supports the adrenal glands and helps the body cope with stress) Ayurvedic herb that is also useful for muscle tension.

Medical herbalist Amanda McQuade Crawford, M.N.I.M.H., Dip.Phyto., of Ojai, California, has found kava-kava effective on a short-term basis. Take 1,500 mg of kava (tablets) every 1–4 hours, not exceeding 6 g over 24 hours, says Crawford. Do not take kava for more than 6 months at 2 doses per day, she notes, adding that kava is not for those under 14 years of age.

Crawford also recommends passionflower (*Passiflora incarnata*) tea, which you can drink indefinitely. To make the tea, put 1 ounce of the herb in 1 quart of boiled water and let steep for 15 minutes. Strain, and drink 1/2 to 1 cup every 1–4 hours as needed. For flavor, you can mix it with other herbal teas such as lemon balm or fennel seed.

Homeopathy

Michael G. Carlston, M.D., a homeopathic physician from Santa Rosa, California, recommends:

If the anxiety is acute and you feel paralyzed by fear, with the classic anxiety feeling that you're going to die, take Aconite napellus 30c or 200c every few hours. When you feel better, stop taking the remedy. Dr. Carlston reports that this is a common remedy for people after a big earthquake or an auto accident.

If the anxiety is acute but less severe, the weak and shaky type of anxiety (shakiness similar to that of flu, for which this remedy is also commonly used), or anxiety in anticipation (as in stage fright), take Gelsemium sempervirens 30c. If stage fright is the source, take the remedy once before your speech or other appearance. You can take repeatedly if needed.

Nutritional Supplements

Naturopathic physician Bradley Bongiovanni, N.D., of Independence, Ohio, recommends the following program of supplements and herbs to ease anxiety; they can be taken on an ongoing basis as maintenance and prevention:

Flaxseed oil: 1,000 mg 3 times daily; this essential fatty acid is needed for nerve transmission.

Magnesium: 250 mg 3 times daily; helps ease muscle tension.

GABA (gamma-aminobutyric acid): 500–1,000 mg 3 times daily; a calming neurotransmitter.

Kava-kava: 200 mg (30 percent lactones [kava's active constituent]) 3 times daily; an anxiolytic (anti-anxiety) herb.

Oatstraw (*Avena sativa*) extract: 2 ml 3 times daily; a nervous system restorative.

Reflexology

Diaphragm, solar plexus, adrenal glands, spine

Stone/Crystal Therapy

There are a number of helpful stones for anxiety, according to Katrina Raphaell, crystal healing therapist and author of the crystal reference series *The Crystal Trilogy*. She cites black tourmaline, amazonite, lepidolite, and rose quartz amethyst. Place the stone on the center of your body at the level of the heart or over your solar plexus (top of the abdomen, below the ribs). Leave it in place for 5 minutes while you visualize your health goal, such as a deep sense of calm with no more anxiety. Do this 3 times daily, as needed. In addition, wear the stone, hold it, or carry it in your pocket for ongoing healing benefits.

Athlete's Foot

See Fungal Infection.

Backache

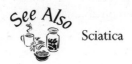 Sciatica

Pain in the upper, middle, or lower back afflicts an estimated 80 percent of Americans at some time in their lives.[1] Among the many causes of backache are poor posture, injury, improper lifting, prolonged sitting, improper footwear, stress, and obesity (the back bears the strain of carrying around extra weight, and weak abdominal muscles force the back to do more of the work in supporting the body's posture and movement). If you suffer from chronic backache or your symptoms do not lessen within a few days of onset of the pain, seek medical help to determine and eliminate the underlying causes. The remedies here can help alleviate those occasional aches and pains in the back that most of us experience.

Essential Oils

Chamomile, Marjoram, and Lavender essential oils have pain-relieving, antispasmodic, sedative, and nervine (nerve tonifying) properties, all of which are beneficial for a backache. Chamomile is also anti-inflammatory. Use one or more of the oils in a bath, added to a carrier oil for massage, and/or on a cold or hot compress applied to the affected area, as needed. Wintergreen, Camphor, and Eucalyptus are warming oils that aid in muscle relaxation. Rub the chosen oil into the sore area, as needed.[2]

Flower Essences

As backache is often due to emotional tension, flower essence therapy is best tailored to the individual's particular emotional blockages, states Patricia Kaminski, a flower essence therapist and educator from Nevada City, California. That said, Arnica Alleve flower oil compresses can be used for symptom relief, she notes. Rub 1–2 tablespoons of Arnica Alleve flower oil on the affected area and cover with a hot or cold compress, depending on the condition. Do 2–4 applications daily, or as needed. Self-Heal can aid the back pain sufferer in looking at the specific healing issues in his or her life, adds Kaminski. Take 4 drops, 2–4 times daily, as needed.

Food Therapy

Eat:

Fiber, low-fat diet.

In addition, for their anti-inflammatory effects, drink green tea and eat pineapple, papaya, ginger, turmeric, and foods rich in omega-3 essential fatty acids (see part 3, "Food Therapy," p. 376), advises Nick Buratovich, N.M.D., a naturopathic physician from Tempe, Arizona. Eat turkey, which is high in pain-relieving tryptophan. You should eat it by itself, not with other foods, to promote uptake of the tryptophan. Eat pineapple and papaya by themselves as well, to get the anti-inflammatory effect of the enzymes these fruits contain. "Also consider that by eating or having these nutritional elements as a regular part of your diet, you better equip your body to deal with a future injury and minimize its effects," says Dr. Buratovich.

Avoid:

Red meat, large meals, dairy.

Dr. Buratovich advises avoiding coffee and other forms of caffeine (aside from green tea) because caffeine blocks endorphin receptors in the brain. As endorphins facilitate pain relief, people who consume a lot of caffeine tend to have a low threshold of pain. Avoid animal products (aside from turkey) because they contain arachidonic acid, which promotes inflammation. You may also want to avoid foods in the nightshade family (see part 3, "Food Therapy," p. 377). In some people, nightshades increase inflammation as an allergic reaction.

Herbal Medicine

"Most back pain originates from kidney and bladder weakness," says herbalist Michael Tierra, L.Ac., OMD. Toxins that those organs can't process get deposited in nearby tissue, notably in the lower back, eventually producing inflammation. For this reason, Dr. Tierra recommends a diuretic (increases urine output) tea to help cleanse the bladder and kidneys. Combine equal parts juniper (*Juniperus communis*) berries, uva-ursi (*Arctostaphylos uva-ursi*), parsley (*Petroselinum crispum*) root, and marshmallow (*Althea officinalis*) root. In a covered pan, simmer 2 ounces of the herbal mixture in 1 quart of water for 15 minutes. Strain, and drink half a cup 3–4 times a day.[3]

Chaparral (*Larrea tridentata*) is an excellent herb for back pain. It is antioxidant and helps cleanse, tone, and rebuild muscle tissue. Add the herb to boiled water, strain, and drink as a tea 3–4 times daily.[4]

As a topical treatment, capsaicin cream (available in commercial preparations) is a potent pain reliever. Capsaicin is derived from cayenne pepper (*Capsicum spp.*). In addition to containing salicylates (aspirin's active component), it is known to interfere with pain perception and stimulate release of endorphins (pain-relieving substances).[5]

Homeopathy

The following homeopathic remedies are commonly indicated for backache, according to Stephen Cummings, M.D., and Dana Ullman, M.P.H.:[6]

Hypericum: If there are shooting pains or you have injured your coccyx.

Nux vom: If the pain is worse with movement, particularly turning over in bed.

Bryonia: If the pain is worse with movement, but turning over in bed doesn't produce more pain.

Rhus tox: If continual movement eases the pain, the back is stiff and painful when still, the pain is worse when getting up in the morning, but improves once you have moved around some, and the pain is worsened by cold and damp and eased by heat; may be accompanied by sciatica.

Take the appropriate remedy at a potency of 6c(x) or 12c(x) every 6 to 12 hours for several days. As your symptoms improve, take the remedy less often. If there is no improvement after 2–3 days of taking the remedy, try a different one.

Nutritional Supplements

For backache, Dr. Buratovich particularly recommends calcium and magnesium, which can be taken alone or with the other supplements below:

Calcium lactate or calcium citrate: These chelated forms of calcium are the most easily absorbed. Take 1,000 mg 3 times daily until back pain is resolved. Calcium is an antispasmodic.

Magnesium glycinate: This form of magnesium is most easily absorbed and less likely to cause the diarrhea some people get when they take magnesium. Take 1,000 mg 3 times daily until back pain is resolved. Magnesium is another antispasmodic.

Bromelain: 2 capsules on an empty stomach 3 times daily until the pain is resolved; an anti-inflammatory enzyme compound found in pineapple.

DLPA (D,L-phenylalanine): 750 mg 3 times daily before meals for 1–3 weeks; a pain-relieving amino acid.

Tryptophan: 2–4 g 3 times daily for up to 1 month. This amino acid has been shown to reduce pain, perhaps by raising the pain threshold, although the exact mechanism is unknown.[7] To ensure uptake, avoid protein for 90 minutes before and after taking.

Reflexology

Treat the spinal area of the foot corresponding to the location of your backache.

Stone/Crystal Therapy

Use amber, double-terminated clear quartz, or green tourmaline to aid in healing a backache, states crystal healing therapist Katrina Raphaell of Kapaa, Hawaii. Place the stone(s) on your back where the pain is located. Leave the stone there for 5 minutes while visualizing your health goal (freedom from back pain, for example). Do this 3 times daily. In between these treatments, wear the stone, hold it, or carry it in your pocket to continue the effects.

Other Remedies

For backache, Amanda McQuade Crawford, M.N.I.M.H., Dip.Phyto., a medical herbalist from Ojai, California, cites the universal anti-inflammatory technique of icing the painful area. Use an ice pack or a cloth so the ice is not directly on the skin. Ice the area for 20 minutes 2 times daily for 2 days. If symptoms worsen, consult a qualified health practitioner.

Bacterial Infection

Bacteria, a class of microorganisms, are normally present throughout our bodies and the environment. Some bacteria are beneficial to the human body and necessary for its proper functioning; for example, the acidophilus bacteria in the intestines aid in the absorption of nutrients. Many other bacteria are pathogenic, meaning disease producing, and can cause mild to serious infection.

A bacterial infection can occur anywhere in the body, from a cut on the skin to an internal organ, as in cystitis (bladder infection) or bronchitis. Symptoms include inflammation of the affected area, which manifests as pain, heat, redness, and swelling, and fever, depending on the degree and kind of infection.

A healthy immune system is equipped to keep harmful bacteria in check and prevent them from producing illness. Weakened immunity, however, allows bacteria to flourish and create infection. Stress, poor nutrition, toxic exposure, lack of exercise, lack of sleep, and overuse of antibiotics and other drugs can all contribute to suppressed immunity. Since we live in a toxic world, lead stressful lives, and eat food grown in depleted soil or a diet of processed food, most of our immune systems are compromised to some degree.

There are numerous natural antibiotics that you can use topically or systemically to treat bacterial infection. In addition, strengthening your immune system can help restore your body's ability to heal itself.

Essential Oils

Specific essential oils are known for their antibacterial effects. In England, where aromatherapy is a more accepted aspect of medical care, particularly in nursing, than it is in the United States, hospitals regularly employ these oils to reduce the microbial breeding ground effect associated with hospitals.[1] Research has demonstrated the especially strong antibacterial properties of Oregano, Savory, Cinnamon, Thyme, Clove, and Tea Tree (*Melaleuca alternifolia*) essential oils against a long list of common pathogens, including *Staphylococcus, Streptococcus,* and *Pneumococcus.*[2]

While Tea Tree essential oil can safely be applied undiluted on the skin, the others are irritating and should not be applied to the skin. The exception is that Thyme and Oregano can be rubbed into the soles of the feet, according to Kurt Schnaubelt, Ph.D., scientific director of the Pacific Institute of Aromatherapy in San Rafael, California. Use a diluted solution, 2–3 drops of essential oil to 1 teaspoon of carrier oil. Thyme and Oregano are well tolerated in this mode of delivery, which is a highly effective way to disperse the essential oils throughout the body, says Dr. Schnaubelt.[3] The other antibacterial oils can be inhaled from the bottle or used in a diffuser. Do not use these oils for steam inhalation.

Other essential oils have been shown to be effective against a smaller selection of microbes: Marjoram works on three bacteria, including *Salmonella pullorum;* French tarragon on four, including *Staphylococcus;* and Eucalyptus on three, including *E. coli* and *Staphylococcus.*[4] Massage with the essential oil in a carrier oil or diffusion is a good method of delivery for these oils. You can also rub them undiluted into the soles of the feet. (For instructions on using essential oils in massage and diffusion, see part 3, "Essential Oils," p. 366–68.)

Flower Essences

Self-Heal and Yarrow Special Formula can serve as the foundational healing agents for a bacterial infection. Other flower essences to address the specific emotions, mental attitude, and environmental conditions of the individual are recommended, states Patricia Kaminski, a flower essence therapist and codirector of the Flower Essence Society.

Self-Heal supports the body's innate healing ability. Yarrow Special Formula strengthens and protects against environmental toxicity and stress. Take 4 drops of each 2–4 times daily, or as needed.

Food Therapy

Eat:

Garlic, onion, turmeric, ginger, seaweed, yogurt, papaya, foods high in vitamin C (see part 3, "Food Therapy," p. 378).

Avoid:

Sugar, soft drinks, caffeine, alcohol, refined foods.

Herbal Medicine

Among the many natural antibiotics in the plant world are the berberine-containing plants goldenseal (*Hydrastis canadensis*), barberry (*Berberis vulgaris*), Oregon grape (*Berberis aquifolium*), and goldthread (*Coptis chinensis, C. trifolia*). Berberine is a potent antimicrobial alkaloid with demonstrated effects against a number of bacteria, including *Salmonella, Staphylococcus,* and *E. coli.* Aloe vera is also strongly antibacterial, proven effective against *Staphylococcus, Streptococcus*, and *E. coli*, among other bacteria.

Other herbs known for their antibacterial properties are echinacea (*E. spp.*), pau d'arco (*Tabebuia avellanedae*), and St. John's wort (*Hypericum perforatum*).[5] Aloe vera juice can be taken internally, and the fresh gel from the plant applied topically to a bacterial infection of the skin. The other herbs can be taken in tincture or capsule form. Goldenseal powder can be mixed with a little water and applied topically, but note that it tends to turn the skin yellow temporarily.

To strengthen the immune system, herbalist Kathi Keville recommends the following formula: combine 1/2 teaspoon each of tinctures of echinacea root, pau d'arco bark, Siberian ginseng (*Eleutherococcus senticosus*) root, licorice (*Glycrrhiza glabra*) root, astragalus (*Astragalus membranaceus*) root, and bupleurum (*Bupleurum spp.*) root. Take the entire amount 2 times daily for 2–3 weeks to boost immunity. During an acute infection or other immune problem, take it 4–6 times daily.[6]

Homeopathy

See the particular type of bacterial infection.

Nutritional Supplements

Colloidal silver, a potent antibiotic, can be an effective treatment for a systemic bacterial infection. Sue Reynolds, M.S.W., L.M.T., a certified herbalist and aromatherapist from Goleta, California, recommends taking 1 teaspoon 3 times daily until you are well. The colloidal silver you use must be under 3 microns in particle size; check the product label before purchasing.

Grapefruit seed extract is a powerful antimicrobial agent, proven effective against bacteria, fungi, viruses, and protozoa.[7] Tablets are a palatable way to take the extract; some people object to the taste and drying sensation of the liquid form. Take as directed for your particular infection. You can also use it topically as an antiseptic spray (see "Cuts and Scrapes").

For any bacterial infection, antioxidants are standard supplements. They neutralize harmful free radicals that proliferate in an infection. Antoxidants include vitamins A, C, and E, beta-carotene, selenium, coenzyme Q10, bioflavonoids, pycnogenol (grape seed extract), the amino acid glutathione, and the enzyme superoxide dismutase. Antioxidants exert more powerful effects when they are taken in combination rather than singly.

Reflexology

Treat the spleen area and the area of the foot corresponding to the part of the body afflicted by bacterial infection, or the part where symptoms are the most pronounced.

Stone/Crystal Therapy

For bacterial infection, bloodstone, peridot, or sulphur can be beneficial, says Katrina Raphaell, crystal healing therapist and founder of the Crystal Academy of Advanced Healing Arts in Kapaa, Hawaii. Place the stone directly on the site of infection. Keep it in place for 5 minutes while visualizing your health goal. Do this 3 times daily. If the infection is systemic, lay the stone over the area most affected, that is, where the symptoms are focused. You can also wear the stone, hold it, or put it in your pocket for ongoing effects.

Other Remedies

For a systemic bacterial infection, cream of tartar can be useful, according to Sue Reynolds. Stir 1/2 teaspoon of cream of tartar into 1/2 cup of warmed water (not microwaved). Continue to stir as you drink. Bacteria thrive in an acid environment, thus alkalinizing the body via cream of tartar creates a hostile environment for bacterial proliferation. The strong alkalinizing effect will throw off your sodium-potassium balance, so half an hour after taking the cream of tartar drink some water or juice with 1/2 teaspoon of salt dissolved in it. Sea salt is preferable and vegetable juice masks the salt taste best. You can take this two-phased remedy 2–3 times in several hours if necessary.

Bad Breath

Though it may seem like a simple, though embarassing or unpleasant, problem, bad breath (halitosis) is not usually a mere condition of the mouth. While it may be the result of tooth decay, gum infection, or poor dental hygiene, it often has its roots in poor diet, digestion, and elimination. In this case, bad breath is actually the smell of putrefied food and bacterial waste in the gastrointestinal tract. The problem can be in the stomach where food is not being broken down properly, or in the intestines where there is an accumulation of toxins due to sluggish elimination or chronic constipation. When this is the cause of bad breath, a mouthwash is obviously only going to provide a temporary masking effect. You need to address the underlying gastrointestinal problems and get rid of the toxic buildup to get rid of your bad breath.

Halitosis can also be caused by through-the-mouth breathing, which dries out the mucous lining of the mouth. People who snore, sleep with their mouth open, or have allergies or another condition involving sinus congestion may suffer from bad breath. Finally, foul mouth odor can be a sign of more serious illness, such as diabetes or liver or kidney problems.

Essential Oils

As a mouthwash for bad breath, add 3–4 drops of Myrrh essential oil to a glass of warm water. Use daily, or as needed.[1]

Flower Essences

Self-Heal can serve as a foundational healing agent for bad breath. Other flower essences to address the specific emotions, mental attitude, and environmental conditions of the individual are recommended, states Patricia Kaminski, a flower essence therapist and codirector of the Flower Essence Society. Self-Heal supports the body's innate healing ability. Take 4 drops 2–4 times daily, or as needed.

Food Therapy

Eat:

Fiber, green vegetables, parsley, sprouts, yogurt/kefir, foods high in vitamin B6 (see part 3, "Food Therapy," p. 378). Drink plenty of water.

Avoid:

Sugar, excess carbohydrates, cheese, red meat, fried foods, yeast bread, caffeine, alcohol, food allergens.

Herbal Medicine

If your bad breath is not due to a dental abscess or other problem of the gums or teeth, "sweetening" the stomach can help, says David R. Field, N.D., L.Ac., a naturopathic physician from Santa Rosa, California. A sour stomach means poor digestion, which is a common cause of bad breath. Increasing the acidity of the stomach enhances digestion and can improve the smell of the breath, explains Dr. Field. This can be accomplished with bitters. These herbs derive their name from their bitter taste, but are known for their numerous beneficial effects on digestion, including increasing the flow of digestive juices, improving the gut environment overall, and even promoting repair of the lining of the stomach.[2]

Dr. Field recommends the bitter herb gentian (*Gentiana lutea*). Put 10 drops of gentian tincture in 1/4 glass of water and drink before each meal. Angostura Bitters, a flavoring used in cocktails and readily available at the supermarket, serves the same purpose, he notes. Use in the same dosage as the gentian tincture. Do this for 2–4 weeks. You will likely notice an improvement in your breath before the 4-week point.

Fennel and cardamom aid in digestion, and are instant breath fresheners. Chew and swallow 3–5 fennel or cardomom seeds after every meal, suggests medical herbalist Amanda McQuade Crawford, M.N.I.M.H., Dip.Phyto., of Ojai, California. You can do this indefinitely. If your bad breath continues unabated after 24 hours of following this treatment, however, you need to consult a qualified health practitioner to determine the underlying cause.

Homeopathy

There are many homeopathic remedies for bad breath, depending on its characteristics and source. Here is a selection from Dr. Barry Rose of the Royal London Homeopathic Hospital:[3]

Aurum met 6c: For bad breath with a putrid or bitter taste and ulcers on the gums; afflicting girls at puberty.

Mercurius 6c: For bad breath with increased saliva production, spongy, sore gums that bleed easily, and a yellow, thick, flabby, teeth-indented tongue.

Pulsatilla 6c: For bad breath when your mouth is dry without thirst and your tongue is yellow or white with a mucus coating.

Silica 6c: For bad breath due to gum infection.

Spigelia 6c: For foul breath with a bad taste and a painful, fissured tongue.

Terebinth 6c: For foul breath that feels cold, accompanied by a sore, dry, red, shiny tongue burning at the tip.

Take the appropriate remedy 4 times daily until your bad breath improves, as needed.

Nutritional Supplements

Liquid chlorophyll is useful in ameliorating bad breath. Sue Reynolds, M.S.W., L.M.T., a certified herbalist and aromatherapist from Goleta, California, suggests taking 1 teaspoon straight or in water

2–4 times daily. You can also chew papaya mints, which contain enzymes that aid in digestion, as needed.

By improving digestion, plant-based digestive enzymes with HCl (hydrochloric acid, a gastric digestive juice) are also useful, according to Dr. Field. Take 1–2 capsules midway through each meal, 3 times daily for 2–4 weeks. Taking the enzymes midmeal aids digestion, but prevents the body from developing a reliance on the supplement for its enzyme supply instead of producing its own.

Reflexology

Stomach, intestines, liver, the head region on the big toes

Stone/Crystal Therapy

Aquamarine is a useful stone for bad breath, according to Daya Sarai Chocron, a vibrational healer based in Northampton, Massachusetts. Hold the stone, wear it, carry it in your pocket, or lay it on your body (anywhere over the line of the gastrointestinal tract, from your lips to your abdomen) for 15–20 minutes daily, as needed.

Other Remedies

Practice good dental hygiene. Flossing every day removes food particles that if left between the teeth can contribute to bad breath.

Bed-Wetting (Childhood)

Clinically known as enuresis, bed-wetting is urination in bed at night after the age when bladder control is usually established; this typically occurs by the age of five. If there is no structural problem, infection, or other organic cause present, conventional medicine tends to view bed-wetting as a psychological problem, born of emotional stress or misguided toilet training. While these may be factors, alternative medicine practitioners have discovered that nutritional deficiencies and food allergies can both play a significant role in a child's inability to control urination.[1] If deficiencies are the problem and they are corrected with nutritional supplementation, the bed-wetting often disappears. The same is true when allergies are involved. By identifying allergenic foods and eliminating them from the diet, the problem is resolved in some children.

Essential Oils

For bed-wetting, aromatherapy authority Robert B. Tisserand recommends Cypress. It has restringent (restraining) effects on body fluids. Put 3–5 drops of the essential oil in a before-bedtime bath or give your child a bedtime massage (5 drops of essential oil per 2 teaspoons of vegetable oil).[2]

Flower Essences

St. John's Wort flower essence taken internally (4 drops 2–4 times daily), accompanied by applications of St. John's Shield to the urogenital area before bedtime, can help prevent bed-wetting, states naturalist Richard Katz of Nevada City, California. When bed-wetting is accompanied by nightmares and/or fear of the dark, he recommends Aspen (4 drops 2–4 times daily).

Food Therapy

Eat:

Celery, foods high in magnesium (see part 3, "Food Therapy," p. 377).

Avoid:

Additives, preservatives, cow's milk, junk food, refined sugar, salty or spicy foods, high-oxalate foods (see part 3, "Food Therapy," p. 377), food allergens.

Herbal Medicine

A tea formula containing herbs traditionally used for urinary problems and to promote bladder control can be effective in the treatment of bed-wetting, says Jody E. Noé, M.S., N.D., a naturopathic physician from Brattleboro, Vermont. It is important to consider possible physiological and psychological factors as well, she notes. Combine equal parts of corn silk (*Zea mays*), oatstraw (*Avena sativa*), and horsetail (*Equisetum arvense*) grass. Use 1 tablespoon of the mixture per 1–1/2 to 2 cups of boiled water. Let steep for 15 minutes, then strain. The dosage is 1 cup 2–3 times daily while the problem persists.

An herbal tincture combination is also effective, according to herbalist Kathi Keville. For "Dry Bed Tincture," combine equal parts of tinctures of St. John's wort (*Hypericum perforatum*) tops, fresh oat berries, corn silk, and plantain (*Plantago major*) leaves. The dosage (for a 50-pound child) is 15 drops 3 times daily.

Keville also cites Russian research demonstrating the efficacy of aloe vera juice: ". . . almost all the children in [the] study not only stopped wetting their beds when they were given aloe, but also became noticeably less irritable." Keville suggests 1/2 to 1 cup of aloe vera juice daily (don't overdo it, she cautions), added to an equal amount of fruit juice.[3]

Homeopathy

In cases of bed-wetting, one of the following remedies can be helpful, says London homeopath Miranda Castro:[4]

Belladonna: If the child sleeps too deeply to wake.
Causticum: If the bed-wetting occurs during first sleep, and the child is whiny or cries easily, doesn't want to go to bed alone, and has restless sleep.
Pulsatilla or Sulphur: If the child generally only wets the bed when sick.
Silica: For the child who wets the bed after a fall or a bout of worms.

Give the appropriate remedy in a 6x or 6c potency 3 times daily (for up to 10 days). Stop giving your child the remedy as soon as there is significant improvement. Repeat the remedy as needed.

Nutritional Supplements

Magnesium, an important mineral in the regulation of muscle contractions, has proven useful in the treatment of bed-wetting. Give your child 200 mg daily for at least a month.[5] Beta-carotene and vitamin E can also be helpful. They normalize the function of the bladder muscles. A typical dosage is 15 mg of beta-carotene daily and 100 IU of vitamin E daily for a 6–12-year-old child.[6] To ensure balance with other nutrients, give the child a good daily multivitamin/mineral supplement as well.

Reflexology

Bladder, ureters

Stone/Crystal Therapy

Use black obsidian as a gemstone remedy for bed-wetting, says vibrational healer Daya Sarai Chocron, of Northampton, Massachusetts. Make sure the stone is too large to be swallowed and place it under the child's pillow. Alternatively, the child can hold the piece of obsidian as he or she drifts off to sleep, or it can be placed near the bed.

Other Remedies

A traditional remedy for bed-wetting is the proverbial spoonful of honey at bedtime.[7]

Black Eye

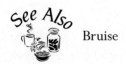 See Also Bruise

A blow to the eye area, nose, or forehead can produce the swelling, bruising, and discoloration around the eye known as black eye. The black-and-blue bruise arises from broken blood vessels (typically capillaries) leaking into nearby tissue.

Essential Oils

To treat a black eye, combine 1 drop each of Geranium and Chamomile essential oils with 2 teaspoons of witch hazel, says aromatherapist Valerie Ann Worwood. Blend it well, then mix it into 1 tablespoon of ice-cold water. Soak cotton pads with the blend and lay them on your closed eyelid and the area around the eye.[1]

Flower Essences

Self-Heal and Five Flower Formula can serve as the foundational healing agents for a black eye. Other flower essences to address the specific emotions, mental attitude, and environmental conditions of the individual are recommended, states Patricia Kaminski, a flower essence therapist and codirector of the Flower Essence Society. Self-Heal supports the body's innate healing ability. Five Flower Formula, which brings immediate calm and emotional neutralizing, is indicated for physical and/or emotional trauma. Take 4 drops of each 4 times daily, or more frequently if needed.

Food Therapy

Eat:

Foods high in vitamins C and K and zinc (see part 3, "Food Therapy," p. 378).

Avoid:

Dairy products.

Herbal Medicine

A prickly pear cactus pad will definitely work better than the old folk remedy of a raw steak on the eye to reduce a shiner. In fact, it can dramatically reduce swelling and later discoloration or even prevent a shiner from developing. A black eye in the making is a condition of congestion resulting from the broken blood vessels and tissue fluid retention that accompany an injury, according to clinical herbalist Michael Cottingham, of Silver City, New Mexico.

A prickly pear pad placed over the closed eye increases circulation movement in the area and relieves the congestion by drawing out moisture. In most cases, 1–2 applications are sufficient. Leave the pad on for 20–30 minutes per application. Change the pad with each application and do the second application right after the first. You can do up to five applications, depending on the severity of the injury, but after the first two applications, separate them by an hour or more. See "Boil" for how to prepare and apply the prickly pear cactus pad.

The ubiquitous "weed" plantain (*Plantago major*), which contains anti-inflammatory compounds, also works well. Crush or chew the leaves to a pulp and apply to the injured area (with the eye closed). Repeat as needed.[2]

Homeopathy

"Arnica is the first thing you think of for any kind of injury," says homeopathic physician Michael G. Carlston, M.D., of Santa Rosa, California. For an injury that will likely become a black eye, he recommends Arnica montana 12c, 4 times a day, to reduce the pain and inflammation. When the symptoms have lessened, cut down to once a day. Do not use arnica gel or ointment, Dr. Carlston advises, because a black eye is a trauma and blood is gathered in the area. You don't want to add to the trauma by rubbing the skin to apply an ointment. He suggests instead that you mix a tincture of arnica montana with a little water, soak some gauze with it, and lay it on the eye for 20 minutes. Do this twice a day.

Nutritional Supplements

Taking vitamin C with bioflavonoids can help strengthen capillary walls. Take 500 mg of each 2 times daily for 2–3 weeks, then reduce to once daily for another month. Proanthocyanidins (PCOs), found in grape seed and bilberry, are potent antioxidants and also help decrease the fragility of capillaries. Take 80 mg of standardized bilberry extract (25 percent PCOs) 3 times daily, or 50–100 mg standardized grape seed extract (90 percent PCOs) 3 times daily.[3]

Reflexology

Eye, face

Stone/Crystal Therapy

Green calcite and green aventurine are helpful for a black eye, says crystal healing therapist Katrina Raphaell of Kapaa, Hawaii. Place the stone directly on the site of impact. Keep it in place for 5 minutes while visualizing your health goal. Do this 3 times daily. You may also want to wear the stone, hold it, or carry it in your pocket for continual healing effects.

Bladder Infection (Cystitis)

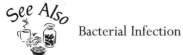 Bacterial Infection

A bladder infection is one kind of urinary tract infection (UTI), although the terms are often used interchangeably. Infection can occur anywhere along the urinary tract, from the urethra (the passageway for urine from the bladder to outside the body) to the bladder to the kidneys. A bladder infection, or cystitis, most often occurs as a result of what is called an ascending infection, meaning it starts in the urethra (urethritis) and moves up to the bladder if treatment doesn't curtail it. If still untreated, it can then travel farther up the tract to the kidneys. As kidney involvement can be quite dangerous, it is important to stop the infection before it travels that far. Infection can also move down the urinary tract to the bladder from the kidneys, but that is not as common as the ascending variety. UTIs are usually bacterial.

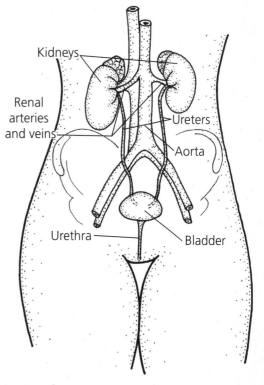

Symptoms of UTI are: burning or painful urination; frequent sensation of needing to urinate, with little output; foul-smelling, dark, and sometimes bloody urine; and pain in the lower abdomen. If you experience lower back pain, there may be kidney involvement. Do not let your UTI go untreated at any stage, and medical assistance is imperative if the kidneys are affected.

Far more women than men get bladder infections, which is likely due to bacterial migration facilitated by the proximity of the urethra to the vagina and anus. Under normal circumstances, the urinary tract can handle the presence of bacteria. Urine both flushes bacteria out of the body and inhibits bacterial growth with its chemical composition. If a person doesn't drink enough water or urinate regularly (as in "secretary's syndrome," when the person "holds it" because they are too busy or forget amidst the pressures of work to go to the bathroom), the bacteria may not get flushed out and infection can result. Or, if the immune system is weak, the bacteria can multiply beyond acceptable levels and cause infection.

Other factors that contribute to cystitis include prolonged sexual intercourse (thus the phrase "honeymoon cystitis"), pregnancy, use of a too-large contraceptive diaphragm (which presses on the bladder and impedes urinary elimination), and chronic constipation (which both impedes urinary flow and weakens immunity).[1]

As with any kind of bacterial infection, treatment of a UTI should both address the infection and strengthen the immune system. Chronic UTIs indicate an ongoing imbalance. Seek medical help in identifying and treating the causes.

Essential Oils

Taking daily baths with a blend of Eucalyptus, Juniper, and Thyme essential oils or a blend of Lavender and Sandalwood (be sure the oil is pure) can help alleviate a bladder infection. Use 6–8 drops of each blend in a tub of hot water.[2]

Flower Essences

When the bladder infection is accompanied by "extreme overwhelm and other symptoms of sensory overload," take Dill, says Patricia Kaminski, an herbalist and flower essence therapist from Nevada City, California. Take 4 drops at least 4 times daily, more often if needed.

Food Therapy

Eat:

Blueberries, watermelon, celery, watercress, parsley, foods high in vitamin C (see part 3, "Food Therapy," p. 378). Drink plenty of water.

There has been some confusion over whether to drink cranberry juice as part of treatment for a bladder infection. While research has shown that drinking cranberry juice changes the walls of the urinary tract so bacteria can't adhere to them,[3] it may make urination more painful because it acidifies the urine. (While it may temporarily be more painful, the acid urine inhibits bacterial growth.) With that proviso, naturopathic physician Kathi Head, N.D., of Sandpoint, Idaho, recommends it for a bladder infection. "In mild cases, cranberry juice alone can take care of it," she states, adding that cranberry juice can be used for prevention as well. The juice must be pure, unsweetened cranberry juice, not the "cocktail" variety. If you are prone to urinary tract infections, drink 2 cups daily as prevention, suggests Dr. Head. During acute infection, drink 2 quarts daily, spread throughout the day. If you get no results in 3 days, then you need to start other treatment, such as the herbs uva-ursi and buchu, she notes.

Avoid:

Sugar, caffeine, alcohol, refined carbohydrates, fried or spicy foods, soft drinks, food allergens, acidic foods such as chocolate, tomatoes, and cooked spinach.

Foods that alkalinize the urine are best avoided, according to David R. Field, N.D., L.Ac., a naturopathic physician from Santa Rosa, California. Bacteria cannot proliferate in acidic urine. Urine-alkalinizing foods include high-calcium foods (see part 3, "Food Therapy," p. 376) and citrus fruit such as oranges. Oranges are an example of the axiom that acidic foods don't necessarily create acidity in the body. Although oranges are quite acidic, they alkalinize the urine. Also avoid high-protein foods, because the more protein there is in the urine, the more food there is for bacteria, says Dr. Field.

Herbal Medicine

For a bladder infection, Amanda McQuade Crawford, M.N.I.M.H., Dip.Phyto., medical herbalist and author of *Herbal Remedies for Women*, recommends uva-ursi (*Arctostaphylos uva-ursi*) leaf tea and/or echinacea (*E. spp.*). To make the tea, use 1 ounce of the herb per 1 pint of boiled water. Steep for 10 minutes. Drink 1/2 cup every 3 hours for 3 days. You can take echinacea in tablet or tincture form. As tablets, take 4 g with water 4 times daily. As tincture, take 2 teaspoons of 1:5 strength tincture in 1 cup of water 4 times daily for 3 days. (1:5 refers to the ratio of the herb to its carrier liquid; you will find the ratio on the label of a product.) If after 3 days of this treatment, you have worsening pelvic pain or a fever, seek medical attention.

Both uva-ursi (also known as bearberry) and buchu (*Agathosma betulina*) have a long history of use for bladder infections. Uva-ursi is most effective in an alkaline environment, so don't drink cranberry juice while you are taking it, advises Dr. Head. Her recommended dosage is 400 mg in capsules 3 times daily for 10 days. The dosage is the same for buchu, but you don't have to worry about cranberry juice with buchu because this herb doesn't require the alkaline environment. In fact, there are cranberry-buchu capsules, combining the herb with cranberry extract.

Drinking horsetail, watermelon, and goldenrod teas is also soothing to the urinary tract, says Dr. Head. If you have pain, taking marshmallow (*Althea officinalis*) root can help, she notes. Take 2 capsules 3 times per day. You can take this with the other herbs.

The following herbal tea formula can resolve a UTI, says naturopathic physician Jody E. Noé, M.S., N.D., of Brattleboro, Vermont. If your urinary problem is not due to an infection, the formula will not help. Combine equal parts of bayberry (*Myrica cerifera*), juniper (*Juniperus communis*) berries, corn silk (*Zea mays*), oatstraw (*Avena sativa*), horsetail (*Equisetum arvense*) grass, and lavender (*Lavandula officinalis*). Use 1 tablespoon of the mixture per 1–1/2 to 2 cups of boiled water. Let steep for 15 minutes, strain, and drink 1 cup 4–5 times daily until the UTI is gone.

Homeopathy

Cantharis 30c, taken 3 times daily, can work quickly for a urinary tract infection, reports Dr. Head, often in only 1 to 3 doses. As soon as you experience significant relief of your symptoms, stop taking the remedy.

Nutritional Supplements

Dr. Head recommends taking vitamin C and magnesium citrate. Take the buffered form of vitamin C, which doesn't acidify the urine as much as regular vitamin C. Take 1/2 teaspoon powder twice daily (that equals about 2,000 mg per day) in water or water with a little unsweetened cranberry juice, for 10 days. Some forms of this vitamin C bubble when you put it in liquid; wait until it finishes bubbling, then drink.

To help alkalinize the urine, which reduces the pain with urination, take 250 mg of magnesium citrate twice daily. Some people get diarrhea from this amount of magnesium. If that occurs, cut the dosage to bowel tolerance (just below the amount that produces diarrhea).

Dr. Field recommends the multifaceted protocol below for a urinary tract infection, to be followed for 1 week:

Cranberry juice concentrate: Dilute the juice concentrate according to the manufacturer's instructions and drink 1 quart of the juice daily. You can take cranberry extract capsules instead (2 capsules 4 times daily), but be sure to drink 1 quart of water daily as well.

Vitamin C: 500 mg every 2 hours until bowel tolerance. Use plain vitamin C, not an ester-C or a calcium ascorbate. Taking vitamin C may make urination more painful, but the marshmallow root is soothing and reduces that effect.

Marshmallow root: Take 30 drops of the tincture in 1/2 cup of cool water 6 times daily; soothes the lining of the urinary tract.

Sitz baths: Mix 1 cup of Epsom salts in half a bathtub of warm water and soak. Do this twice daily. You can also use a sitz bath (a special tub that allows you to immerse your pelvic region in water with your legs out of the tub) or a washtub big enough for you to sit in with water up to your navel.

Reflexology

Kidneys, bladder, ureters

Stone/Crystal Therapy

Blue sapphire and nephrite are beneficial stones for a UTI, while gem silica and kyanite are specifically indicated for a bladder infection, according to Katrina Raphaell, crystal healing therapist and founder of the Crystal Academy of Advanced Healing Arts in Kapaa, Hawaii. Place the stone on the lower abdomen. Leave it there for 5 minutes while visualizing your health goal. Do this 3 times daily. In addition, wear the stone, hold it, or carry it in your pocket to continue the healing benefits.

Other Remedies

Wear cotton underwear. Shower, rather than take baths, and especially avoid bubble baths. Urinate after sexual intercourse. Wipe yourself from front to back following urination; wiping from back to front risks the transferral of bacteria from the anus or vagina to the urethra.

Blister

A blister is a collection of fluid beneath the outer surface of the skin in response to irritation, a burn, allergic reaction, an insect bite, or other trauma to the skin. Since the interior of a blister is a sterile environment and the fluid collects to protect the tissue beneath it, it is best not to pop the blister, which opens the damaged tissue to infection.

Essential Oils

Apply Lavender essential oil directly on the blister, says Patricia Davis, founder of the London School of Aromatherapy in London, England. Apply several times daily, as needed. If the blister is on your foot, you can put a few drops of Lavender on a piece of gauze and use it to cover the blister and protect it a bit from shoe rubbing. After the initial Lavender treatment, you can combine equal parts of Lavender and Benzoin in the direct application. Benzoin helps the skin heal.[1]

Flower Essences

Add Lavender flower essence and Lavender essential oil to Self-Heal cream, and apply to a blister to speed healing, says Richard Katz, naturalist and founder of the Flower Essence Society. Add 4–6 drops of the flower essence and 8 drops of the essential oil to 1 ounce of Self-Heal cream. Apply 2–4 times daily until the blister is healed.

Food Therapy

Eat foods high in vitamins A and C (see part 3, "Food Therapy," p. 378).

Herbal Medicine

A pad from the prickly pear cactus can heal new blisters quickly by drawing out their contents, states Michael Cottingham, a clinical herbalist from Silver City, New Mexico. It does so without breaking the skin, but to be safe, do not use in cases where breaking the blister may cause further damage. It doesn't do much for old blisters because there is little moisture left in them for the prickly pear to draw out. See "Boil" for instructions on using a prickly pad. You can tailor the size of pad you break off the cactus to the size of the area you need to treat and cut it into the appropriate sized pieces. In most cases, 1–2 applications, 20–30 minutes each, is sufficient to drain the blister, after which it dries up. Change the pad with each application and do the second right after the first.

Calendula (*Calendula officinalis*) cream applied topically can also aid the healing process of a blister.

Homeopathy

Maesimund B. Panos, M.D., cites these homeopathic remedies to help resolve blisters:[2]

Cantharis: If there is raw burning pain eased by cold applications.
Urtica: If the blister is accompanied by burning heat.

Take the appropriate remedy in a 6x potency 3–4 times daily. As symptoms improve, decrease the frequency. Stop taking the remedy when the improvement is well established.

Nutritional Supplements

Cut open gel capsules of vitamin A and/or E and spread the oil on the blister for their antioxidant and skin-healing properties. If you only have the vitamins in tablet form, you can crush a tablet and mix it with a little water or oil to make a paste.[3]

Stone/Crystal Therapy

Use celestite or anyhydrite, recommends crystal healing therapist Katrina Raphaell of Kapaa, Hawaii. Place the stone directly on the blister. Keep it in place for 5 minutes while visualizing your health goal. Do this 3 times daily. You can also wear the stone, hold it, or carry it in your pocket for ongoing effects.

Other Remedies

Cider vinegar, honey, and cornstarch are good kitchen remedies for a blister. You can mix the vinegar and honey together and apply it, or use them singly. Blend the cornstarch with warm water or vegetable oil and apply.[4]

Body Odor

Body odor results from the interaction of bacteria and the secretions of the underarm sweat glands. Regular bathing reduces the presence of bacterial waste, which has an unpleasant odor. Like bad breath, however, heavy body odor often has its roots in poor diet, digestion, and elimination. The smell emitted through the skin reflects the accumulation of toxins (putrefied food and bacterial waste) in the intestines. Deodorant and antiperspirants only mask the problem temporarily, if at all. For a lasting solution to this type of body odor, you need to address the underlying gastrointestinal problems and get rid of the toxic buildup in your body. In addition to chronic constipation, parasites, diabetes, liver disease, and zinc and/or magnesium deficiency can cause body odor.[1]

Essential Oils

Benzoin, Bergamot, Clary, Cypress, Eucalyptus, Lavender, Neroli, and Patchouli essential oils all counteract body odor, states aromatherapy authority Robert B. Tisserand.[2] Essential oils that aid the body in detoxifying may also be beneficial. These include Birch, Fennel, Garlic, Juniper, and Rose.[3] Use 1–3 of the oils at a time in massages, baths, or diffusions.

Flower Essences

To address body odor on a deep level, take Crab Apple and Self-Heal to detoxify and balance the system, recommends flower essence therapist Patricia Kaminski of Nevada City, California. Take 4 drops of each 2–4 times daily.

Food Therapy

Along with cleansing your internal environment, modifying your diet is "the most beneficial thing you can do to get rid of body odor," states naturopathic physician Linda Rector Page, N.D., Ph.D.[4]

Eat:

Fiber, fresh vegetables, yogurt/kefir, parsley, sprouts, foods high in magnesium and zinc (see part 3, "Food Therapy," pp. 377, 378). Drink plenty of water to help keep the body flushed of toxins that can contribute to body odor.

Avoid:

Fried foods, red meat, heavy sweets, caffeine.

Herbal Medicine

Antibacterial herbs such as licorice, thyme, oregano, rosemary, and coriander can help reduce body odor, says herbalist James A. Duke, Ph.D. Licorice has the most significant antibacterial activity of these, but all will likely provide some benefit. Dr. Duke suggests making a strong tea of one or more of the herbs, soaking a washcloth with it, and holding it against the underarms for a few minutes. Adding sage may produce an antiperspirant effect.[5]

Homeopathy

Consult a homeopath for individualized, constitutional treatment.

Nutritional Supplements

Liquid chlorophyll can help decrease body odor, notes Sue Reynolds, M.S.W., L.M.T., a certified herbalist and aromatherapist from Goleta, California. Take 1 teaspoon straight or in water 2–4 times daily. She also recommends zinc at a dosage of 25 mg 1–3 times daily. Adjust the dose as needed for effect; some people require less than others.

Magnesium supplementation is also beneficial in many cases. Magnesium deficiency is rampant in the United States, due to the standard American diet of processed foods. Typical dosages range from

250 to 500 mg daily. After initial supplementation, you may find that eating foods high in magnesium is sufficient to maintain a more pleasant body odor.

As a potent antimicrobial, grapefruit seed extract (GSE) makes an effective deodorant because it controls bacteria that contribute to body odor, says clinical nutritionist Allan Sachs, D.C., C.C.N. It also exerts mild antiperspirant action via its astringent properties, he notes. Combine 1/2 ounce of GSE with 10 ounces of water in a spray bottle. You can add calendula and/or arnica tincture as well. Spray the underarms as needed. You can also use it on your feet to control odor. Be careful to avoid getting the spray in your eyes.[6]

Reflexology

Intestines, stomach, solar plexus

Stone/Crystal Therapy

Wolfeite is a crystal remedy for body odor, according to Melody, author of the crystal reference series *Love Is in the Earth*. Apply as an elixir under the arms daily on an ongoing basis. (For instructions on making an elixir, see part 3, "Stone/Crystal Therapy," p. 403.)

Other Remedies

Apple cider vinegar used as an underarm deodorant can eliminate body odor.[7]

Boil

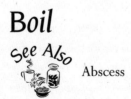 See Also Abscess

A boil, or furuncle, is a painful nodule in the skin resulting from subcutaneous inflammation. The areas of the body most typically afflicted are the face, neck, underarms, and buttocks. A boil begins as a red, painful bump, followed by the formation of a pustule in its center. The deep inflammation produces a core of blood clots. The core is characteristic of a boil and the source of the pain. Resolution of a boil involves expulsion of the core or its reabsorption by the body. A carbuncle is a cluster of boils.

Staphylococci bacteria, entering the skin by way of the hair follicle, are the common source of the infection, but deeper causes of recurrent boils include poor diet, toxic blood or colon, allergies, suppressed immunity, and thyroid disorders.[1]

You should not attempt to burst a boil, as that may spread and deepen the infection. Applying warm compresses can ease the pain and speed drainage of a boil. To avoid spreading the infection to others, do not share clothing, towels, or bedding.

Essential Oils

The potent antibacterial Tea Tree (*Melaleuca alternifolia*) oil is helpful for boils. Make a compress by putting 2–3 drops of the essential in 1 cup of warm water and soaking a cotton ball or cotton cloth with the blend. Lay the compress on the boil and leave it on for 10–15 minutes. Do this 4 times daily.[2]

Flower Essences

See Abscess.

Food Therapy

Eat:

Leafy greens, foods high in vitamin A and zinc (see part 3, "Food Therapy," p. 378).

Avoid:

Sugar, refined carbohydrates, greasy food, and food allergens.

Herbal Medicine

For a boil at any stage, prickly pear cactus provides an excellent remedy, according to Michael Cottingham, a clinical herbalist from Silver City, New Mexico. As it is useful for many health ailments, he recommends growing it as a houseplant if your climate precludes growing it outside. It doesn't harm the cactus to break off one of its pads.

A pad from the prickly pear is a powerful anti-inflammatory and hypotonic, which is a sucking and drawing substance, explains Cottingham. The nature of the cactus is to seek moisture, pull it in, and hold it. The pad acts on a boil as it does in nature, seeking out the weakest point on your skin, which is the boil, then drawing out and sucking up its fluid contents—the pus and inflammatory products.

To prepare the pad, knock off the prickles using a potholder or thick glove. Then use tongs to hold the pad over a flame (a burner on a gas stove is easiest, but a candle or a lighter will work) and burn off the spine of the pad. This is the part running around the edge. Hold the pad under running cold water to flush away the burned parts. Then cut it in half. Cut one of the pieces crosswise to expose the gooey inside of the pad. Make sure it's not too hot, and then place one of these pieces, gooey side down, on your boil. Leave the other pieces in the sun or in the oven near the pilot light to keep them warm. In many cases, one half-hour application is enough, but more infected boils may require several applications.

Use a fresh piece of pad every half-hour. Keep applying the pads until the inflammation and pus are gone, instructs Cottingham. As you probably now have a picture of how this works, you can see that you don't need a big pad for a single small boil. You can tailor the size of pad you break off the cactus to the size of the area you need to treat and cut it into the appropriate sized pieces.

Birch (*Betula spp.*) bark tea is also useful in resolving boils. Simmer 1 cup of bark in 1 quart of water for 10–15 minutes, strain, and drink the tea throughout the day. Continue the practice until your boils are healed.[3]

Homeopathy

For boils, Drs. Andrew Lockie and Nicola Geddes recommend:[4]

Belladonna: for the early stages of a boil, when it's beginning to form, and the surrounding skin is hard, swollen, dry, burning, red, and painful; take 30c every hour for up to 10 doses.

Hepar sulph: for the later stages of a boil, when pus is present, the boil is near bursting, and it is sensitive to even slight touch; take 6c every hour for up to 10 doses.

Nutritional Supplements

Vitamin A and zinc can be effective in resolving a boil, according to nutritional medicine specialist Allan Magaziner, D.O. His recommended daily dosage is 10,000 IU of vitamin A and 15–20 mg of zinc, taken until the boil is gone. If you have a tendency to develop boils, cut these dosages in half and take as a preventive, maintenance protocol, says Dr. Magaziner.[5]

Reflexology

Treat the area of the foot corresponding to the part of the body where the boil is located.

Stone/Crystal Therapy

For a boil, apply petrified palm, states Melody, author of the crystal reference series *Love Is in the Earth*. Use hypoallergenic tape to secure the stone on or near the boil. Leave it on for 2–3 days, until the condition is resolved.

Other Remedies

A potato poultice is an easy and effective treatment for a boil or abscess, according to naturopathic physician Susan Roberts, N.D., of Portland, Oregon. Grate potato, put it in gauze, and hold on the affected area for 15 minutes. Do this 4 times daily, using fresh potato each time, until the boil is resolved. The potato draws out the infection.

Bone Fracture (Healing Support)

Once you have received medical attention for a bone fracture, natural therapies can ease the pain and speed healing of the broken bone.

Essential Oils

"Helichrysum is aromatherapy's arnica," says medical aromatherapist Julia Fischer of Northern California. In cases of injury to bones, tendons, or ligaments, it aids healing, reduces swelling, pain, and inflammation, and stimulates circulation in the area, which aids all of the other processes. For a doubly powerful remedy, Fischer recommends a liniment of Helichrysum essential oil in an arnica base oil (an oil infused with the herb arnica) or arnica tincture. Blend 10–15 drops of Helichrysum and 1 ounce of the base oil or tincture. Apply to the affected area 4–5 times daily. You can reduce the number of treatments per day after the initial healing phase if you want, but you should continue applying the liniment on a daily basis until the bone is healed, usually about 6 weeks.

Flower Essences

As flower essence support for healing a bone fracture, use Comfrey, says naturalist Richard Katz of Nevada City, California. Take 4 drops under the tongue 4 times daily until the bone is healed.

Food Therapy

Eat:

Lean protein, foods high in calcium, phosphorus, and vitamin D. (For a list of foods containing these nutrients, see part 3, "Food Therapy," p. 376-378.)

Avoid:

Sugar, red meat, caffeine, soft drinks, excess salt, acid-forming foods (see part 3, "Food Therapy," p. 376).

Herbal Medicine

As healing support for a bone fracture, an herbal blend taken in capsule form is very effective, says David Winston, A.H.G., a clinical herbalist and consultant from Washington, New Jersey. "I have yet to see a fracture that doesn't heal in half the time with this formula." To make the blend, put the following herbs in a coffee or seed grinder or a blender in the proportions indicated:

Nettle (*Urtica dioica*) leaf: 2 parts of the dried herb

Horsetail (*Equisetum arvense*): 1 part of the dried herb

Alfalfa (*Medicago sativa*): 1 part of the dried herb

Dandelion (*Taraxacum officinalis*) leaf: 1 part of the dried herb

Oatstraw (*Avena sativa*): 1 part; this herb is optional

When you take the lid off the blender, there will be a cloud of dust. Be careful not to inhale it. Fill empty capsules with the powder. Take 2 capsules 2–3 times daily until the bone is healed.

Homeopathy

When you have any injury, the first remedy to use is Arnica montana, says homeopathic physician Michael G. Carlston, M.D., of Santa Rosa, California. For bone fracture, take Arnica montana 30c every hour or two at first for discomfort and pain. As the pain gets less, cut back to taking it a few times a day, instructs Dr. Carlston.

When the bone fracture is especially affected by motion, when you get pain from motion and want to hold the injured part, use Bryonia alba 30c every hour or two at first, then a few times a day. This is in addition to the Arnica montana.

Symphytum officinale (derived from the herb comfrey, also known as "knitbone" because of its bone-healing properties) and Calcarea phosphorica are helpful for the long term, for the healing of the bone. Once you are past pain being the issue, take 12c or 30c of either once or twice a day until the bone is healed.

Nutritional Supplements

Along with taking a regular multivitamin/mineral, Paul Reilly, N.D., L.Ac., a naturopathic physician and acupuncturist of Seattle, Washington, recommends the following nutritional supplement protocol as healing support for a bone fracture:

Microcrystalline hydroxy hepatite: A specially processed form of bone meal. "When they think of healing bones, most people think about calcium, but this works better. It contains calcium as well as other bone factors." Take 500 mg 3 times daily with food.

Vitamin D: 1,000 IU daily; helps the body absorb calcium.

Vitamin K: 2 mg daily; helps calcium bind to the bone.

Vitamin C: 2,000–3,000 mg daily; It's a good practice to take this on an ongoing basis as part of your total health program. "This is the amount of vitamin C that animals make daily. The human body cannot manufacture vitamin C, but must get it from food or supplements."

Take the above supplements until the bone fracture is healed.

Reflexology

Treat the area of the foot corresponding to the part of the body where the bone fracture is located. If it is in the foot, do not use reflexology.

Stone/Crystal Therapy

Green calcite, black (and blue) kyanite, hematite, and malachite support the healing of bones, says Katrina Raphaell, crystal healing therapist and founder of the Crystal Academy of Advanced Healing Arts in Kapaa, Hawaii. Place the stone directly on the site of the fracture. While visualizing your health goal, leave the stone in place for 5 minutes. Do this 3 times daily. In between these treatments, wear the stone, hold it, or carry it in your pocket to continue the effects.

Bone Spur (Heel Spur)

A bone spur typically refers to a pointed growth consisting of calcium deposits on the heel bone (calcaneus), so it is also known as a heel or calcaneal spur. Those afflicted may experience pain while walking or standing, or they may have no symptoms. For those with pain, it may be associated with stress on the Achilles tendon, which hiking, jogging, or improper footwear can produce.[1] Excess weight, arthritis, tendonitis, and neuritis are associated with bone spurs.[2] A high intake of oxalate foods (peanuts and chard, among others) resulting in a high level of oxalic acid in the body may also contribute to bone spur formation. Excessive levels of oxalic acid interfere with the absorption of calcium, leading to calcium deposits in the form of bone spurs.[3]

Essential Oils

For a liniment to relieve the pain of a bone spur, combine 2 drops each of essential oils of Helichrysum, *Eucalyptus citriodora* (lemon eucalyptus), and Birch with 2 droppersful (2 ml) of arnica tincture or St. John's wort tincture, recommends medical aromatherapist Julia Fischer of Northern California. In addition to warming, analgesic properties, this mixture is anti-inflammatory and helps calm nerve endings. Gently rub the liniment into the afflicted area as needed.

Flower Essences

Self-Heal can serve as a foundational healing agent for a bone spur. Other flower essences to address the specific emotions, mental attitude, and environmental conditions of the individual are recommended, states Patricia Kaminski, a flower essence therapist and codirector of the Flower Essence Society. Self-Heal supports the body's innate healing ability. Take 4 drops 2–4 times daily, or as needed.

Food Therapy

Eat:

Fiber, foods high in magnesium (see part 3, "Food Therapy," p. 377). Drink black cherry juice.

Avoid:

Citrus, sugar, alcohol, coffee, excess salt, high-oxalate foods (see part 3, "Food Therapy," p. 377).

Herbal Medicine

Joanne B. Mied, N.D., a naturopath, herbalist, and iridologist from Novato, California, has found hydrangea (*Hydrangea arborescens*) root capsules very effective for bone spurs. (Note that hydrangea leaves are poisonous, but the roots are not.) Take 9 capsules (325 mg each) daily until the pain is gone. Then cut back to 6 capsules daily. If the pain returns, go back up to 9. Drink lots of water, at least 8 glasses (8 ounces each) a day.

Homeopathy

For a bone spur, Dr. Barry Rose of the Royal London Homeopathic Hospital advises Hekla lava 12c. Take the remedy 2 times a day until your symptoms improve.[4]

Nutritional Supplements

"Vitamin C applied topically has the ability to lessen or completely alleviate pain from a heel spur," states holistic nutritionist Cathy Sparks, Ph.D. Combine vitamin C powder (no more than 15 g) with enough water to form a paste, spread it on a gauze pad, and tape the pad to the afflicted heel. Do this for a few days, until the pain abates. Dr. Sparks notes that the vitamin C is absorbed through the heel and provides needed collagen and elastin (important components in connective tissue such as ligaments and tendons) to the extremely tight tendon involved in a heel spur. Do not be alarmed if your heel turns brown; the brown comes right off with washing.[5]

Other helpful supplements include betaine HCl, calcium, and magnesium. Many people are deficient in stomach acid (hydrocloric acid, or HCl), which is necessary for proper uptake of calcium. Ensuring absorption helps prevent calcium deposits in body tissue. Take betaine HCl as directed by the manufacturer. Likewise, ensuring that you are getting a proper ratio of calcium and magnesium, which function in concert with each other, can also help prevent deposits. A typical dosage is 1,500 mg of calcium and 750 mg of magnesium. The chelate form of these minerals is more easily absorbed by the body.[6]

Reflexology

Do not use reflexology on an injured or painful foot.

Stone/Crystal Therapy

By promoting the excretion of excess minerals from a joint, whiteite may be helpful for a bone spur. You can keep the stone in place over the affected area by covering it with an adhesive bandage.

Obviously, don't wear shoes when you have it in place, or wear back-less shoes. Alternatively, place the stone on the bone spur area and rest quietly several times a day for 10–15 minutes.[7]

Other Remedies

Dr. Mied has seen a number of patients whose bone spurs were caused by working out on a skiing exercise machine, which involved impact on the heel. When they stopped using the machine, they had no further problems with bone spurs.

Bronchitis and Other Upper Respiratory Infection

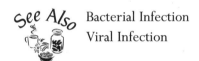 See Also

Bacterial Infection
Viral Infection

Bronchitis, or inflammation of the mucous membrane of the bronchi (the two large branches of the trachea) in the lungs, is one type of upper respiratory infection (URI). URI is a general term for any infection of the nasal passages, pharynx, and bronchi.

Bronchitis can be caused by viral or bacterial infection, irritation of the airways by dust or fumes, or allergies. Acute bronchitis, also known as a chest cold, frequently follows the common cold or a bout of flu and can turn into pneumonia. Symptoms include fever, a cough that is dry at first and later produces mucus, and body aches.

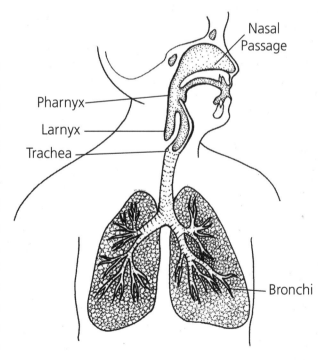

Nasal Passage

Pharynx

Larnyx

Trachea

Bronchi

Chronic bronchitis is caused by frequent irritation of the airways. Allergies, smoking, recurrent acute bronchitis, and prolonged stress can contribute to this chronic condition. It is characterized by increased mucus secretion and buildup, thickening of the bronchial walls, and a cough that lasts for three months out of the year. Chronic bronchitis increases the risk of respiratory infection.

If the mucus from your lungs is yellow or bloody, you have a fever higher than 102 degrees, or the bronchitis lasts for more than 5 days, seek medical help.

The remedies below can be used for other upper respiratory infections in addition to bronchitis.

Essential Oils

As a steam treatment for bronchitis, Paul Reilly, N.D., L.Ac., a naturopathic physician and acupuncturist from Seattle, Washington, recommends putting 30 drops of Eucalyptus essential oil in a pot of boiled water (removed from heat). Then drape a towel over your head and the pot and breathe in the aromatic steam for 5–10 minutes twice daily. Both the heat and the eucalyptus are beneficial. Eucalyptus is an antiviral and works in the lungs to thin mucus.

Flower Essences

Yerba Santa is the flower essence indicated for bronchitis, especially when a history of respiratory infection can be traced to early childhood onset and accompanying trauma, states Patricia Kaminski, a flower essence therapist and educator from Nevada City, California. Take 4 drops under the tongue 4 times daily until your symptoms subside.

Food Therapy

Eat:

Garlic, cayenne, horseradish, foods high in vitamin C (see part 3, "Food Therapy," p. 378). Drink plenty of fluids (diluted vegetable juices, soups, herbal tea, green tea).

Avoid:

Sugar (and limit fruit and fruit juices), fried food, mucus-forming foods (dairy, chocolate, eggs, junk food).

Herbal Medicine

Since acute bronchitis is typically viral or bacterial and self-limiting, meaning it runs its course without treatment, the focus of remedies should be on supporting the body to help healing occur more rapidly, states Dr. Reilly. To this end, he suggests the following herbs:

Hyssop (*Hyssopus officinalis*) and thyme (*Thymus vulgaris*) tea: Both herbs help to relieve cough and clear mucus. Thyme is also an antimicrobial. Use 3 parts of hyssop to 1 part of thyme. Put 1 teaspoon of the mixture in a cup of boiled water, steep for a few minutes, strain, and drink. Drink 3–4 cups daily. You can add this mixture to green tea if you like.

Grindelia (*Grindelia camporum*): Helps relieve cough and clear mucus; 1 teaspoon of the herb per cup of boiled water, steep. Drink 3–6 cups daily. You can combine this tea with the hyssop and thyme tea.

Echinacea (*E. spp.*) and goldenseal (*Hydrastis canadensis*): Use a 50:50 mix of these immune-supporting herbs. Take 2 capsules 3 times daily.

Take these herbs until you have been free of symptoms for 2–3 days (you can cut the doses in half when you are feeling better). For most people, this protocol, along with the essential oil treatment, homeopathic remedy, and nutritional supplements, resolves bronchitis quickly.

Clinical herbalist Michael Cottingham, of Silver City, New Mexico, notes that lavender flower tea is an excellent remedy for children (and adults) with bronchitis. Lavender (*Lavandula officinalis*) improves respiration because it has antispasmodic and bronchial-dilating properties. It is also a nervine, promoting whole-body relaxation, which increases circulation and generally aids in healing. To make the tea, put 1/4 teaspoon of the flowers in 1 cup of boiled water, cover, let steep for 10–15 minutes, and then strain.

With respiratory conditions in children, the most effective approach is "relentless pursuit," says Cottingham. To that end, give your child 2–3 teaspons of the tea every half hour for the first 2 days. Decrease the dosage to 1 teaspoon every hour or two on the third to fourth days. This may be difficult, but 2 teaspoons every half hour or hour for the first 3 days will resolve the condition in 80 percent of children, according to Cottingham. He notes that Mexican grandmothers routinely use this remedy on their grandchildren to great effect. Lavender is extremely safe for infants, so there is no need to be concerned about giving them this much.

Adults should use 1 heaping teaspoon of lavender flowers per cup of water. If the taste is too strong, you can dilute the tea slightly or add honey and lemon. Drink a cup of tea up to 5 times daily for a week, or as needed. If you are prone to respiratory infections, it is a good idea to drink lavender tea on a regular basis to strengthen your lungs.

Homeopathy

Dr. Reilly cites two homeopathic remedies as most commonly useful for bronchitis:

Phosphorus: Reduces the likelihood of bronchitis turning into pneumonia.
Kali bich: Take this remedy if you are coughing up a lot of mucus.

Take the remedy in a 6x or 12x potency, under the tongue, 2–4 times daily.

Nutritional Supplements

As part of his total protocol for bronchitis, Dr. Reilly uses the following supplements for immune support (in addition to a regular multivitamin/mineral):

Vitamin C: Take more vitamin C than you usually do; up the dosage to 3,000–5,000 mg daily.
Vitamin A: 10,000–20,000 IU daily. (If you are pregnant or there is any chance you could become so, don't take any more than a total of 5,000 IU daily.)
Zinc: 60 mg daily.
Thymus extract: 200–300 mg 3 times daily.

Keep taking these supplements until you have been free of symptoms for 2–3 days. As with the herbal remedies, you can cut the doses in half when you are feeling better.

Reflexology

Lungs, solar plexus, spleen

Stone/Crystal Therapy

Rose quartz, kunzite, amazonite, and green aventurine can be beneficial for bronchitis, according to crystal healing therapist Katrina Raphaell of Kapaa, Hawaii. Place the stone on your chest over the place in your lungs where you feel the most distress. While visualizing your health goal, leave the stone in place for 5 minutes. Do this 3 times daily. For added benefit, also wear the stone, hold it, or carry it in your pocket.

Bruise

A bruise, or contusion, is an injury from impact that produces discoloration of the skin, without breaking the surface. The discoloration—"black and blue"—is due to broken blood vessels (usually capillaries), which leak blood into local tissue. A black eye is one form of bruise. Excess weight, anticlotting medications, and nutritional deficiencies are associated with easy bruising.

Essential Oils

Rub Helichrysum essential oil onto the bruise or area likely to bruise. "If you can get the oil on before the bruise shows up, it may prevent it," states naturopathic physician Boyer B. Cole, N.M.D., of Cottonwood, Arizona. For already existing bruises, it can reduce swelling and take away the pain and color; it even works for older bruises, according to Dr. Cole. Apply the Helichrysum 3–4 times daily for 1 day. For a small bruise, use the essential oil neat (straight, undiluted). For a larger area, it can be expensive to use pure oil, so dilute it in a base oil such as almond or olive oil. Use a ratio of 1:5 (essential oil:base oil).

Flower Essences

To speed healing and relieve the pain of a bruise, apply Arnica Alleve flower oil 2–4 times daily, recommends Richard Katz, founder of the Flower Essence Society.

Food Therapy

Eat:

Green vegetables, citrus, green tea, foods high in vitamins C and K. (For a list of foods containing these nutrients, see part 3, "Food Therapy," p. 378.)

Avoid:

Dairy products

Herbal Medicine

A comfrey root poultice can help a bruise heal more quickly, according to herbalist Teresa Boardwine of Washington, Virginia. Comfrey (*Symphytum officinale*) is a potent tissue-healing herb with the active constituent allantoin, a substance that promotes cell proliferation. To make the poultice, first prepare a decoction by simmering 1/2 cup of comfrey root in 1 quart water for 30 minutes. Strain off the tea and set aside. Tie the comfrey root in a cotton handkerchief or single-layer (unlined) cotton baby diaper. Place the pack on the affected skin, and leave on for 30 minutes to 1 hour. When the pack cools, put the herbs back in the tea water to rehydrate, then reapply. This poultice has a cooling effect on the bruised area. Note: Do not drink the tea; for external use only.

Homeopathy

The following remedies are indicated for bruises, states London homeopath Miranda Castro:[1]

Arnica: "The number one remedy for bruises," may prevent a bruise if taken right after injury; indicated for swelling without discoloration, although it can speed the healing of an already formed bruise.

Bellis: For bruises with bumps and lumps remaining.

Ledum: Indicated for discoloration; give Ledum if Arnica has failed to prevent the formation of the bruise.

Sulphuric acid: For blue-black, slow-to-heal bruises; will complete the healing of bruises that do not respond to Arnica or Ledum.

Take the appropriate remedy in a 6c or 12c potency every 1–8 hours, as needed. Discontinue the remedy when there is improvement. Repeat if necessary.

Nutritional Supplements

To speed healing of a bruise, the following supplements are beneficial, according to naturopathic physician Nick Buratovich, N.M.D., of Tempe, Arizona:

Vitamin C: 1–2 g three times daily for 1–3 weeks; promotes skin healing.

Bioflavonoids: These anti-inflammatory plant substances also help stabilize capillary membranes. Quercetin or citrus bioflavonoids are the best form to take. Take 1–3 g daily for 1–3 weeks.

Vitamin K: 70–140 mcg daily, in 3 divided doses; increases clotting, which helps limit blood seepage into tissue.

Reflexology

Treat the area of the foot corresponding to the part of the body where the bruise is located or is likely to appear.

Stone/Crystal Therapy

For treatment of bruises, Melody, author of the crystal reference series *Love Is in the Earth*, recommends an elixir of purpurite or scolecite applied to the area 3 times daily for 2–3 days. Euclase placed upon the bruise can also ease discomfort. Attach the stone with hypoallergenic tape and leave it on for 2–3 days. (For instructions on making an elixir, see part 3, "Stone/Crystal Therapy," p. 403.)

Other Remedies

A poultice made of green clay or French green clay can actually prevent a bruise from forming or reduce its severity if you apply it soon after the injury, says Teresa Boardwine. Clay is a drawing agent, and can help pull out the cellular debris and waste products of injury and inflammation. Put 1/4 cup of the clay in a small dish, cover it with water to 1/2 inch above it. Let it sit for 20 minutes to allow the clay to soak up the water. Stir the paste and apply it to the injured area. When the clay is hard, reapply. Do this 4–5 times total. If the injury is a turned ankle or an ankle kicked during team sports, you can wrap the poulticed area with gauze and an elastic bandage.

Bunion

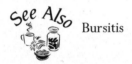 Bursitis

A bunion is a protrusion at the base of the big toe, an enlargement of the joint that connects the toe to the foot. The enlargement, caused by inflammation and thickening of the bursa in the joint, can also push

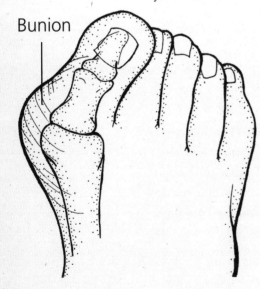

Bunion

the big toe out of alignment so it leans toward or overlaps the second toe. Heredity and joint diseases such as arthritis are contributing factors, but the main culprit in most cases of bunions is the habitual wearing of tight shoes, particularly high heels, that force the toes together.

Essential Oils

To alleviate the pain and swelling of a bunion, aromatherapist Valerie Ann Worwood recommends a two-part treatment done twice a day. Blend 1 teaspoon each of Tagetes and Jojoba essential oils. As the first step, rub 3 drops of the mixture into the affected foot, particularly the bunion and the ball of the foot. Next, massage the entire foot with the following essential oil blend: Tagetes (10 drops), Carrot (5 drops), and German chamomile (15 drops) in 2 tablespoons of vegetable oil.[1]

Flower Essences

Self-Heal can serve as a foundational healing agent for bunions. Other flower essences to address the specific emotions, mental attitude, and environmental conditions of the individual are recommended, states Patricia Kaminski, a flower essence therapist and codirector of the Flower Essence Society. Self-Heal supports the body's innate healing ability. Take 4 drops 2–4 times daily, or as needed.

Food Therapy

Eat:

Green vegetables.

Avoid:

Fried food, saturated fats.

Herbal Medicine

For a bunion, Karen Vaughan, E.M.T, A.H.G, a clinical herbalist from Brooklyn, New York, suggests a threefold treatment plan: use plastic inserts or an orthopedic brace (see "Other Remedies" following), don't wear high heels, and apply violet (*Viola odorata*) leaf poultices to ease the inflammation and relieve the pain of a bunion in the acute stage. Violet is high in salicylates (the active ingredient in aspirin is derived from salicylates) and other anti-inflammatories. To prepare the violet leaf poultice, put a handful of fresh leaves in the blender and chop up fine. Add just enough water to make a goop. Tie it up in a handkerchief and lay it on the bunion, with the plastic insert between your toes in place. Cover with a plastic bag to avoid violet stains and wrap the whole with an elastic bandage. Leave it on overnight and repeat as needed.

If you do all of the above and the bunion doesn't improve, you might want to see an acupuncturist, says Vaughan. Bunions are often related to disturbances of the spleen meridian (energy pathway in the body), which acupuncture can treat, she notes.

St. John's wort (*Hypericum perforatum*) oil or cream or comfrey (*Symphytum officinale*) cream applied twice daily can help relieve the pain and inflammation of a bunion, says herbalist Penelope Ody. Use as needed.[2]

Homeopathy

For a bunion with tearing pain in the big toe, Dr. Barry Rose of the Royal London Homeopathic Hospital in London, England, cites Benzoic acid 30c. Take the remedy 3 times a day on 1 day each week. This eases the pain and seems to retard the development of the bunion, says Dr. Rose.[3]

Nutritional Supplements

Anti-inflammatory supplements, such as bromelain, grape seed, or pine bark extract, and flaxseed oil, are helpful for bunions. Bromelain is an enzyme compound found in pineapple. Take 250–500 mg on an empty stomach 2–3 times daily. Take 25–50 mg of grape seed or pine bark extract 2–3 times daily, also on an empty stomach. The dosage for flaxseed oil is 1 tablespoon daily.[4]

Reflexology

Do not do reflexology on an injured or painful foot, or on a foot problem.

Other Remedies

Using an orthopedic brace for a bunion is very important, notes Karen Vaughan, as it holds the big toe in a more normal position, instead of allowing its slant toward the second toe to worsen. You can get plastic inserts or larger braces designed for the purpose at drugstores or orthopedic Web sites. Vaughan also observes that people with bunions are typically out of alignment in movement, so can benefit from deep body work such as polarity therapy or rolfing to correct the problem.

Home physical therapy is good for bunions as well. Exercise the toes and the toe joints by picking up marbles or other small objects with your toes.[5]

You may want to consider acupuncture, because bunions are often associated with imbalances in the pancreas and thyroid.[6] Treatment of the spleen/pancreas meridian (energy pathway) can help correct these imbalances.

Burn

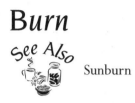

See Also   Sunburn

A burn is tissue damage caused by heat or fire. (Chemicals and electricity can also burn tissues; seek medical attention immediately.) Burns are rated by degree of severity.

First-degree burns involve superficial damage, affecting only the epidermis, or outer layer of the skin, and produce redness and mild pain. Most cases of sunburn are first-degree burns.

Second-degree burns damage tissue in the epidermis and the next layer of skin, the dermis; redness, blisters, and more severe pain accompany second-degree burns.

Third-degree burns destroy the epidermis and dermis and damage tissue beneath the skin; the skin may be charred. In the case of a third-degree burn, a second-degree burn larger than a quarter in size, or an electrical burn, get medical care immediately.

Common wisdom used to dictate the application of butter or other grease to burns. You should definitely discard this practice, along with the notion that ice water can take the heat out quickly. Using ice water on your burn can actually make it worse. Run cool water over the burn instead.[1]

Essential Oils

Kurt Schnaubelt, Ph.D., scientific director of the Pacific Institute of Aromatherapy in San Rafael, California, recommends Lavender or German Chamomile essential oil for a burn. Apply 1–3 drops or the amount needed to cover the surface area of the burn. Do this frequently in the first 2–3 hours after being burned. Continue until the pain or swelling goes down. Seek medical attention if symptoms persist.

For second-degree burns, Julia Fischer, a medical aromatherapist practicing in Northern California, relies on a combination of oils. First, apply 1 drop each of Tea Tree (*Melaleuca alternifolia*) and Lavender essential oils to cleanse the wound. Then blend the following:

Helichrysum essential oil: 9 drops
Spike Lavender essential oil: 6 drops
Sage essential oil: 6 drops
Rosemary Verbenone essential oil: 6 drops
Rose hip seed fatty oil: 1 teaspoon (5 ml); this is a carrier oil that has
    been infused with rose hip seed
Sunflower vegetable oil: 5 teaspoons (25 ml)

Apply enough of this mixture to cover the area of the burn, 3 times daily, until the burn is healed. Gradually reduce the application to 2 times daily, then once a day, to help the skin complete its recovery. Protect the burn from direct sun exposure throughout.

Flower Essences

Applying Self-Heal flower essence cream and St. John's Shield flower oil to a burn 2–4 times daily helps restore the damaged tissue, notes Patricia Kaminski, an herbalist and flower essence therapist from Nevada City, California. Mix 1–2 tablespoons of the oil with 1 ounce of the cream, or apply them alternately. You can also alternate these two applications with a lavender formula (see "Blister," p. 46). Continue treatment until the burn is healed.

Food Therapy

Eat:

Green and yellow vegetables, flaxseed (grind in a coffee or herb grinder and sprinkle on salads, cereal, and other food). Drink plenty of water.

Avoid:

Sugar.

Herbal Medicine

To aid in healing and protect from infection, Paul Reilly, N.D., L.Ac., a naturopathic physician and acupuncturist from Seattle, Washington, recommends the following protocol:

Use aloe vera or calendula (*Calendula officinalis*) to help heal the tissue: Aloe vera gel is well known as a treatment for burns. The fresh gel right out of the plant is the most effective, while the stabilized gel you buy is second-best—a distant second—and the long-lasting aloe vera gel typically shelved with suntan lotions is not even in the running, notes Dr. Reilly. The stabilized gel doesn't keep well, which makes growing aloe as a house or garden plant even more advisable. Break off a piece of the plant, open it up, and apply the gel directly on your burn, once or twice a day until it is healed.

For calendula, use the succus form, says Dr. Reilly. Succus refers to the juice expressed from calendula petals. You can buy calendula succus as a tincture (a succus contains more plant extract and less alcohol than a regular tincture). Apply this to the burn 2–3 times daily.

You can apply one or the other of these remedies as often as hourly, if you like. In any case, treatment should be most intensive on the first day. You can cut back to 1–3 times daily for the next few days, then once a day after that.

Use tea tree (*Melaleuca alternifolia*) ointment to protect from infection: Apply once a day; tea tree oil is a potent antibacterial agent.

Michael Cottingham, a clinical herbalist from Silver City, New Mexico, notes that prickly pear cactus pads can do wonders for a second-degree burn with blisters in the early stages (just forming). Prickly pear can pull the moisture from the blisters and the skin can then return to normal, circumventing the usual healing process. There is no point in using prickly pear in the later stages of blistering because the skin has already started decaying. In most cases, 1–2 applications is sufficient. Leave the pad on for 20–30 minutes per application. Change the pad with each application and do the second right after the first. You can do up to five applications, depending on the severity of the injury, but after the first two applications, separate them by an hour or more. See "Boil" for how to prepare and apply the prickly pear cactus pad.

Homeopathy

To ease the pain of a burn, take Urtica urens or Apis mellifica, says Dr. Reilly. Take a 6x or 12x potency as often as needed, even every 15 minutes when the pain is acute. As the pain reduces, reduce the frequency. Keep taking until the pain is gone; do not continue the remedy when you no longer have pain.

Nutritional Supplements

To aid in healing a burn, you can use supplements both topically and internally. Here are Dr. Reilly's protocols:

Topical application: Choose either the vitamin oil or the DMSO detailed here or one of the herbal remedies above.

Break open vitamin E and vitamin A capsules, or use liquid supplements if you have them. Use 3 parts vitamin E to 1 part vitamin A. Spread the oil blend on your burn, 2–3 times daily for the first couple of days. As with the herbal remedies, you can apply the vitamins as often as hourly. Treatment should be most intensive on the first day.

As an alternative, you can dab liquid DMSO (dimethyl sulfoxide) on the burn with a cotton ball, 2–3 times daily or more frequently if you like. Buy a 30 percent solution or dilute it down. For example, if you can only find a 90 percent solution, use 2 parts water to 1 part DMSO to bring it down to 30 percent. DMSO can repair damaged tissue and speed healing.

Oral supplements: All of these are important nutrients for the skin. Take them in addition to your regular multivitamin/mineral until the burn is healed.

Vitamin A: Take extra vitamin A along with your regular multivitamin; 10,000–25,000 IU daily (if you are pregnant or suspect you are, don't take any more than a total of 5,000 IU daily).

Zinc: 60 mg daily.

Vitamin C: 5,000 mg daily, taken in 2–3 doses.

Flaxseed oil: 1 tablespoon daily.

Stone/Crystal Therapy

For burns, use angelite, larimar, or blue calcite, says crystal healing therapist Katrina Raphaell of Kapaa, Hawaii. Place the stone on the burn, or as near the burn as possible if it is painful to situate the stone directly on it. Keep it in place for 5 minutes while visualizing your health goal. Do this 3 times daily. In between treatments, wear the stone, hold it, or carry it in your pocket to continue the healing effects.

Bursitis

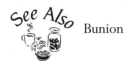 Bunion

Shoulder Joint

Bursae

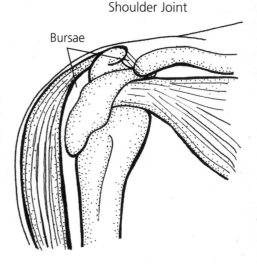

This painful condition is inflammation of a bursa, a fluid-filled sac found in joints and other areas where friction occurs. Bursae act as cushioning pads between tendons and bones, and tendons and ligaments. Pain, restricted movement, and calcium deposits in the joint can accompany bursitis. Common forms of bursitis include frozen shoulder, tennis elbow, housemaid's knee, and bunion. Strain and injury are the typical causes of bursitis.

If you suffer from chronic bursitis, consult a doctor.

Essential Oils

Daily baths and/or massages of the sore area with Lavender oil can ease the pain and inflammation of bursitis. Use as needed.[1] (For instructions on how to use essential oils in baths and massages, see part 3, "Essential Oils," p. 366–68.)

Flower Essences

Self-Heal can serve as a foundational healing agent for bursitis. Other flower essences to address the specific emotions, mental attitude, and environmental conditions of the individual are recommended, states Patricia Kaminski, a flower essence therapist and codirector of the Flower Essence Society. Self-Heal supports the body's innate healing ability. Take 4 drops 2–4 times daily, or as needed.

Food Therapy

Eat:

Small meals, lean protein, steamed greens, fiber, pineapple (eaten by itself), alkalinizing foods and foods high in vitamin B12. (For a list of foods containing these nutrients, see part 3, "Food Therapy," p. 376, 378.)

Avoid:

Greasy or fried foods, food allergens, nightshade vegetables, acid-forming foods (see part 3, "Food Therapy," pp. 376, 377).

Herbal Medicine

For bursitis, David Winston, A.H.G., a clinical herbalist from Washington, New Jersey, uses the following combination of oral and topical treatments to reduce inflammation and relieve pain:

Oral tincture blend: Combine the herbs below in the proportions noted and take 5 ml (roughly 1 teaspoon) of the blend 3 times daily for 2 months.

2 parts turmeric (*Curcuma longa*) tincture; anti-inflammatory

2 parts meadowsweet (*Filipendula ulmaria*) tincture; anti-inflammatory

2 parts sarsaparilla (*Smilax spp.*) tincture; anti-inflammatory

1 part ginger (*Zingiber officinale*) tincture; anti-inflammatory

1–2 parts black cohosh (*Cimicifuga racemosa*) tincture; this pain-relieving herb is used for conditions such as muscular arthritis and fibromyalgia

Immune support: take a strong antioxidant such as grape seed extract (pycnogenol); use according to the manufacturer's directions.

Topical treatment: Combine equal parts of infused oils of arnica (*Arnica montana*), St. John's wort (*Hypericum perforatum*), and lobelia (*Lobelia inflata*) seed, with a few drops of essential oil of Sweet Birch. (Note that an infused oil is distinct from an essential oil or herbal tincture. It is the herb in a carrier oil such as olive oil, rather than an extract or an essential oil preserved in alcohol or glycerin. Some infused products are labeled olive oil extract.) Lightly massage the blend into the affected joint twice daily, for as long as needed. (This oil blend is available as Compound Arnica Oil from Herbalist and Alchemist; see David Winston's listing under "Herbal Medicine" in Appendix B: Resources.)

Homeopathy

Homeopathic physician Michael G. Carlston, M.D., of Santa Rosa, California, recommends the following homeopathic remedies:

Bryonia: If your bursitis is characterized by aversion to motion, the desire to hold the sore area, and improvement with warmth.

Rhus tox: If the bursitis feels better when you persist in moving the joint through the initial pain and stiffness (like a rusty hinge loosening if you move it back and forth), is aggravated by wet weather, and is sensitive to cold.

Ruta: If your bursitis is similar to that described for Rhus tox, but there is less improvement with motion.

Take the appropriate remedy at a 12c or 30c potency, 2–3 times daily. If the bursitis was acute in onset, rather than coming on gradually, take the remedy 4 times per day. This is especially true of the bursitis for which Bryonia is the remedy. Reduce the frequency gradually as there is improvement. Don't continue taking the remedy when the condition is resolved.

Nutritional Supplements

For bursitis, David R. Field, N.D., L.Ac., a naturopathic physician based in Santa Rosa, California, recommends this program of supplements and herbs, to be followed for 2–4 weeks:

Vitamin B6: 100 mg daily; supports nerve function; B6 deficiency has been implicated in repetitive motion injuries.[2]

Bromelain: 400 mg 3 times daily on an empty stomach; an anti-inflammatory enzyme compound found in pineapple.

Curcumin: 400 mg 3 times daily; the active, anti-inflammatory component of turmeric.

Jamaican dogwood (*Piscidia erythrina*): 200 mg 3 times daily; anti-inflammatory.

Flax oil: 1 tablespoon per 100 pounds of body weight daily; anti-inflammatory.

For a topical treatment, gently massage Peppermint or Lavender essential oil into the affected area as needed.

Reflexology

Treat the adrenal glands and the area of the foot corresponding to the joint afflicted by bursitis.

Stone/Crystal Therapy

Place midnight lace obsidian on the affected area, says Melody, author of the crystal reference series *Love Is in the Earth*. Keep the stone in place with hypoallergenic tape. Leave it on for 1–2 days, then remove for 1–2 days. Repeat this cycle 3 times total, then use as needed.

Canker Sore

An ulcer in the mouth or on the lips, a canker sore (aphthous ulcer) starts as a red mark, in the center of which a white head develops and eventually bursts. The pain of canker sores is exacerbated by acidic foods. Canker sores are distinct from cold sores, which are caused by the herpes simplex virus I and tend to recur in the same spot. Canker sores are "creeping" ulcers, and occur in various spots on the gums, inner lips, and inner walls of the cheeks. The formation of canker sores may involve an autoimmune (abnormal immune) response to bacteria normally found in the mouth. Allergies, certain foods, stress, and fatigue can trigger an outbreak.

Essential Oils

Naturopathic physician Boyer B. Cole, N.M.D., of Cottonwood, Arizona, suggests the following blend of essential oils as an effective remedy for canker sores:

Eucalyptus citriodora: 10 drops
Helichrysum: 5 drops
Bergamot: 5 drops
Lavender: 10 drops
Geranium: 5 drops
Lemon: 5 drops

Combine these essential oils in 1/2 ounce of vegetable glycerin (available at health food stores; do not use the pharmaceutical variety). Using your finger or a cotton swab, dab the blend on your canker sore(s) 3–4 times daily. Wash your hands afterward. Keep applying until the sore dries out. "This blend can cut the healing time in half," says Dr. Cole.

Flower Essences

Self-Heal and Yarrow Special Formula can serve as the foundational healing agents for canker sores. Other flower essences to address the specific emotions, mental attitude, and environmental conditions of the individual are recommended, states Patricia Kaminski, a flower essence therapist and codirector of the Flower Essence Society. Self-Heal supports the body's innate healing ability. Yarrow Special Formula strengthens and protects against environmental toxicity and stress. Take 4 drops of each 2–4 times daily, or as needed.

Food Therapy

Eat:
Steamed vegetables, soup, yogurt, complex carbohydrates (see note regarding wheat below).
Avoid:
Acidic foods (citrus, tomatoes, chocolate, coffee, black tea), alcohol; limit animal protein.
If you have recurrent canker sores, food allergies may be the problem, states Paul Reilly, N.D., L.Ac., a naturopathic physician and acupuncturist from Seattle, Washington. Wheat and gluten (a component of wheat, but also found in rye, barley, and oats) are common

culprits. Try cutting them out of your diet, along with any other foods you know or suspect you might be allergic to, and see if that reduces or eliminates your canker sore episodes.

Herbal Medicine

Licorice (*Glycrrhiza glabra*) tea can soothe canker sores, states Dr. Reilly. Sip 2–3 cups slowly throughout the day, retaining the tea in your mouth for a few seconds before swallowing each mouthful. To make licorice tea, use 1 teaspoon of licorice root per 1 cup of water, cover, simmer for 15–20 minutes, and strain.

You can also use deglycyrrhizinated licorice (DGL), available in a powder, to make a mouthwash, says naturopathic physician Donald J. Brown, N.D. Combine 200 mg of powdered DGL with 200 ml of warm water. Gargle and swish this blend in your mouth for 2–3 minutes before spitting it out. Do this in the morning and again at night for 1 week. Alternatively, add a little myrrh (*Commiphora molmol*) tincture or the powdered form to warm water for a different antimicrobial mouthwash. Gargle and rinse in the same way as with the DGL mouthwash, but do it 3–4 times daily.[1]

Homeopathy

The following homeopathic remedies are commonly indicated for canker sores, state naturopathic physicians Robert Ullmann, N.D., and Judyth Reichenberg-Ullmann, N.D.:[2]

Nat mur: This and Borax are the most common remedies for canker sores; indicated for sores inside the mouth and on the lips that burn when food touches them, accompanied by dry lips with a crack in the middle of the lower lip.

Borax: Most common remedy for infants and children, especially indicated if thrush (an overgrowth of the yeast-like fungus *Candida albicans* in the mouth) is present too and for sensitive, hot sores that bleed when touched.

Mercurius: If there is bad breath, a metallic taste in the mouth, excess salivation, spongy and bleeding gums, and worsening of symptoms with heat and cold.

Sulphur: If the mouth is hot and dry, the face and lips are red, the pain
of the sores is burning, and there is a craving for sweets, fat, alcohol, and spicy food.

Take the appropriate remedy in a 30c potency every 4 hours, or
6c every 1–4 hours, until your symptoms improve. Stop taking the
remedy if the symptoms resolve; repeat if the symptoms return. If
there is no improvement with 3 doses, you probably are not using the
correct remedy.

Nutritional Supplements

Dr. Reilly has found the following to be effective in treating
canker sores:

Zinc lozenges: Suck on a zinc lozenge (containing 5–10 mg of zinc)
every few hours.

Acidophilus rinse: Open 2 capsules of acidophilus or use 1/4 teaspoon
powder, add to 2 ounces of water, swish the mixture around in the
mouth, and swallow. Don't drink anything else right away. Do this
twice daily.

Vitamin B12 drops: Put 3–5 mg (3–30 drops depending on the
strength of the product) of vitamin B12 in drop form in your
mouth, swish it around, then swallow. As with the acidophilus,
don't drink anything else right away. Do this twice daily.

Reflexology

Face

Stone/Crystal Therapy

Daya Sarai Chocron, a vibrational healer and author of *Healing
with Crystals and Gemstones*, recommends amber for a canker sore. Hold
the stone, wear it, carry it in your pocket, or lay it on or near the sore
for 15–20 minutes daily, as needed. If the sore is inside your mouth, lay
the stone on the outside, over the place where the sore is.

Cold Sore (Fever Blister)

Occurring on the outer lips or gums, a cold sore manifests as a painful bump that turns into an inflamed blister, from which pus may or may not seep. A cold sore is also called a fever blister because it often develops after a fever, flu, infection, or cold. The lowered immunity after illness (or from chronic allergies) leaves the body vulnerable to the herpes simplex virus I that causes cold sores. As with canker sores, stress can also trigger a cold sore outbreak. As a herpes by-product, cold sores are highly contagious.

Essential Oils

For a cold sore on the lips or around the mouth, Geranium, Melissa, Lavender, or Tea Tree (*Melaleuca alternifolia*) essential oil can be effective, according to Kurt Schnaubelt, Ph.D., scientific director of the Pacific Institute of Aromatherapy in San Rafael, California. Apply 1 drop of one of these oils topically to the sore, 6 times per day for 3–5 days or until the lesion disappears. If dryness or irritation results from application of the undiluted oil, mix the essential oil with hazelnut or sweet almond oil (the essential oil should be 10 percent of the mix), and continue application in the same way.

For cold sores inside the mouth, put 1 drop of Creeping Hyssop on the blister 3–6 times per day, for up to 3 days, says Dr. Schnaubelt. Note: Do not confuse Creeping Hyssop (*Hyssopus officinalis decumbens*) with Hyssop (*Hyssopus officinalis*). They have very different properties. Creeping Hyssop is an antiviral that you can safely use on your own. Hyssop, on the other hand, can be toxic and should only be used under the guidance of a qualified practitioner.

The following blend of essential oils can cut the healing time for a cold sore in half, according to naturopathic physician Boyer B. Cole, N.M.D., of Cottonwood, Arizona. Here is his recipe:

Eucalyptus citriodora: 10 drops
Helichrysum: 5 drops
Bergamot: 5 drops
Lavender: 10 drops

Geranium: 5 drops

Lemon: 5 drops

Combine these essential oils in 1/2 ounce of vegetable glycerin (available at health food stores; do not use the pharmaceutical variety). Using your finger or a cotton swab, dab the blend on your cold sore 3–4 times daily. Wash your hands afterward. Keep applying until the sore dries out.

Flower Essences

Pansy flower essence, taken internally and used topically, can help resolve a cold sore, says Richard Katz, naturalist and founder of the Flower Essence Society. Take 4 drops under the tongue 4 times daily. Add Pansy to Self-Heal cream (6–10 drops per 1 ounce of cream) and apply to the affected area 2–4 times daily. Continue treatment until your cold sore is resolved.

Food Therapy

Eat:

Fresh sauerkraut, seaweed, fish, yogurt/kefir, plain baked potatoes and other high-lysine foods (see part 3, "Food Therapy," p. 377). Drink plenty of water.

Avoid:

Sugar, refined carbohydrates, red meat, soft drinks, alcohol, caffeine, chocolate, nuts and other high-arginine foods (see part 3, "Food Therapy," p. 376), acidic foods such as citrus.

Herbal Medicine

For a cold sore, naturopathic physician Jody E. Noé, M.S., N.D., of Brattleboro, Vermont, recommends treating it topically and taking an antiviral herbal formula internally to help the body fight the herpes virus. Combine equal parts of the following tinctures: licorice (*Glycrrhiza glabra*), goldenseal (*Hydrastis canadensis*), lomatium (*Lomatium dissectum*), osha (*Ligusticum porteri*), dandelion (*Taraxacum officinalis*), passionflower (*Passiflora incarnata*), astragalus (*Astragalus membranaceus*), and lemon balm (*Melissa officinalis*). As soon as a cold sore begins to develop, start taking 1 dropperful of this tincture blend every hour. After 24 hours, decrease the dose to 1/2 teaspoon 2–3 times daily. Continue until the cold sore is resolved. Apply the tincture topically on the cold sore as well, as often as needed.

For a simple topical solution, blend 5 drops (1–2 drops if the sore is particularly raw) of grapefruit seed extract (GSE) and 50 drops of vegetable glycerin. Use a cotton swab to dab the solution on the cold sore 2–3 times daily. "GSE, with its antiviral and astringent properties, can often combat this condition by inactivating the virus and drying up the lesion, sometimes in a matter of hours," states Allan Sachs, D.C., C.C.N.[1]

Homeopathy

The following are common homeopathic remedies for cold sores:[2]

Nat mur: For recurring fever blisters on the lips made worse by emotional stress, sun exposure, and acute illness or fever.

Rhus tox: For swollen, red, itchy, "angry" fever blisters on the lips made worse by cold or damp and fever.

Sepia: For periodic fever blisters on the lower lip with chapped or cracked skin and crusty lesions, which are typically associated with menstruation, so occur monthly, or yearly in the spring.

Take the appropriate remedy at a 30c potency 2–3 times daily for 3 days.

Nutritional Supplements

The following antiviral supplements and herbs are useful in treating and preventing cold sores, according to Bradley Bongiovanni, N.D., a naturopathic physician from Independence, Ohio; take/use all until the cold sore is healed:

Vitamin C: 1,000 mg 3 times daily.

Vitamin E: 400 IU twice daily.

Pycnogenol: 100 mg 3 times daily; powerful antioxidant derived from grape seed.

Selenium: 200 mcg twice daily.

Olive leaf extract: 1,000 mg twice daily.

Monolaurin: 300 mg 3 times daily; a fatty acid ester (compound) found in breast milk, which breaks down the protective coating of viruses; more effective when used with olive leaf extract.

Apply Melissa (*Melissa officianalis*) extract topical cream to the cold sore 3 times daily.

The amino acid lysine has been shown to be effective in reducing the severity and frequency of herpes outbreaks. Research suggests that lysine inactivates the virus.[3] Apply lysine cream topically; follow the manufacturer's instructions.

Reflexology

Face

Stone/Crystal Therapy

Turquoise is a good gemstone for cold sores, states vibrational healer Daya Sarai Chocron, of Northampton, Massachusetts. Hold the stone, wear it, carry it in your pocket, or lay it on or near the sore for 15–20 minutes daily, as needed. If the sore is inside your mouth, lay the stone on the outside, over the place where the sore is.

Colic (Infant)

Colic, or severe abdominal pain, in infants usually occurs during the first three months of life. Typical symptoms include inconsolable crying, irritability, a need for movement, and pulling the legs up against the body. Infant colic is caused by gas in the intestines as a result of feeding problems, which include swallowing air while feeding, allergies to infant formula, allergies to something in the nursing mother's diet, and insufficient burping.

Essential Oils

An essential oil "Tummy Rub" can help ease colic, says herbalist Kathi Keville. Combine essential oils of Lemongrass (6 drops), Chamomile (1 drop), and Fennel (1 drop) in 2 ounces of vegetable oil. You can use Lemon Balm essential oil in place of the Lemongrass, but it's quite expensive. Gently rub some of the blend on the child's stomach every hour, or as needed.[1]

Flower Essences

To ease colic, put 1 drop of Chamomile flower essence under your baby's tongue 4 times daily, says flower essence therapist Patricia Kaminski of Nevada City, California. This is quite effective on its own, but massaging the baby's stomach 2–4 times a day with Calendula Caress flower oil (which also contains chamomile) is highly soothing as well.

Food Therapy

Bland, light food is best for a colic-prone baby, says Alan Christianson, N.M.D., a naturopathic physician from Scottsdale, Arizona. As babies have a weak system when it comes to breaking down proteins, casein in dairy products and gluten and gliadin from wheat frequently become allergens (allergy-causing substances) and can contribute to colic, explains Dr. Christianson. Removing dairy and wheat products from the baby's diet, along with eggs, nuts, and soy, which are also common allergens, may relieve the colic. Since casein passes through breast milk, the nursing mother should eliminate dairy from her diet as well. She may also want to avoid gas-producing foods such as onions, garlic, and the *Brassica* family of vegetables (see part 3, "Food Therapy," p. 376).

Herbal Medicine/Nutritional Supplements

A gruel remedy as a preventive measure for colic can be quite effective, according to Dr. Christianson. Make a gruel with the following ingredients, preparing the cereal according to the product directions, but using the proportions indicated here: 1 / 2 part cereal, 2 parts water, 1 teaspoon of either licorice (*Glycrrhiza glabra*) root powder or slippery elm (*Ulmus rubra, U. fulva*) powder, 1/2 teaspoon of the amino acid glutamine, and a pinch of either cloves or cardamom to add some taste (cardamom can also help with digestion). Give the baby a teaspoon of this gruel at every feeding.

Lavender (*Lavandula officinalis*) flower tea is great for infants with colic, says Michael Cottingham, a clinical herbalist from Silver City, New Mexico. It aids in digestion and stimulates the immune system. To make the tea, put 1/4 teaspoon of the flowers in 1 cup of boiled water, cover, let steep for 10–15 minutes, and then strain. Give your baby 2 teaspoons of the tea 3–4 times daily for 2 weeks. When you are nearing the time of day that your baby normally gets colicky, you can increase that dose to up to 5 teaspoons. After the initial 2 weeks, which is sufficient time to begin tissue healing and for the baby's body to begin reversing the colic pattern, use the tea as needed if the colic recurs. Give the tea for 1–2 days after a colic recurrence.

At the same time, if the mother is breast-feeding, she can drink the tea (1/2 teaspoon of the flowers per 1 cup of boiled water), 2 cups daily for 2 weeks, then drink 2–4 cups weekly as long as she is breast-feeding. This will transmit lavender to the infant through the breast milk as well. Lavender also increases milk flow, but not excessively. The herb is extremely safe for infants, notes Cottingham, so there is no need to be concerned about giving them this amount.

Joanne B. Mied, N.D., a naturopath and herbalist based in Novato, California, has found a combination tincture of catnip (*Nepeta cataria*) and fennel (*Foeniculum vulgare*) effective in treating colic. Give the child 5–10 drops of the tincture every 15 minutes or half-hour until he or she calms down. "If it doesn't work in three to four hours, it's not going to," notes Dr. Mied.

Homeopathy

Michael G. Carlston, M.D., a homeopathic physician practicing in Santa Rosa, California, recommends the following remedies, with the proviso that if there is no improvement, you should seek medical help:

Use Colocynthis if your baby is angry and the abdominal pain of colic seems to be eased in a doubled-up posture or when you put the baby on your shoulder. Use Chamomilla if the baby wants to be carried and you have to keep moving to keep the baby at all calm—the walking up and down the hall syndrome. For either, use a 12c or 30c potency in the midst of an episode. Crush 2 pellets betweeen two clean spoons, and sprinkle in the baby's mouth. Repeat as needed, up to every half hour. These remedies act as a preventive as well, notes Dr. Carlston. They can decrease both the severity and frequency of episodes after this treatment. Do not continue giving your baby the remedy once the colic is resolved, however.

Dr. Christianson has also found homeopathic remedies to be useful in cases of colic, and since they taste like little sugar pills, they are easy to administer to children. He suggests Hyland's Calm's Forte or Calcarea carbonica 3x or 6c; give 2–3 pellets of one or the other 2–3 times daily during an acute episode.

Reflexology

Stomach, intestines

Stone/Crystal Therapy

For colic, black tourmaline is useful, states Katrina Raphaell, crystal healing therapist and founder of the Crystal Academy of Advanced Healing Arts in Kapaa, Hawaii. Place the stone in the baby's bath water. You can also put the stone in the infant's crib, as long as the baby is too young to move around. As an extra measure of caution, use a stone large enough that the baby can't swallow it, in the unlikely event that he or she gets hold of the stone.

Other Remedies

A gentle massage of the baby's abdomen may ease the spasms of colic.

Common Cold

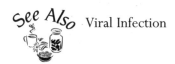 See Also Viral Infection

Most people are well acquainted with the symptoms of the respiratory infection known as the common cold: stuffy and runny nose, sneezing, mucus buildup and discharge, watering eyes, headache, perhaps a sore throat and cough. The passages between the nose and the sinuses can become blocked, producing the stuffy, full feeling of sinus congestion.

As with other viral infections, if your immune system is strong, you are less likely to catch a cold. A cold can be viewed as a way for the body to expel toxins, waste, and microorganisms that have built up to the point that the immune system cannot handle them normally.[1] For this reason, you should not use a decongestant; it interferes with the body's cleansing process. If you are someone who tends to turn to antibiotics as a solution to infection, be forewarned that antibiotics have no effect on viral infections.

Treatment for the common cold should include a protocol of immune support to aid the body in restoring its natural internal balance.

Essential Oils

Antiviral essential oils used in cases of a light cold or at the first sign of a cold coming on can stop a full-blown cold from developing, according to Kurt Schnaubelt, Ph.D., scientific director of the Pacific Institute of Aromatherapy in San Rafael, California. He recommends an inhalation formula of *Eucalyptus radiata* (5 ml), *Eucalyptus globulus* (2.5 ml), and Ravensare (2.5 ml) essential oils. Inhale with an electric diffusor for 5–10 minutes 6 times a day. Or sprinkle 5 drops of the formula on a cloth and inhale it directly, 2–3 times an hour when the condition is acute.[2]

Flower Essences

Self-Heal and Yarrow Special Formula can serve as the foundational healing agents for a cold. Other flower essences to address the specific emotions, mental attitude, and environmental conditions of the individual are recommended, states Patricia Kaminski, a flower essence therapist and codirector of the Flower Essence Society. Self-Heal supports the body's innate healing ability. Yarrow Special Formula strengthens and protects against environmental toxicity and stress. Take 4 drops of each 2–4 times daily, or as needed.

Food Therapy

Eat:

Garlic, cayenne, horseradish, curry, foods high in vitamin C (see part 3, "Food Therapy," p. 378). Drink plenty of fluids (diluted vegetable juices, soups, herbal tea, green tea).

Combine grated horseradish with some apple cider vinegar and mix it in your food at every meal, suggests herbalist and nutritionist James Kusick. Start with just a little and build up to 1/4 teaspoon or more at each sitting.[3]

Avoid:

Sugar (and limit fruit and fruit juices), bread, fried food, and mucus-forming foods (dairy, chocolate, eggs, junk food).

Herbal Medicine

"If you start treatment when a cold is first coming on, it's easy to knock out," says naturopathic physician Alan Christianson, N.M.D., of Scottsdale, Arizona. He strongly recommends a Chinese patent formula, Yin Chao. Containing a blend of Chinese medicinal herbs including lonicera and forsythia, it has a diaphoretic (promotes sweating and cleansing) effect and is "the simplest, most efficient cold treatment I know." You can get it over the counter in Chinese medicine stores and now in many health food stores. It comes as a vial of wafers. Chew the wafers or crush them into powder and make a tea. Take a wafer every few hours, so that you go through 1 vial in the course of a day. Do this for 2–3 days.

Although Dr. Christianson also recommends the increasingly popular cold remedy echinacea, he cites the fresh juice as more effective than the tincture (the juice is available at health food stores or via the Internet). Take 1 teaspoon of the juice 2 times daily for 3–7 days. It is not the case, he notes, that echinacea should not be used long-term. That idea has been perpetuated by a mistranslation of a German research article. In fact, the herb is fine to use long-term, but 3–7 days is about what you need to knock out a cold, states Dr. Christianson.

Herbalist Teresa Boardwine of Washington, Virginia, finds echinacea (*E. angustifolia* and/or *E. purpurea*) tincture effective when taken in large doses at the first sign of a cold—sneezing or sniffles—or when people around you have colds. Whole plant tincture is preferable, she notes, as all the parts of the plant have active constituents. Take a dropperful (30 ml) 5 times per day for 5 days. This can often knock the cold out before it gets started, says Boardwine.

If your symptoms persist or you have a head cold that is already under way, Boardwine recommends a tea of equal parts of the following dried herbs (with a little less eucalyptus): eyebright, elder, eucalyptus, peppermint, and yarrow. Pour 1 quart boiled water over a rounded 1/4 cup of the herb mixture. Cover and let steep for 20 minutes. Strain the tea and put in a thermos or bottle to drink throughout the day. Drink 1 quart of tea and another quart of plain water daily for up to 10 days. Along with this, take a clove of garlic daily; you can chop it up, put it on a spoon, and take it down like a pill. Garlic is antimicrobial, so eat it in your diet as well.

If your phlegm is green, take 1 capsule of goldenseal root 3 times daily, but not for more than 3 days. Goldenseal (*Hydrastis canadensis*) should be used on a short-term basis, notes Boardwine.

Homeopathy

The following are among the many homeopathic remedies indicated for the common cold, according to Maesimund B. Panos, M.D.:[4]

Allium cepa: if there is sneezing, streaming eyes and nose, the nasal discharge makes the nose and upper lip sore, and symptoms improve outside.

Euphrasia: If there is a flowing watery discharge from the nose and eyes that makes the eyes, but not the nose sore, the discharge increases at night and when you are lying down, and a cough worsens during the day but improves when lying down.

Nat mur: If the cold begins with sneezing and a watery or egg-white-consistency discharge that irritates the nose, the nose is stuffed up, smell and taste are impaired, and there may be a cough, bursting headache, and/or fever blisters.

Nux vom: For the early stages of a cold, if there are sneezing spells, a runny nose during the day and a stuffed-up nose at night, sore throat, irritability, susceptibility to being chilled, and symptoms worsen in cold air.

Pulsatilla: For a "ripe" cold with thick yellow discharge, a stuffed-up nose at night and indoors, runny nose outdoors, chapped lips, fever without thirst, weepiness, craving for the open air, and improvement with motion.

Take the appropriate remedy in a 6x potency every 2–4 hours. As symptoms improve, decrease the frequency. Stop taking the remedy when the improvement is well established.

Nutritional Supplements

Natural medicine practitioner David Carroll recommends the following supplement protocol for both colds and flu. He emphasizes that you should start taking supplements as soon as you notice symptoms. Once the cold is full-blown, the supplements don't have as great an effect, although they still aid the body in healing.[5]

High-potency vitamin B complex: At the first sign of symptoms, take as directed; take as a preventive as well.

Vitamin C: Beginning at the first sign of symptoms, take 1,000 mg every 2 hours for 3 days.

Vitamin A: Beginning at the first sign of symptoms, take 10,000 IU every 2 hours for 3 days. *Or* on the first day of symptoms, take 7 tablets (10,000 IU each) at night before going to bed. "This massive dose will often prevent the cold from developing at all," states Carroll. Caution: Stop taking vitamin A if you get dizzy, nauseous, or have other symptoms after taking it.

Calcium lactate: Beginning at the first sign of symptoms, take 200 mg every 4 hours for 3 days.

Bee pollen (optional): If bronchial complaints accompany your cold, take granules or tablets as directed; bee pollen is antimicrobial and full of nutrients.

Zinc lozenges have become a ubiquitous remedy for colds. Dr. Christianson recommends them when the cold symptoms include a sore throat, but otherwise tends to rely on other remedies (see "Herbal Medicine"). Take 30 mg daily as lozenges; be careful not to exceed 45 mg daily.

Reflexology
Nose, throat, head, chest

Stone/Crystal Therapy
Peridot and sulphur are beneficial stones for the common cold, says crystal healing therapist Katrina Raphaell of Kapaa, Hawaii. Place the stone at the site or sites of distress: against the nose, over the sinuses, on the upper chest. Leave the stone there for 5 minutes while visualizing your health goal. Do this 3 times daily. Wear the stone, hold it, or carry it in your pocket for ongoing healing effects.

Other Remedies
Washing your hands frequently during cold and flu season can reduce the likelihood of contracting illness from the many viruses to which most of us are exposed.

Rest. It may seem an obvious remedy, but many people don't apply this simple treatment when they have a cold.

Conjunctivitis (Pinkeye)

Conjunctivitis is a common ailment of childhood, but can occur in adults as well. It involves inflammation of the conjunctiva, the mucus membrane lining the eyelids, and is known as pinkeye because dilated blood vessels in the whites of the eyes give them a pink or red hue.

Symptoms begin with watery eyes and progress to painful inflammation with a pus-like discharge that can cause the eyelids to stick together after a night of sleep or other prolonged period of the eyes being closed.

While pinkeye can be caused by allergies, eye irritation or injury, or bacterial infection, most cases are viral in nature and contagious.

Essential Oils

Essential oil should not be used in the eyes, states Kurt Schnaubelt, Ph.D., scientific director of the Pacific Institute of Aromatherapy in San Rafael, California. However, you can use a hydrosol, aromatic water that is a coproduct of the essential oil distillation process. Dr. Schnaubelt specifically recommends Green Myrtle hydrosol for conjunctivitis. Spray it directly into the eyes up to 6 times per day, while irritation persists.

Medical aromatherapist Julia Fischer of Northern California recommends putting a pinch of goldenseal powder in Lavender hydrosol and letting it sit for 10 minutes. Strain the liquid through an unbleached coffee filter. With an eye cup, hold the solution on one eye for a few seconds. Do both eyes, but use fresh solution for each eye and rinse the eye cup between applications. This helps prevent the spread of the infection from one eye to the other. Do this procedure 4–5 times daily until the condition subsides.

Flower Essences

Self-Heal and Yarrow Special Formula can serve as the foundational healing agents for conjunctivitis. Other flower essences to address the specific emotions, mental attitude, and environmental conditions of the individual are recommended, states Patricia Kaminski, a flower essence therapist and codirector of the Flower Essence Society. Self-Heal supports the body's innate healing ability. Yarrow Special Formula strengthens and protects against environmental toxicity and stress.

Food Therapy

Eat:

Yogurt, protein, vegetables, foods high in vitamins A and C (see part 3, "Food Therapy," p. 378).

Avoid:

Sugar, fried foods.

Herbal Medicine

As conjunctivitis is a self-limiting condition, meaning it runs its course with or without intervention, Alan Christianson, N.M.D., a naturopathic physician from Scottsdale, Arizona, tends to focus treatment on providing relief and aiding the healing process. To that end, he recommends an eye wash. To 1 ounce of contact saline solution add 10 drops of goldenseal (*Hydrastis canadensis*) tincture and 5 drops of eyebright (*Euphrasia officinalis*) tincture. Goldenseal is an antimicrobial and soothes mucous membranes, while eyebright works to lessen oversecretion of mucus.

Treat both eyes, even if you have the condition in only one; it tends to spread easily. You can use an eye cup or a pair of old swim goggles. Keep the liquid in contact with the open eye for 1 minute. With the goggles, put the wash in each side of the glasses, lean forward and press the goggles to your face to create a seal, then tilt your head back, and let the wash bathe your eyes. Do the eye wash 3 times daily. If you do not want to do the eye wash, use an eyedropper to put 2–3 drops of the preparation in each eye, 3 times daily. Eye washing is more effective, however.

Homeopathy

"The vast majority of conjunctivitis cases are readily treated by homeopathy," states homeopathic physician Roger Morrison, M.D.[1] Pulsatilla nigricans is a common remedy for both allergic and infectious conjunctivitis. Some of the indications for this remedy are: in the case of infection—red conjunctiva with thick yellow or green discharge, worse in heat or warm rooms and better outside and with the application of cold; in the case of allergy—red, teary, burning, itchy eyes, accompanied by a strong desire to rub them and a sensation as of a hair in the eye. Take at a 30c potency 3 times daily. If the remedy is the correct one, you should see a response within 24 hours of starting the remedy.

Nutritional Supplements

Proanthocyanidins (PCOs) from grape seed or white pine bark are potent antioxidants and aid in tissue healing. Naturopathic physician Linda Rector Page, N.D., Ph.D., recommends taking 100 mg of PCOs twice daily. She also recommends taking zinc at a rate of 50 mg twice daily, and putting 1 drop of castor oil in each eye 3 times daily. Continue this program until your conjunctivitis is resolved.[2] Note that long-term use of zinc can result in a copper deficiency, so it's important to take it only on a short-term basis.

Reflexology

Eyes, sinuses

Stone/Crystal Therapy

For conjunctivitis, Daya Sarai Chocron, a vibrational healer based in Northampton, Massachusetts, recommends emerald or malachite. Hold the stone, wear it, carry it in your pocket, or lay a stone on each of your eyelids or near each eye for 15–20 minutes daily, as needed until the condition is resolved.

Other Remedies

A potato poultice is an easy and effective treatment for conjunctivitis, according to naturopathic physician Susan Roberts, N.D., of Portland, Oregon. Grate potato, place it on a square of gauze, draw the ends together to form a sack, and hold it on the affected eye (closed) for 15 minutes. Do this 4 times daily, using fresh potato each time, until the condition is resolved. The potato draws out the infection.

Constipation

Constipation has become an American malady, largely due to the standard American diet of processed foods. Infrequent, incomplete, or difficult bowel movements characterize constipation. Many alternative medicine doctors cite two to three bowel movements per day as optimal for health. Many Americans do not have even one daily bowel movement, often simply as a result of not getting enough fiber in the diet, not drinking enough water, and not getting enough exercise.

If the intestines do not empty waste every day, detrimental toxins can begin to accumulate.[1] A toxic colon may be a contributing factor in the development of serious disorders, such as diabetes, thyroid disease, and ulcerative colitis, among others.[2]

Essential Oils

For constipation, Julie Oxendale, C.M.T., an aromatherapist based in San Francisco, California, recommends Patchouli, which is an intestinal cleansing oil. Put 30 drops of Patchouli essential oil in 2 tablespoons of a carrier oil. Rub the abdomen with this blend, moving in a clockwise direction (as you're looking down at your stomach, twelve o'clock is at the top, and three o'clock to the left). Do this once daily for a week, as needed.

Flower Essences

Self-Heal can serve as a foundational healing agent for constipation. Other flower essences to address the specific emotions, mental attitude, and environmental conditions of the individual are recommended, states Patricia Kaminski, a flower essence therapist and codirector of the Flower Essence Society. Self-Heal supports the body's innate healing ability. Take 4 drops 2–4 times daily, or as needed.

Food Therapy

Eat:

Fiber, celery, lettuce, yogurt, prunes, foods high in magnesium (see part 3, "Food Therapy," p. 377). Drink plenty of water.

Avoid:

Sugar, fried foods, dairy, limit coffee and alcohol (they are dehydrating).

Although many people think of eating fruit when they are constipated, nutritionist Ann Louise Gittleman, N.D., C.N.S., M.S., advises only moderate intake of fruits because they contain sugar. She suggests eating a small sweet potato or a half cup of beans if you are constipated. To prevent and alleviate constipation, eat more fiber-rich vegetables (celery, carrots, lettuce, and other leafy greens). As a general practice, Dr. Gittleman recommends eating 10 almonds daily, as well as ground flaxseed. You can sprinkle the latter on your cereal or other food. Or you can use ground flaxseed as a substitute for butter or margarine in your pancake or muffin batter. It's a 3:1 ratio; that is, use 3 tablespoons of ground flaxseed in place of 1 tablespoon of butter.

Herbal Medicine

Here is a formula from renowned master herbalist Raymond Christopher, M.H., N.D., which is indicated for all bowel complaints, including constipation. It promotes regularity and tones the intestines.[3]

Dr. Christopher's Lower Bowel Tonic
Cascara sagrada (*Rhamnus purshiana*): 2 parts
Barberry (*Berberis vulgaris*) root: 1 part
Rhubarb (*Rheum palmatum*) root: 1 part
Goldenseal (*Hydrastis canadensis*): 1 part
Raspberry (*Rubus idaeus*) leaves: 1 part
Lobelia (*Lobelia inflata*): 1 part
Ginger (*Zingiber officinale*) root: 1 part

Use the powdered form of all of these herbs, mix the powders together, and put the blend in gelatin capsules. Take 2 capsules, 3 times daily, as needed for constipation.

Homeopathy

There are numerous homeopathic remedies for constipation. If it is a common problem for you, you may want to consider consulting a homeopath for individualized, constitutional treatment. That said, Dr. Barry Rose of the Royal London Homeopathic Hospital cites the following common remedies for constipation:[4]

Alumina 6c: If stool is soft and sticky or hard and dry with difficult defecation.

Graphites 6c: If stool is large, smelly, and comprising many lumps held together by mucus, with pain in passing.
Lycopodium 6c: If stool is hard, dry, and painful to pass.
Nux vom 6c: If incomplete stool is passed, so rectum feels unemptied; accompanied by feeling chilly and irritable.
Silica 6c: If the stool is hard and slips back after partial expulsion.
Sulphur 6c: If the stool is smelly, hard, dry, and black, there is anal irritation and pain and burning with defecation.

Take the appropriate remedy 3 times daily until your symptoms improve. At that point, reduce the dosage to 2 times daily for 3 days, then once daily for 3 more days, after which you should stop taking the remedy.

Nutritional Supplements

Magnesium and flaxseed oil are two important supplements for constipation, according to Dr. Gittleman. Magnesium carries water into the intestinal tract and therefore assists in elimination. Many of us are magnesium deficient. Stress, coffee, diuretics, birth control pills, and menstruation all draw this important mineral from the body. If you are taking calcium, you need to take an equal amount of magnesium or up to double the amount; in other words, the dosage of magnesium to calcium should range from a 1:1 to a 2:1 ratio. Taking a multivitamin/mineral supplement with your additional magnesium may supply these needs.

Take 400–800 mg of magnesium daily, divided into 3 doses. (Adjust your calcium supplementation accordingly; for example, if you take 400 mg of magnesium daily, you should be getting 200–400 mg of calcium daily.) Adjust your magnesium dosage to bowel tolerance. This means that if your stools become too loose, cut back the amount of magnesium you are taking to the point at which your stools are not too loose. Take magnesium on an ongoing basis.

Taking a daily fiber supplement is also a beneficial ongoing practice if you are prone to constipation, says Dr. Gittleman. She prefers flaxseed oil as a fiber source. It acts as an intestinal lubricant and is a gentle source of insoluble fiber for "sweeping" the intestines. Take 1–2 tablespoons of flaxseed oil in water in the morning. Drink it a half hour to an hour before breakfast. Adjust the dosage as needed. However, don't assume that more is better, Dr. Gittleman cautions. Too much fiber escorts minerals out of the body.

You can also take psyllium powder to get your bowels moving. Add 1 teaspoon to a glass of water and drink; drink additional water after taking, at least 1–2 glasses.[5]

Reflexology

Colon (all), liver, gallbladder, lower back, solar plexus, adrenal glands

Stone/Crystal Therapy

For constipation, use magnisite, citrine, aquamarine, or green tourmaline, states Katrina Raphaell, crystal healing therapist and founder of the Crystal Academy of Advanced Healing Arts in Kapaa, Hawaii. Place the stone on your abdomen. If you feel distress in a specific area of the abdomen, put the stone over that spot. While visualizing your health goal, leave the stone in place for 5 minutes. Do this 3 times daily. In between treatments, wear the stone, hold it, or carry it in your pocket to continue the healing effects.

Cough

The causes of coughing are numerous. It may be simply to clear the throat of an irritating dust, smoke, vapor, or other inhaled substance. Or coughing may be a by-product of a wide range of illnesses, from infections and allergies to heart disease and cancer.

Coughs can be categorized as productive (producing mucus; also termed effective) or nonproductive (dry). This division is useful in determining the cause and the appropriate treatment.

As with colds, it is unwise with a cough involving respiratory tract inflammation to use a medication that suppresses it, especially if the cough produces mucus.[1] In that case, coughing is the body's mechanism to clear the lungs.

Essential Oils

If you have an incessant cough, but no infection, so there is no clear treatment, try Lavender essential oil. It works amazingly well to stop a cough, according to clinical herbalist Michael Cottingham, of Silver City, New Mexico. Simply open the bottle and take a deep breath of lavender. Breathing lavender opens up the bronchial tubes because the herb is an antispasmodic, and all essential oils are vasodilators, meaning they open the blood vessels and increase blood flow.

Flower Essences

Self-Heal and Yarrow Special Formula can serve as the foundational healing agents for a cough. Other flower essences to address the specific emotions, mental attitude, and environmental conditions of the individual are recommended, states Patricia Kaminski, a flower essence therapist and codirector of the Flower Essence Society. Self-Heal supports the body's innate healing ability. Yarrow Special Formula strengthens and protects against environmental toxicity and stress. Take 4 drops of each 2–4 times daily, or as needed.

Food Therapy

Eat:

Foods high in vitamin C (see part 3, "Food Therapy," p. 378). Drink plenty of water.

Avoid:

Mucus-forming foods (dairy, chocolate, eggs, junk food).

Avoid all sugar because it suppresses the immune system, says Susan Roberts, N.D., a naturopathic physician from Portland, Oregon. "And that includes fruit and fruit juices," she adds. Dr. Roberts advises allowing the body to rest by giving it a break from the work of digestion. With that in mind, keep your diet close to a fast, meaning liquids and soups (miso especially, because it is so nourishing). Hot liquids act as a cough suppressant, she says. Though cold liquids might feel soothing to the throat, they are actually not helpful for a cough.

Herbal Medicine

Herbal authority James A. Duke, Ph.D., recommends licorice (*Glycrrhiza glabra*) and slippery elm (*Ulmus rubra*), both of which are soothing to the mucous membranes and have a long tradition as cough remedies. Use 1 teaspoon of dried licorice root per cup of water, simmer for 10 minutes, strain, and drink up to 3 cups of the tea daily. Dr. Duke cautions not to use it on a long-term basis; it can cause headaches and result in water retention, among other symptoms. Make slippery elm tea in the same way as licorice root tea. Commercial throat lozenges containing slippery elm are also an option.[2]

Homeopathy

The following are some of the many homeopathic remedies for cough, according to Stephen Cummings, M.D., and Dana Ullman, M.P.H.:[3]

Bryonia: If the cough is dry, spasmodic, painful, worse with deep breathing, warm rooms, and during the day, and improved by warm drinks or open air.

Rumex: If the cough is dry, shallow, set off by tickling in the throat, and worsened by inhaling cold air.

Phosphorus: Indicated for all types of cough, especially those accompanied by chills or laryngitis and hoarseness.

Pulsatilla: If the cough is accompanied by thick, yellow-green phlegm, worse with exertion, warm rooms, and lying down, and improved in the open air.

Causticum: If the cough is accompanied by laryngitis or the feeling that you can't cough deeply enough to expectorate the mucus in your lungs; worse with cold and waking in the morning and better during the day and with cold drinks.

Kali carb: If the cough comes in spasms that are most severe from 2 to 5 A.M., is worsened by cold air, exertion, and lying down, and the throat has the sensation of a splinter caught in it.

Take the appropriate remedy at a potency of 6c(x) or 12c(x) 3–4 times daily. As your symptoms improve, take the remedy less often. If there is no improvement after 2–3 days of taking the remedy, you are probably not taking the correct one for your cough.

Nutritional Supplements

To help resolve a cough, Dr. Roberts recommends vitamin C and a combination tincture of echinacea and goldenseal. Take 2,000–3,000 mg of vitamin C daily, in divided doses throughout the day for at least a week. Take a dropperful of the tincture every 2 hours for the first 24 hours, then 4 times daily for a week, if needed.

Reflexology

Throat

Stone/Crystal Therapy

Aquamarine, rose quartz, kunzite, amazonite, or green aventurine can help ease a cough, says crystal healing therapist Katrina Raphaell of Kapaa, Hawaii. Place the stone directly over the site of distress; for example, your throat or your chest. Keep it in place for 5 minutes while visualizing your health goal. Do this 3 times daily. You may also want to wear the stone, hold it, or carry it in your pocket for ongoing benefits.

Cuts and Scrapes

With minor household injuries such as a cut or scrape, you might be tempted to reach for a tube of antibiotic cream or a conventional antiseptic. If you use these products, you are needlessly exposing yourself to more chemicals in a world where we get plenty without self-infliction. There are a number of safe and often more effective natural alternatives to treat cuts and scrapes. Not only can they prevent infection, they also promote healing of the skin.

Essential Oils

After washing the cut or scrape, apply Tea Tree (*Melaleuca alternifolia*) essential oil as a natural disinfectant, says Sue Reynolds, M.S.W.,

L.M.T., a certified herbalist and aromatherapist from Goleta, California. Research has demonstrated that Tea Tree has significant antiseptic properties.[1]

Flower Essences

Applying Self-Heal cream to a cut or scrape aids tissue recovery, states naturalist Richard Katz of Nevada City, California. Apply directly on the injury 2–4 times daily for as long as needed.

Food Therapy

Eat:

Foods high in vitamins C and K and zinc. (For a list of foods containing these nutrients, see part 3, "Food Therapy," p. 378.)

Avoid:

Sugar and dairy.

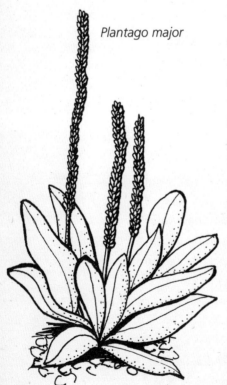

Plantago major

Herbal Medicine

"Grapefruit seed extract's powerful germ-fighting ability makes it an ideal antiseptic alternative," says Allan Sachs, D.C., C.C.N. In addition, it facilitates tissue repair. "Healing time is often remarkably short with the proper use of GSE." Dr. Sachs suggests keeping the following preparation on hand for household accidents. Mix 1/2 ounce of GSE with 8 ounces of distilled water and store in a spray bottle. For an even more potent solution, add a small amount of an extract of one of the powerhouse herbal healers such as calendula (*Calendula officinalis*), goldenseal (*Hydrastis canadensis*), echinacea (*E. spp.*), or plantain (*Plantago major*). Shake well before using, then spray the cut or scrape liberally with the solution every few minutes as you're washing out the wound. End with the spray, and repeat as needed.[2]

Fresh plantain is useful for scrapes and grit in the knee, reports Chanchal Cabrera, M.N.I.M.H., A.H.G., a medical herbalist from Vancouver, British Columbia.

Not only is it a powerful drawing agent, but it is also antimicrobial, has pain-relieving properties, and promotes healing. In addition, it grows everywhere, so is readily at hand when emergency first aid is needed.

As a drawing agent, plantain will pull out dirt, slivers, or other debris in the wound. It contains vitamin A and zinc, both of which aid healing, plus allantoin, a wound-healing substance that promotes cell proliferation.

Pick fresh plantain leaves. Mash them into a pulp by chewing them, using a mortar and pestle, or putting them in a blender or herb grinder. Place the pulp over the cut or scrape and wrap gauze around it. If you're in the woods, you can use a bandanna or other piece of clothing in place of the gauze. Leave the plantain on the wound for an hour, then check to see if it has pulled matter out of the wound. Leave the poultice on day and night, changing it daily, until the wound has sufficiently healed, which means it is closed over and looks clean.

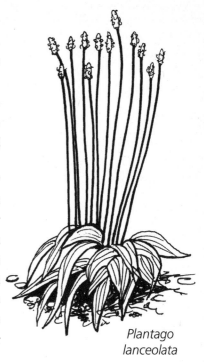

Plantago lanceolata

Homeopathy

"Calendula is the chief homeopathic medicine for wounds," states Maesimund B. Panos, M.D. She recommends using calendula lotion to gently clean an abrasion, and calendula or hypericum lotion for a cut. If the cut requires dressing, moisten a gauze pad with calendula or hypericum lotion and bandage it in place. Leave the dressing on the cut for the first day or so, moistening it with more lotion periodically. Do not change the dressing during that time.

If a cut becomes inflamed, take Hepar sulphuris calcareum 3 times a day for 2–3 days.

Dr. Panos adds the caution, "Never apply Arnica tincture or lotion to an open wound; it will usually irritate the skin severely."[3]

Nutritional Supplements

Nick Buratovich, N.M.D., a naturopathic physician from Tempe, Arizona, recommends the following supplements as support for skin healing to be taken until the cut or scrape heals:

Vitamin C: 1–2 g three times daily. If you take only one supplement, take vitamin C. It promotes skin healing because it increases the production of collagen, an important protein in the skin.

Bioflavonoids: These anti-inflammatory plant substances also help stabilize capillary membranes. Quercetin or citrus bioflavonoids are the best form to take. Take 1–3 g daily.

Vitamin A or beta-carotene: 25,000 IU 4 times daily; speeds skin healing. Although vitamin A can be toxic when taken at high doses for a prolonged period, the dosage here, taken on a short-term basis, will not produce toxicity.

Vitamin E: 200–400 IU 2 times daily; increases circulation and speeds wound healing.

Vitamin K: 70–140 mcg daily, in 3 divided doses; increases blood clotting.

Zinc: 30–60 mg 2 times daily; speeds wound healing.

Stone/Crystal Therapy

Place carnelian near the cut or scrape for 15–20 minutes daily, as needed, or hold the stone, wear it, or carry it in your pocket until the wound is healed, says vibrational healer Daya Sarai Chocron of Northampton, Massachusetts.

Dandruff

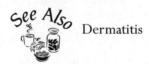 See Also Dermatitis

The proliferation of scaly white flakes of dead skin in scalp and other body hair seems to indicate a dry skin condition, but dandruff is frequently a result of the opposite. Also known as seborrheic dermatitis of the scalp or seborrheic dandruff, this type of dandruff is a by-product of overactive sebaceous glands, the glands in hair follicles that secrete oily sebum. This is why dandruff is a common complaint in adolescence, when those glands tend to be more active. An overproduction of sebum clogs the glands, which then secrete even more sebum in an effort to clear the passages. Scaly flakes and itchy skin ensue.

Another type of dandruff is pityriasis (sicca or capitis), which is more of a dry skin condition. The cause of this type is unknown, but it is more easily controlled through dietary changes and frequent hair washing and brushing.[1]

Essential Oils

Jojoba and Rosemary essential oils can alleviate dandruff, according to Sue Reynolds, M.S.W., L.M.T., a certified herbalist and aromatherapist from Goleta, California. Massage 2 drops of each into the scalp after washing hair.

Flower Essences

Self-Heal can serve as a foundational healing agent for dandruff. Other flower essences to address the specific emotions, mental attitude, and environmental conditions of the individual are recommended, states Patricia Kaminski, a flower essence therapist and codirector of the Flower Essence Society. Self-Heal supports the body's innate healing ability. Take 4 drops 2–4 times daily, or as needed.

Food Therapy

Eat:

Protein, vegetables, fiber, yogurt/kefir, foods high in sulphur (see part 3, "Food Therapy," p. 378).

Avoid:

Sugar, fried or processed food, allergenic foods.

Nutritionist Ann Louise Gittleman, N.D., C.N.S., M.S., advocates getting off of fat-free diets if you have dandruff because essential fatty acids (EFAs) are very important for the health of skin and hair. EFAs are our body's internal moisturizer to prevent dryness from occurring, she says. Foods rich in EFAs are therefore helpful for dandruff. Eat nuts and seeds: almonds, walnuts, pecans, and sunflower, sesame, and pumpkin seeds. Eat avocado, with lemon to help digest it.

Herbal Medicine

Dandruff is a sign of systemic imbalance, says herbalist David L. Hoffman, M.N.I.M.H. As an alterative herb, burdock (*Arctium lappa*) can help bring the body back into balance when taken internally. It is especially indicated for skin conditions characterized by scaly skin. To make a tea, add 1 teaspoon of burdock root to 1 cup of water, boil, then simmer for 10–15 minutes, and strain. Drink 1 cup 3 times daily. If you prefer, you can take burdock tincture instead (2–4 ml 3 times daily).[2]

As an external treatment for dandruff, rinse your hair daily with rosemary (*Rosmarinus officinalis*) tea or nettle (*Urtica dioica*) tea.[3] To make either tea, use 3 teaspoons of the dried herb per cup of boiled water, cover, and let stand for 10–15 minutes. Massage into the scalp at each use.

Homeopathy

The following are some of the remedies that may help alleviate dandruff, according to Dr. Barry Rose of the Royal London Homeopathic Hospital:[4]

Arsenicum 6c: If your scalp itches intolerably and more so at night, the scalp is sensitive, rough, covered with dry scale, and looks dirty, and there are circular bare patches.

Badiagia 6c: If your scalp is sore and very dry.

Kali mur 6c: For dandruff with eczema on other parts of your body.

Kali sulph 6c: For dandruff with scalp ringworm.

Medorrhinum 6c: If your scalp itches intensely and more so at night, and your hair is very dry.

Sanicula 6c: If the dandruff is profuse and scaly.

Thuja 6c: If the dandruff is white and scaly, the skin on your face is greasy, and your hair is dry and falls out easily.

Take the appropriate remedy 3 times daily until your dandruff improves.

Nutritional Supplements

For dandruff, Ann Louise Gittleman recommends zinc, selenium, and essential fatty acids.

Zinc: Take 30–45 mg daily (split into two doses). It is best to take zinc with food, as it causes nausea in some people. Taking zinc picolinate or a chelated form of zinc reduces the likelihood of nausea. (Sufficient zinc in the body can also help reduce split ends.)

Selenium: Take 200–400 mcg daily.

Essential fatty acids: Take 1–2 tablespoons of flaxseed oil daily.

Reflexology

Head

Stone/Crystal Therapy

Zincite (natural) used as an elixir mixed with your shampoo can help resolve dandruff, according to Melody, author of the crystal reference series *Love Is in the Earth*. Do 3 shampoos, then use as needed. (For instructions on making an elixir, see part 3, "Stone/Crystal Therapy," p. 403.)

Other Remedies

A vinegar hair rinse can help eliminate dandruff, according to Ann Louise Gittleman. With dandruff, the acid mantle, or protective pH covering, of the scalp is out of balance. A vinegar rinse can help restore the pH. Mix 1/2 cup water and 1/2 cup apple cider vinegar. Soak the scalp and hair with the rinse. Leave on for a couple of minutes, then wash it out with water only, no shampoo. You can also leave the rinse in your hair and not wash it out. Use this rinse when you wash your hair, as long as dandruff is present.

Dental Abscess

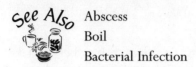

See Also   Abscess
            Boil
            Bacterial Infection

A dental abscess, also known as a gumboil, is an abscess (a collection or pocket of pus in a cavity formed by disintegrating tissue and surrounded by inflamed tissue) occurring in the gum next to a tooth, typically near the root. The gum appears swollen and red, and the area is tender to extremely painful. The face over that area of gum may be affected as well, with swelling and redness. Causes of a dental abscess include infection, injury, and denture friction or pressure.

Essential Oils

A blend of essential oils can resolve a dental abscess within days, says naturopathic physician Boyer B. Cole, N.M.D., of Cottonwood, Arizona. Combine the following essential oils in the amounts indicated:

Geranium: 20 drops
Myrrh: 20 drops
Lemon: 10 drops
Thyme Linalol or Moroccan Thyme (*Thymus satureioides*): 10
     drops; use these types of Thyme essential oil because
     standard thyme can be irritating.

Apply the blend directly on the affected area of the gums 3 times daily. If the abscess doesn't resolve in a few days, consult a dentist.

Flower Essences

Self-Heal and Yarrow Special Formula can serve as the foundational healing agents for a dental abscess. Other flower essences to address the specific emotions, mental attitude, and environmental conditions of the individual are recommended, states Patricia Kaminski, a flower essence therapist and codirector of the Flower Essence Society.

Self-Heal supports the body's innate healing ability. Yarrow Special Formula strengthens and protects against environmental toxicity and stress. Take 4 drops of each 2–4 times daily, or as needed.

Food Therapy

Eat:

Garlic, yogurt, foods high in vitamins A and C. (For a list of foods containing these nutrients, see part 3, "Food Therapy," p. 378.)

Avoid:

Sugar, soft drinks, fried or processed food.

Herbal Medicine

Medical herbalist Chanchal Cabrera, M.N.I.M.H., A.H.G., of Vancouver, British Columbia, has found the following program useful for dental abscesses:

Herbal mouth rinse: For an astringent antimicrobial rinse for the gums, combine equal parts of tinctures of the herbs salvia (cooking) sage, rosemary, myrrh, goldenseal, echinacea, bloodroot, and peppermint (for flavoring). Add 1 teaspoon of this blend to 1/2 cup of water. Swish it around in your mouth for 1 minute, then gargle. It's fine to swallow the mixture. Do this 2–3 times a day (3–4 during acute stage) or as often as you can. Myrrh works on contact, so do not rinse your mouth out afterward. Continue the procedure for as long as there is pain, swelling, and inflammation.

The rinse is helpful for receding gums, too, says Cabrera. A commercial preparation of this mouth rinse, called Orcln, is available through the Gaia Garden Herbal Dispensary and Clinic in Vancouver, British Columbia (see Cabrera's listing under "Herbal Medicine" in Appendix B: Resources). Note: The herbal mouth rinse is not intended to be used in lieu of dental treatment.

Pain relief: To relieve pain, put a drop or two of essential oil of clove on a cotton ball, place it on the abscess, and leave it on for 15–30 minutes. Do this 2–3 times a day. Stop if irritation results.

Immune support: Take echinacea tincture at a dosage of 1 teaspoon 3–4 times daily, for 3–4 weeks. The common view that echinacea should be taken only for brief periods because the body builds up a resistance to it is erroneous, states Cabrera. She explains that a mistranslation of the German in a German study of echinacea is behind the misunderstanding. (See "Nutritional Supplements," below.)

Myrrh and propolis can resolve a dental abscess in some cases, says Amanda McQuade Crawford, M.N.I.M.H., Dip.Phyto., director of the Ojai Center of Phytotherapy in Ojai, California. Use 1/2 teaspoon each of tinctures of myrrh (*Commiphora molmol*) and propolis (resin collected by bees from under tree bark). Swish the mixture around in your mouth for 1 minute and then spit it out. You can also swallow it to strengthen immunity, but you should not do so on an empty stomach. Some people find the propolis hard on the stomach lining. Do this every 4 hours for 3–6 days, until your symptoms decrease. Then reduce the treatment to twice daily for another 3–6 days. If the infection does not clear in a week or gets worse, you need to seek medical care, advises Crawford.

Homeopathy

Homeopathic physician Michael G. Carlston, M.D., of Santa Rosa, California, recommends the following:

Silica: If the dental abscess doesn't produce much pain.
Hepar sulph: If the abscess is painful, take 6c, 12c, or 30c. Take 2 or 3 pellets. It is likely that you'll need to take it 4 times a day.

Take the appropriate remedy in a 6c, 12c, or 30c potency. During the acute stage, take 2 or 3 pellets, or a couple of drops if you are taking the remedy in drop form, 2 to 3 times per day. Dental abscesses respond slowly. You may have to continue the remedy for weeks. As your symptoms lessen, reduce the frequency of dosage. Don't keep taking the remedy when the dental abscess is gone.

Nutritional Supplements

Chanchal Cabrera has found that the lozenge form of zinc is quite helpful for a dental abscess; suck on lozenges to give you 30–50 mg of zinc per day. Note: do not take zinc on a long-term basis as it can cause copper deficiency.

Applying liquid chlorophyll to the affected area can help resolve a dental abscess, according to naturopathic physician Linda Rector Page N.D., Ph.D. Take it internally as well, at a dosage of 3 teaspoons daily, she says.[1]

Grapefruit seed extract (GSE) has powerful germ-fighting abilities and also facilitates tissue repair, says Allan Sachs, D.C., C.C.N. For a mouthwash to treat a dental abscess, break open 1 capsule of GSE, pour the powder into 6–8 ounces of water, and mix well. Swish the blend around in the mouth, then rinse thoroughly. GSE comes in liquid form, but it has quite a bitter taste, notes Dr. Sachs.[2] Use the mouthwash daily until the dental abscess is resolved.

Reflexology

Teeth

Stone/Crystal Therapy

For a dental abscess, lay aquamarine or clear crystal on the outside of the cheek over the problem tooth for 15–20 minutes daily, as needed, recommends Daya Sarai Chocron, a vibrational healer and author of *Healing with Crystals and Gemstones*. You can also hold the stone, wear it, or carry it in your pocket until the abscess is resolved.

Depression

The word "depression" comes from the Latin *depressio,* a pressing down. That is the overriding sensation of the mental-emotional state of depression. Those afflicted feel flat, unable to summon enthusiasm for activities, people, and events they normally love. Other symptoms include fatigue, sleep problems, loss of sex drive, loss of appetite or the reverse, difficulty concentrating, feelings of worthlessness, lack of motivation, and social withdrawal.

Depression ranges from mild to clinical, in which the depressed person suffers from numerous of the above symptoms (and possibly recurrent thoughts of suicide or death as well) for at least a month.

Clinical depression is beyond the scope of the treatments discussed here.

The causes of depression, aside from a normal response to loss or grief, are many. They include imbalances in brain neurotransmitters (the chemical "messengers" of the brain), nutritional deficiencies, allergies, hormonal imbalance, stress, thyroid disorders, heavy metal toxicity, certain prescription drugs, and lack of sunlight. The latter form of depression is known as seasonal affective disorder, or SAD. The winter months, when there is less sunlight, can trigger depression in people who suffer from SAD. The use of full-spectrum lighting, the artificial light that most closely resembles sunlight, can help combat this disorder.

Essential Oils

Patricia Davis, founder of the London School of Aromatherapy in London, England, makes a very important point regarding essential oils for depression, a point overlooked by many practitioners. While there is a significant list of essential oils with antidepressant activity, it is necessary to look deeper to discover the oil that is an appropriate remedy for your variety of depression. If your depression is accompanied by fatigue and lethargy, the antidepressant oils that also have sedative properties are not the ones you will want to use. Conversely, if your depression is characterized by irritability, sleep problems, and restlessness, you will want a sedative rather than stimulating antidepressant essential oil. Bergamot, Geranium, Melissa, and Rose are nonsedating antidepressant oils, says Davis, while Chamomile, Clary Sage, Lavender, Sandalwood, and Ylang Ylang are sedative antidepressant oils. For depression accompanied by anxiety, Davis recommends Neroli essential oil. Massages and baths are good methods of delivery because they are in themselves therapeutic for depression.[1] (For instructions on how to use essential oils in baths and massages, see part 3, "Essential Oils," pp. 366–368.)

Flower Essences

Like anxiety, depression is a huge area of treatment in flower essence therapy, says Patricia Kaminski, a flower essence therapist and educator from Nevada City, California. Here are the highlights among dozens of possible flower essence remedies:

Borage: For depression accompanied by grief.
Pine: For depression accompanied by a sense of loss, regret, and excessive melancholia.
St. John's Wort: When depression is seasonal, accompanied by insomnia, or due to spiritual imbalance.
Gorse: For loss of optimism or loss of hope for the future.
Scotch Broom: When depression is influenced by world events or other surrounding context.
Wild Rose: For depression accompanied by suicidal tendencies.
Mustard: For depression with frequent mood swings.

Take 4 drops of the appropriate flower essence for your depression, 2–4 times daily, or more often during acute episodes. You can continue taking the remedy as needed.

Food Therapy

Eat:

Protein, seafood, whole grains, nuts, spinach, foods high in tryptophan (low-fat dairy, bananas, soy, turkey), foods high in magnesium and calcium (see part 3, "Food Therapy," pp. 376, 377).

Avoid:

Sugar, caffeine, alcohol, processed foods, aspartame, allergenic foods.

Consider increasing your protein intake if it is low, says naturopathic physician Alan Christianson, N.M.D., of Scottsdale, Arizona. "Garden-variety depression is not biochemical as often as we think." Chronic low protein intake and digestive problems are more commonly the cause than a biochemical imbalance is. Keeping fat intake low and eating more frequent meals to help stabilize blood sugar are also helpful dietary practices, he notes.

Herbal Medicine

St. John's wort (*Hypericum perforatum*) has become popular as an herbal antidepressant, and clinical studies have proven its efficacy for mild to moderate depression.[2] Dr. Christianson recommends taking 300 mg of the standardized herb 3 times daily. It may take 4 weeks before you feel the effects. Do not take St. John's wort in combination with prescription antidepressants. In people who are sensitive to the sun, the herb can produce greater sensitivity and make it easier for them to get sunburned. This is especially true for those taking more than the recommended dosage.

For an antidepressant tea, combine equal parts of St. John's wort, damiana (*Turnera aphrodisiaca, T. diffusa*), oatseed (*Avena sativa*), and vervain (*Verbena officinalis*). Use the aboveground parts of the herbs. Add 1 ounce of the blend to 2 cups of boiled water, cover, and let stand for 10 minutes. Strain and drink up to 3 cups a day, as needed for depression.[3]

Nutritional Supplements

The following supplements can be effective in lifting depression, says Dr. Christianson:

SAMe or SAM (S-adenosylmethionine): Manufactured in the body from the amino acid methionine, SAMe is involved in many metabolic processes, including the production of brain chemicals. People suffering from depression may not produce enough SAMe, so supplementation can be helpful. Gradually build your dose up to 400 mg, 4 times daily. A starting dose can be 100–200 mg, 4 times per day. Look for products that were manufactured according to German GMP standards or were tested in clinical European trials. These are the quickest acting, have the lowest incidence of side effects, and have no interaction with prescription drugs. The drawback of SAMe is that it's quite costly. A full daily dose runs $10–$12.

5-HTP (5-hydroxy tryptophan): This is a plant extract that behaves like the amino acid tryptophan in the body. Tryptophan is a precursor to the neurotransmitter serotonin, which regulates mood. A low-protein diet can result in a deficit of tryptophan. Take 50–150 mg of 5-HTP 3 times daily. It may take a few weeks for effects to be felt. Some people experience slight nausea.

Homeopathy

Your depression may best be treated by a constitutional homeopathic remedy. You may want to consult a homeopath for individualized treatment. However, the following are two common remedies for depression, as cited by Drs. Andrew Lockie and Nicola Geddes:[4]

Ignatia: If there is depression with greatly fluctuating moods, inappropriate behavior such as suddenly crying or laughing for no reason, a tendency to hold in emotions, sensitivity to noise, and self-blame for all that goes wrong, and worsened by strong smells, coffee, stimulants, being cold, and being warmly dressed.

Pulsatilla: If the depression is accompanied by extreme tearfulness, self-pity, crying over the smallest upset, yearning for reassurance and comforting, and lack of self-esteem and willpower, and is made worse by heat, stuffy rooms, rich, fatty foods, and twilight.

Take the appropriate remedy in a 6c potency 3 times daily for up to 14 days.

Reflexology

Brain/head, solar plexus, endocrine system

Stone/Crystal Therapy

There are a number of stones that are useful as healing aids in depression, according to Katrina Raphaell, crystal healing therapist and author of the crystal reference series *The Crystal Trilogy*. She cites citrine, black tourmaline, smoky quartz, lepidolite, pink tourmaline, and pink calcite. Place the stone on the center of your body at the level of the heart or over your solar plexus (top of the abdomen, below the ribs). Leave it in place for 5 minutes while you visualize health. Do this 3 times daily, as needed. In addition, wear the stone, hold it, or carry it in your pocket for ongoing healing effects.

Dermatitis (Eczema)

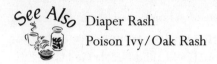 **See Also** Diaper Rash
Poison Ivy/Oak Rash

Dermatitis—literally, inflammation of the skin—is characterized by redness, itching, scaling, flaking, lesions, and thickening of the skin. The word "eczema" is now used synonymously with "dermatitis," but eczema is more a description of the symptoms than a distinct diagnosis.[1]

A common form of dermatitis, atopic dermatitis, may involve hereditary and allergic components. The lesions typically appear at the knees, wrists, and elbows. Research has found decreased prostaglandin levels in people with this type of dermatitis.[2] Prostaglandins are complex fatty acids with hormone-like actions. They are involved in inflammatory processes, among other functions. The body cannot produce prostaglandins without sufficient essential fatty acids (see "Nutritional Supplements" below).

Another common type, contact dermatitis, is a reaction to an irritant on the skin, such as poison ivy resin or a detergent. As people have varying degrees of sensitivity to substances, with one person reacting strongly to a mild soap, for example, while another person has no reaction to the same soap, one could argue that some cases of contact dermatitis also involve allergies (to call them "sensitivities" may be verbal hair-splitting).

Essential Oils

Kurt Schnaubelt, Ph.D., scientific director of the Pacific Institute of Aromatherapy in San Rafael, California, recommends several topical essential oil formulas, depending on the type of dermatitis. For dry eczema, combine essential oils of Lavender (1 ml), Palmarosa (1 ml), and Calophyllum (10 ml) in 6 teaspoons of Rose Hip seed oil. Apply to the affected area 3–4 times daily until the condition is resolved. This blend relieves itchiness and stimulates skin healing, says Dr. Schnaubelt. For weeping eczema, combine essential oils of Thyme (thujanol type, 1 ml), Eucalyptus citriodora (1 ml), and Calophyllum (10 ml) in 6 teaspoons of Rose Hip seed oil. Use in the same way as the dry eczema formula.[3]

Flower Essences

To ease dermatitis, use Self-Heal cream and St. John's Shield flower oil topically, recommends Richard Katz, founder of the Flower Essence Society. Apply 2–4 times daily, alternating the cream and the oil, until your symptoms subside.

Food Therapy

Eat:

Fiber, dark green leafy vegetables, cold-water fish (salmon, mackerel), flaxseed and olive oils, nuts (except peanuts), seeds, avocado, turmeric, biotin-rich foods (soy, garlic, sesame), foods high in potassium (see part 3, "Food Therapy," p. 377)

Avoid:

Refined foods, fried foods, alcohol, shellfish, margarine, dairy, red meat, peanuts, gluten (protein in wheat, rye, barley, and oats).

"Food allergies are almost always a component in eczema," says Paul Reilly, N.D., L.Ac., a naturopathic physician and acupuncturist from Seattle, Washington. Eliminating common allergens such as milk, wheat, corn, eggs, and dairy may produce improvement in your skin condition, he notes, although he recommends working with a qualified practitioner to identify your allergies.

Herbal Medicine

Dermatitis indicates the need to help the body cleanse, observes herbalist Teresa Boardwine of Washington, Virginia. "It's an outer manifestation of something the body can't process, such as antigens [allergenic substances]. Eczema is almost an allergy symptom in itself. In children, it often occurs as a result of an allergy to cow's milk."

She suggests the alterative herbs (herbs that help restore the body to a healthy state) nettle and yellow dock to help the body flush toxins via the urine.

Nettle (*Urtica dioica*) is an herb you can ingest as tea and as a food indefinitely. Highly nutrititious, nettle is a whole-body tonic. Make the tea (infusion) by pouring boiled water over the herb (1 tablespoon herb per 1 cup of water), covering, and letting steep for 15–20 minutes. Strain, and drink 1 cup of tea 3 times daily. Boardwine suggests making fresh nettle a regular part of your diet. You can cook it like spinach, but don't eat it raw (the formic acid it contains can give you a sting).

Yellow dock (*Rumex crispus*) helps cleanse the liver, notes Boardwine. Take as tincture (15 drops in a little water) or capsules (1 capsule) twice daily before meals. Yellow dock is a bitter, which means that it stimulates the digestive juices. The herb is also a bit of a laxative, so don't be concerned if your stools get a little loose.

Boardwine also recommends an external wash of calendula tea for dermatitis. Steep 1 tablespoon of calendula (*Calendula officinalis*) in 1 cup of water for 15–20 minutes. Strain the tea and rinse the affected area with it as often as possible. During acute dermatitis, you should do this a minimum of 3–4 times daily. For maintenance, use the rinse once daily.

Dr. Reilly recommends the following herbal program for dermatitis, used in combination with his dietary provisos and nutritional supplement protocol:

Topical: Use chamomile (*Matricaria recutita*) or lavender (*Lavandula officinalis*) to make a tea; 1 teaspoon of either herb to 1 cup of boiled water. Let the tea cool, then use a cotton ball to apply it to itchy areas 2–4 times per day.

Internal: Use ground dandelion (*Taraxacum officinalis*) and burdock (*Arctium lappa*) roots to make a tea; 1/2 teaspoon of each powder to 1 cup of boiled water. Drink 1–2 cups daily.

Homeopathy

Atopic dermatitis is best treated by a constitutional homeopathic remedy. You may want to consult a homeopath for individualized treatment.

That said, the following are remedies commonly indicated for eczema/dermatitis:[4]

Graphites: If the skin is rough, hard, and cracked with a discharge the consistency of honey; often used for infants with eczema.

Kali mur: If there are blisters containing white fluid.

Kali sulph: If it is "weeping eczema."

Nat mur: If the skin is raw and inflamed.

Sulphur: If the skin is hot, extremely itchy, and bleeds easily when scratched.

Take the appropriate remedy in a 6x or 6c potency 3 times daily, or more often during acute eruption. Stop taking the remedy when your symptoms improve. You can restart it if the improvement doesn't last, but you shouldn't take the remedy on an ongoing basis.

Homeopathic calendula cream can also provide relief; apply topically as needed.

Nutritional Supplements

The following supplemental protocol can be beneficial for dermatitis and should be taken in addition to your regular multivitamin/mineral, says Dr. Reilly:

Digestive enzymes and HCl: "People with dermatitis usually have weak digestion," notes Dr. Reilly. Supplementing with pancreatic enzymes and hydrochloric acid (digestive acid of the stomach) can aid digestion. Use a combination product, with 200–250 mg of pancreatic enzymes and 5 grains of HCl per capsule. Pancreatin comes in different strengths; 8–10x is the strongest, 4x half as strong. Take the most concentrated form you can find in order to reduce the number of capsules needed. Take 1–3 capsules in the middle of every meal. If you take them before or after the meal, they may cause heartburn.

Essential fatty acids (EFAs): Use EPA (eicosapentaenoic acid, an omega-3 EFA) and borage oil. Dr. Reilly prefers borage oil to evening primrose oil as a source of GLA (gamma-linolenic acid, an omega-6 oil) because it is less expensive and works better, in his opinion. Take 1 capsule (300–500 mg) of EPA and 1 capsule (300 mg) of borage oil at every meal. You can take up to a total of 10 g of the combined oils per day.

Zinc and vitamin B6: Take 30–50 mg of zinc picolinate and 50 mg of vitamin B6 daily; the body needs these nutrients to absorb essential fatty acids and convert them into prostaglandins.

Quercetin: This bioflavonoid helps reduce allergic symptoms. Take 500 mg with each meal. You can omit this supplement from the program, if you like.

The above protocol takes 2–3 weeks to start working, so be patient.

Follow the dietary, herbal, and nutritional supplement recommendations as a package program for 6 weeks, then evaluate the results. If it is working, you can start trying to reduce the dosages of what you are taking. Cut the dosages by 25 percent the next month. If you don't have a flare-up of your skin condition, reduce the dosages by another 25 percent the following month. The goal is to find the maintenance level for you: that is, the amounts that keep your dermatitis from recurring. In many cases, one-quarter of the dosages given here is sufficient for long-term maintenance.

Reflexology
Endocrine glands, lymphatic system, kidneys, solar plexus

Stone/Crystal Therapy
Phosphorite and wavellite are beneficial for dermatitis, says Melody, author of the crystal reference series *Love Is in the Earth*. Treat the affected area with phosphorite elixir 3 times daily for 3 days, then as needed. Tape wavellite on the affected area with hypoallergenic tape; leave it on for 4 days. (For instructions on making an elixir, see part 3, "Stone/Crystal Therapy," p. 403.)

Diaper Rash

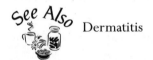 Dermatitis

A form of contact dermatitis, diaper rash is characterized by redness with or without small pimples in the groin area. The causes include friction, detergent or soap residue in diapers, or prolonged contact with urine and feces. In the last case, the skin does not have an opportunity to dry out, but remains damp much of the time. In addition, the ammonia in the urine is the contact irritant and can "burn" the skin.

Essential Oils
For diaper rash, naturopathic physician Boyer B. Cole, N.M.D., of Cottonwood, Arizona, has found an essential oil blend effective. Mix the following essential oils with 1/2 ounce of olive oil:

Lavender: 20 drops
German Chamomile: 5 drops
Geranium: 4 drops

When changing a diaper, apply this blend topically in the diaper area after cleaning the baby. Use for as long as the rash persists. The olive oil is protective against the irritation of urine, explains Dr. Cole, while the Geranium is astringent (protects, cleanses, and works against inflammation) and the Lavender and Chamomile promote tissue healing.

Julia Fischer, a medical aromatherapist practicing in Northern California, offers another daily diaper rash regimen. Put 1 drop of Lavender essential oil in your baby's daily bath. Dry your baby well after the bath, and apply an essential oil formula to the affected area. To prepare the formula, combine:

German Chamomile essential oil: 6 drops
Lavender essential oil: 3 drops
Tea Tree (*Melaleuca alternifolia*) essential oil: 1 drop
Calendula fatty oil: 6 teaspoons (30 ml).

Calendula fatty oil is a carrier oil that has been infused with the herb calendula. It is important to use a fatty-oil-based formula for diaper rash rather than a mineral oil or beeswax-based salve, as they are occlusive (clogging) to the skin.

Optional: dust the area lightly with kaolin (white) clay to which you've added powdered lavender flowers (1 teaspoon of lavender powder to 2 ounces of clay).

Flower Essences

Calendula Caress flower oil applied topically each time you change the baby's diapers can ease diaper rash, according to Patricia Kaminski, an herbalist and flower essence therapist from Nevada City, California.

Food Therapy

Diaper rash is typically a low-grade fungal infection, says Alan Christianson, N.M.D., a naturopathic physician from Scottsdale, Arizona. Giving your baby more protein, which helps stabilize blood sugar, creates an environment less hospitable to fungus. Avoid sugar, which feeds fungus, advises Dr. Christianson. If you are giving your baby infant formula, make sure it does not contain any sugars. Acidic foods such as tomatoes and citrus fruit may also contribute to or exacerbate diaper rash. If the diaper rash appears after a change in the diet of either the child or the breast-feeding mother, try eliminating the new food.

Herbal Medicine

Aloe vera gel is another soothing topical application for diaper rash. Aloe is well-known for its skin-healing properties. Apply with each diaper change.

Homeopathy

As in other therapeutic modalities, calendula officinalis is a diaper rash solution in homeopathy, according to Maesimund B. Panos, M.D. She cites the effectiveness of homeopathic calendula ointment, which has a lanolin base. In her practice, she is often consulted by mothers who have tried all the other ointments without success. They try calendula ointment and soon report that the rash has disappeared, says Dr. Panos.[1]

Nutritional Supplements

Giving the baby probiotics can help resolve diaper rash, says Sue Reynolds, M.S.W., L.M.T., a certified herbalist and aromatherapist from Goleta, California. These beneficial bacteria normally reside in the body and keep fungus in check, preventing overgrowth. When the balance of microflora has been thrown off by antibiotics (they wipe out the good bacteria in the body along with the harmful bacteria) or too much sugar in the diet, supplementing with probiotics can restore the proper balance and inhibit fungus. Purchase a product containing *Lactobacillus acidophilus* and the other probiotics baby's bodies need. These are available in a commercial mixture in powder form; some products also contain FOS (fructo-oligosaccharides) which, as a "food" for the beneficial bacteria, increases the effectiveness of the combination. Put a little of the powder on the baby's tongue daily. If the baby is breast-feeding, apply some to the mother's nipples as well.

Other Remedies

A simple remedy for diaper rash is a sea salt bath, notes Joanne B. Mied, N.D., a naturopath and herbalist based in Novato, California. Put 1/2 to 1 cup of sea salt in a small bath of warm water. Keep your child playing in the water for 20 minutes. Rinse afterward. Do this daily until the redness of the diaper rash disappears.

As detergents and diaper material can be factors in diaper rash, Julia Fischer advises using only cotton diapers washed in natural, non-detergent soap or unscented castile soap.

Let your baby go bare bottomed periodically during the day to give the skin air exposure and relief from the constant presence of diapers.

Diarrhea

The abnormally fluid and frequent stools of diarrhea can be caused by a wide range of factors and ailments. Intestinal parasites, viruses, bacteria, and other microorganisms can produce diarrhea, as can food poisoning or a change in food and water (as in traveler's diarrhea). Allergies and stress can also be factors. Colitis and other gastrointestinal disorders are more serious causes of diarrhea.

Diarrhea is an effective way for the body to get rid of toxins, so it is best to let simple cases of diarrhea run their course. If diarrhea lasts longer than a few days, it is important to discover the cause and get appropriate treatment.

Many people stop drinking water in the mistaken notion that this will help solidify their stools. It won't, and it is easy for someone (especially a child or small person) with diarrhea to become dehydrated. Drinking plenty of fluids should be a primary part of your treatment approach.[1]

Essential Oils

Myrrh and Geranium essential oils tone tissue and can be an effective treatment for diarrhea, according to naturopathic physician Boyer B. Cole, N.M.D., of Cottonwood, Arizona. Mix equal parts of olive oil and essential oils (a blend of 50 percent Myrrh and 50 percent Geranium). Take 2 drops of this mix orally every half-hour, up to 16 drops over a day. Do not continue for more than 1 day. If this treatment does not resolve your diarrhea within that time period, you should consider other approaches.

Flower Essences

Self-Heal can serve as a foundational healing agent for diarrhea. Other flower essences to address the specific emotions, mental attitude, and environmental conditions of the individual are recommended, states Patricia Kaminski, a flower essence therapist and codirector of the Flower Essence Society. Self-Heal supports the body's innate healing ability. Take 4 drops 2–4 times daily, or as needed.

Food Therapy

Eat:

Dried blueberries, miso soup, turmeric, garlic, ginger, yogurt/kefir, bananas, tapioca, rice, mashed potatoes, cooked carrots.

Avoid:

High-fiber food, sugar, caffeine, alcohol, dairy (aside from yogurt), fatty or fried foods, food allergens (a common cause of diarrhea).

Herbal Medicine

Marshmallow (*Althea officinalis*) is a helpful remedy for diarrhea, states Joanne B. Mied, N.D., a naturopath and herbalist practicing in Novato, California. Take 5 capsules (450 mg each) right away in an acute episode, then 5 capsules every 2 hours until the diarrhea is gone. As a healing aid to the intestines after the diarrhea is resolved, you can continue taking the marshmallow at a dosage of 3 capsules 3 times daily; finish out the bottle of 100 or so capsules. Marshmallow absorbs the toxins and infection causing the diarrhea, and is soothing to the whole intestinal tract, explains Dr. Mied.

Homeopathy

For diarrhea, Michael G. Carlston, M.D., a homeopathic physician from Santa Rosa, California, recommends the following remedies:

Phosphorus: If diarrhea is explosive and watery, with blood (seek medical help if blood doesn't go away immediately), and the person is anxious and thirsty, especially for cold drinks.

Arsenicum: Diarrhea similar to that of Phosphorus, but the person is more restless, thirsty for warm drinks rather than cold, and fearful rather than anxious.

Sulphur: Similar to Arsenicum, but the diarrhea is burning and the person is less fearful.

Carbo veg: When there is gas along with the diarrhea.

Take the appropriate remedy at a 12c or 30c potency when the diarrhea occurs. At the next episode, take another dose.

Nutritional Supplements

For diarrhea, naturopathic physician Alan Christianson, N.M.D., of Scottsdale, Arizona, recommends a fiber supplement, activated charcoal, probiotics, and a nutrient-rich shake, as detailed below:

Psyllium fiber: Contrary to what you might think, fiber is very helpful for diarrhea. Rather than making it worse, it binds with metabolic waste and bacteria and works to resolve it more quickly. Put 2 teaspoons of psyllium fiber in 16 ounces of water. Let it sit for 10 minutes, then drink. Do this 1–2 times daily.

Activated charcoal: This works similarly to fiber, binding with toxins and speeding their removal from the body. Take 30 capsules or 2 tablespoons of liquid daily for 2 days, if needed.

Probiotics: These beneficial bacteria, of which *Lactobacillus acidophilus* is probably the most well known, are normally found in the intestines. Supplementation can aid in resolving diarrhea by restoring the proper balance of intestinal bacteria. There is an issue with the quality and purity of acidophilus products. Be sure to get powder or capsules that require refrigeration. Take 5–10 billion organisms daily in 2–3 divided doses for a week. (The product will tell you how many organisms are in a specified amount.) Don't take long-term because it can disrupt the balance of other bacteria.

Shake: This nutrient-packed shake is also easy on the gut. Make a full blender of the shake to drink throughout the day. Combine hydrolized whey or lactalbumin protein powder, water, banana, papaya, or other soft fruit, 3 tablespoons of almond oil or coconut oil, and 10–30 g of the amino acid glutamine.

Reflexology

Ascending and transverse colon, liver, diaphragm, adrenal glands

Stone/Crystal Therapy

Black tourmaline or green aventurine are healing stones for diarrhea, states crystal healing therapist Katrina Raphaell of Kapaa, Hawaii. Place the stone on your abdomen. If you feel the distress of diarrhea in a specific area of the abdomen, put the stone over that spot. Leave the stone there for 5 minutes while visualizing your health goal. Do this 3 times daily. In between treatments, wear the stone, hold it, or carry it in your pocket to continue the healing effects.

Dizziness (Vertigo)

Also known as vertigo, dizziness involves light-headed unsteadiness with a sensation of whirling or falling when one is still. The sensation may be so strong that nausea and even vomiting ensue. Vertigo arises when the central nervous system receives conflicting messages from the eyes, inner ear, muscles, and skin pressure receptors. Serious disorders such as a brain tumor or neurologic disease can produce vertigo, so if your dizziness is prolonged, seek medical assistance. Less serious causes of dizziness are ear infections (including labyrinthitis), nutritional deficiencies, allergies, excess ear wax, and stress.

Essential Oils

Orange essential oil can help ease dizziness, as it exerts a stabilizing effect on the nervous system. Use it in a diffuser, inhale it from the open bottle, or sprinkle a few drops on a handkerchief or tissue and inhale it that way, as needed.[1]

Flower Essences

Take Indian Pink flower essence to relieve dizziness, says Richard Katz, naturalist and founder of the Flower Essence Society. Take 4 drops under the tongue as often as once per hour during an acute episode. If the dizziness occurred after an accident or other trauma, continue taking 4 drops 2–4 times daily for a month. (If there is any possibility that you have suffered a head injury, consult your doctor.)

Food Therapy

Eat:

Small and frequent meals/snacks to keep blood sugar stable.

Avoid:

Sugar, refined carbohydrates, fried foods, caffeine, alcohol.

Herbal Medicine

Ginkgo (*Ginkgo biloba*) and hawthorn (*Crataegus oxyacantha*) can alleviate dizziness, according to Sue Reynolds, M.S.W., L.M.T., a certified herbalist and aromatherapist from Goleta, California. Both herbs are vasodilators and as such promote blood circulation in the brain, which can ease vertigo. Take 6–9 capsules of the herbs in combination daily, as needed.

Herbalist James A. Duke, Ph.D., offers an anti-dizziness recipe he calls "Stomach Settler Tea." Mix 4 teaspoons of ginger with dashes of ground pumpkin seed, celery seed, chamomile flowers, fennel, orange rind, peppermint, and spearmint. Steep in boiled water for 15 minutes.[2]

Homeopathy

The following are common homeopathic remedies for acute vertigo:[3]

Bryonia: If the vertigo attacks are severe, with the sensation of sinking into or through the bed, and worsened by trying to get up or any motion; preventing the dizziness requires lying completely still without even moving the eyes; often follows an illness involving a fever.

Calc carb: If the vertigo is worse with exertion, walking, turning the head too fast, or sudden motion.

Cocculus: If the vertigo is characterized by the sensation of the room turning, intense nausea, and the necessity to lie still to prevent dizziness, and made worse by any attempt to get up from the bed or even lift the head, riding in a vehicle, looking at a moving object, drinking wine or alcohol, or missing even a few minutes of needed sleep.

Silica: If the vertigo is associated with stopped ears and sinusitis and worsened by motion, walking, stooping, looking up, lying on the back or left side, and being in a vehicle.

Take the appropriate remedy in a 30c potency 2 times daily for 2–3 days. If it is the correct remedy, you will generally experience improvement in that time.

Nutritional Supplements

The following supplements can be beneficial for vertigo, according to James F. Balch, M.D., and Phyllis A. Balch, C.N.C.:[4]

Vitamin B3 (niacin): 100 mg 3 times per day; promotes circulation in the brain and lowers cholesterol.

Vitamin B complex (high stress): Take as directed; essential for normal functioning of the brain and central nervous system.

Vitamin C: 3,000–10,000 mg daily, in divided doses throughout the day; antioxidant and aid to circulation.

Vitamin E: 400–800 IU per day, gradually increasing dosage; aids circulation.

Reflexology

Eyes, ears, cervical spine, neck

Stone/Crystal Therapy

Crystal can help restore equilibrium, notes vibrational healer Daya Sarai Chocron, of Northampton, Massachusetts. Hold the stone, wear it, carry it in your pocket, or lay it on your body (on your forehead, stomach, or other location) for 15–20 minutes daily, as needed.

Ear Infection

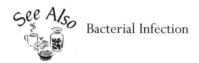 **See Also** Bacterial Infection

Outer ear infection (otitis exterma), also known as swimmer's ear, is the most common kind of ear infection. It affects the canal from the eardrum to the outside of the ear, and its symptoms include discharge, low fever, redness, swelling, and pain that is exacerbated by touching the ear.

Ear infections are a common affliction of childhood; the infection is often otitis media, or inflammation of the middle ear, also known as glue ear due to the buildup of fluid involved. Symptoms include stabbing, dull, or throbbing pain in the ear; fever; and irritability. A child may pull at the ear in an effort to alleviate the pressure created by the fluid accumulation. A middle ear infection often follows an upper respiratory viral or bacterial infection because the nose and throat are connected to that part of the ear via the eustacian tubes.

Allergies and a diet high in mucus-forming foods (notably dairy products) can contribute to chronic ear infection.

Note that pain in the ear may not involve an infection; it can also arise from injury such as a ruptured eardrum. The symptoms are strong, sharp pain followed by sudden drainage. If you suspect that you have a ruptured eardrum, do not use eardrops or any other substance in the ear and consult your doctor.

Essential Oils

"Lavender is particularly useful for ear, nose, and throat infections, and is a useful alternative to Chamomile for infantile ear infections," states aromatherapy authority Robert B. Tisserand.[1] Use the oils singly or in combination in baths, massages, a diffuser placed in the sickroom at night, or hot compresses applied to the ear region, or sprinkle a few drops on a tissue or handkerchief and tuck it under the patient's pillow.

Flower Essences

For those with a chronic history of ear troubles such as ear infection, Mullein flower essence can be useful, says Patricia Kaminski, a flower essence therapist and educator from Nevada City, California. She notes that it is not a direct treatment for an ear infection but, rather, addresses the pattern. Take 4 drops 2–4 times daily for a month or longer.

Food Therapy

Eat:

Garlic, protein (aside from the typical food allergens below).

Avoid:

Sugar (all forms, including undiluted fruit juice, honey, and dried fruit), food additives, oranges, peanut butter, common food allergens (dairy, wheat, eggs, and soy).

"If you took children off of dairy, it would probably clear seventy-five percent of ear infections," says Kathi Head, N.D., a naturopathic physician from Sandpoint, Idaho.

Herbal Medicine

A combination formula of mullein and garlic oil is a well-known herbal remedy for ear infections, and widely available commercially. Herbalist Teresa Boardwine of Washington, Virginia, suggests putting the vial of oil in a cup of warm water to warm it before using. Lie on your side, put 3 drops in your ear (1 drop for children), then massage the ear and pull it away from the head to help the oil go deep into the canal. Wait five minutes, then put a cotton ball in the ear to hold the oil in. Turn over and do the other ear. Do this every other night for 2 weeks. If you or your child suffer ear infections seasonally, as with swimming in the summer or chronic otitis media in the winter, you can use the oil preventively. During the problem season, put 1 drop in each ear (same dosage for children and adults) every other night.

For ear, nose, and throat (ENT) infection, Boardwine recommends wild indigo root tincture. With short-term, intense usage, wild indigo (*Baptisia tinctoria*) has quite strong antimicrobial effects, specifically for ENTs. Use as recommended by the manufacturer of the individual brand. A typical dosage is 10–20 drops of tincture 3 times daily, for no more than 5 days.

Homeopathy

Children respond well to homeopathy, and it is easy to give to them. Choose the remedy according to the symptoms. Dr. Head cites the following remedies as the most common for ear infection in children:

Pulsatilla: If the child is whiny, clingy, and wants to be held, has a cold, and there is a yellow discharge from the nose.
Belladonna: With a high fever; red eardrums; red cheeks; hot, dry head.
Chamomilla: If there is lot of pain, high-pitched screaming, the child wants something but nothing seems to satisfy her/him.

Give the child the appropriate remedy (only one) at a 30c potency, 2–3 pellets under the tongue, 3 times daily; separate from any food, water, or other substance in the mouth by 20 minutes before and after (same for adults). Sometimes it takes only one dose. As soon as there is improvement, stop the remedy. If you don't see a change after a day, you should consider other treatment.

Nutritional Supplements

For adults, taking a high-potency multivitamin/mineral to support immunity is a good idea as a general practice, says Dr. Head. In addition to your regular supplement, she recommends the following for an ear infection; take for 1–2 weeks:

Vitamin C: 1,000 mg 3 times daily.

Zinc/copper: 30 mg of zinc per day, with 2 mg of copper daily to balance it; the two minerals work in ratio to each other.

Beta-carotene: 50,000 IU daily.

For children, Dr. Head has found that the herbal and homeopathic remedies are the best approach because they are easy to administer. You can give children some vitamin A and C along with that. The following supplements are also useful, but keep in mind that too many pills can make treating children a difficult process.

The bioflavonoid quercetin is useful for both prevention and treatment of an ear infection; for adults, 400–500 mg twice daily; for children, 100 mg twice daily.

For glue ear, the amino acid NAC (N-acetyl cysteine) is an excellent supplement. It is both antioxidant and mucolytic (able to break down mucus). The daily dosage is 25 mg per 2.2 pounds (1 kilo) of body weight; for example, a 110-pound adult should take 1,250 mg per day. Divide your daily dosage in half and take in two doses. Be warned, however, says Dr. Head, that NAC is not easy to get down a 3-year-old because it is bitter tasting. She generally recommends it for adults and children older than 6.

Reflexology

Ear, throat, neck

Stone/Crystal Therapy

For an ear infection, tape a piece of frondelite behind the ear for 2–3 days, recommends Melody, author of the crystal reference series *Love Is in the Earth*.

Other Remedies

Teresa Boardwine has found the old folk remedy of salt in a sock soothing for ear infections, especially in children. Put rock salt or coarse sea salt in a cast iron skillet and heat until the salt is holding the heat. Pour the salt into a sock (athletic tube socks work well). Tie off the open end if you like. Touch it to your skin to make sure it's not burning hot. Hold the salt sock against the bone behind the ear (the mastoid process) until the ear area is sufficiently warmed. You'll know when you've had enough because it will stop feeling soothing and become uncomfortable.

Another traditional folk remedy can also be effective, according to Joanne B. Mied, N.D., a naturopath and herbalist based in Novato, California. Bake an onion (leaving the skin on it) in a 350-degree oven for 35 minutes. Let it cool until you can hold it without burning. Rest the stalk (as opposed to the root) end of the onion in the opening of the ear; do not stick the stalk down into the ear. Dr. Mied reports that a friend tried this on her daughter and within 10 minutes the pain of the little girl's earache was gone.

Eczema

See Dermatitis.

Edema (Water Retention)

Edema, also known as water retention or dropsy, involves the accumulation of fluid in between the cells of body tissues, resulting in swelling and bloating. Edema usually refers to subcutaneous (under the skin) fluid accumulation. The problem may simply result from insufficient water intake; in this case, water retention is the body's camel-like attempt to compensate for the lack of fluids. Allergies are another common cause of water retention.[1] Toxic overload may be involved, as the accumulation of fluid is the body's mechanism to dilute the toxins and thus render them less harmful.[2] Circulatory or lymphatic problems, kidney disorders, inflammatory conditions, sodium retention, electrolyte imbalance, and premenstrual syndrome can also produce edema.

Essential Oils

For premenstrual water retention, massages with Geranium, Juniper, and/or Rosemary essential oils in the week to 10 days before your period can be helpful, according to Patricia Davis, founder of the London School of Aromatherapy.

For puffy ankles and legs due to prolonged standing or in advanced pregnancy, Davis recommends daily leg massages with Pine essential oil, which stimulates the lymphatic system. Use long strokes from the ankles up the legs, not downward. "[This] will really reduce the swelling," says Davis, "although it is always more effective to have the massage carried out by a trained therapist."

You can also use Pine massages for swollen lower extremities caused by air travel. Cypress, Geranium, or Myrtle, other essential oils that stimulate the lymphatic system, are indicated as well, says Davis.[3]

Detoxifying essential oils can help the body get rid of the accumulation of toxins that may be causing the edema, notes Davis. Oils for this purpose include Fennel, Juniper, and Lemon. Use them in massage, baths, or diffusion.

Flower Essences

Self-Heal can serve as a foundational healing agent for edema. Other flower essences to address the specific emotions, mental attitude, and environmental conditions of the individual are recommended, states Patricia Kaminski, a flower essence therapist and codirector of the Flower Essence Society. Self-Heal supports the body's innate healing ability. Take 4 drops 2–4 times daily, or as needed.

Food Therapy

Eat:

Foods high in vitamin C and potassium. (For a list of foods containing these nutrients, see part 3, "Food Therapy," pp. 377, 378.)

Get plenty of bioflavonoids, which are believed to strengthen cell walls and hence prevent leakage, by eating blueberries, huckleberries, cranberries, pickled beets, carrots, and other foods with strong colors, says Karen Vaughan, E.M.T, A.H.G, a clinical herbalist from Brooklyn, New York. Also eat fresh nettle leaves, which you can cook like spinach.

Eating watermelon is a wonderful way to reduce edema, says Susan Roberts, N.D., a naturopathic physician from Portland, Oregon, who specializes in women's health care. She advises the women in her practice who suffer from water retention during pregnancy to eat half a watermelon a day, and they have found it quite helpful. "Watermelon is an incredible diuretic," explains Dr. Roberts. A diuretic promotes urinary flow, which helps the body get rid of the excess fluid of edema.

Avoid:

Sugar, coffee, starchy foods, alcohol, MSG (monosodium glutamate), food allergens, excess salt, high protein intake.

Herbal Medicine and Other Remedies

As a lymphatic flusher, meaning a substance that promotes drainage of the lymph system, cleavers (*Galium aparine*) is a useful herb for edema, states medical herbalist Chanchal Cabrera, M.N.I.M.H., A.H.G., of Vancouver, British Columbia. She recommends taking cleavers as a tea. To make an infusion, pour boiled water over the herb (1 teaspoon of dried cleavers per cup of water or 1 ounce of the herb per pint of water), cover the mixture, and let it steep for 10 minutes. Drink 2–3 cups daily; the more the better.

It is important to determine the cause of your edema so you know what treatment to apply and whether heart disease or other more serious problems are involved, says Karen Vaughan. Although treatment will vary depending upon the individual, here is her general protocol for mild leg edema after more serious illnesses have been ruled out:

• Drink peppermint tea. You can use commercial peppermint tea bags or make your own tea: use 1 tablespoon of peppermint to a cup of boiled water, steep for 15 minutes. In Chinese medicine, peppermint is used to treat an energy condition frequently associated with lower leg edema.

• If you are tired and thin with edema in your legs and feet, take buffered vitamin C (1,000–2,000 mg daily) and eat foods high in bioflavonoids (see previous "Food Therapy").

• Drink nettle (*Urtica dioica*) leaf, corn silk (*Zea mays*), or phelloden-dron, huang bai (*Phellodendron amurense*) bark tea. You need to find which herb works best for you. In general, if it's not working for an acute condition within 3 days, it's probably not the right herb. Try one of the others. Nettle is an astringent and a tonic (nourishing to the body) that exerts diuretic effects. Corn silk is a mild diuretic. Both the nettle and corn silk teas are made with 1–2 tablespoons of the herb per cup of boiled water. Steep for 15 minutes, strain, and drink 3–4 cups daily until symptoms have been gone for a few days.

To make the phellodendron bark tea, boil 1/3 cup of crumbled bark in 1 quart of water for 15–30 minutes. Strain and drink in the same way as the other teas. Phellodendron bark isn't used much in the United States, but is available in Chinese herbal stores or through herbal Web sites. It works much like goldenseal to clear heat and dry dampness, and since it has a special affinity for the lower body, it is useful for lower limb edema. Note: Do not confuse phellodendron with the houseplant philadendron, which is poisonous.

• Don't take strong diuretics; they tax the kidneys.

• Drink plenty of water. People tend to cut down on water consumption, thinking that it will only make their edema worse. But you often need to drink more, not less, water when you are suffering from edema.

• Get sufficient exercise.

Homeopathy

Edema is best treated by a constitutional remedy. Consult a home-opath for individualized treatment. In the meantime, the following remedies may help alleviate water retention, according to Dr. Barry Rose of the Royal London Homeopathic Hospital:[4]

Acetic acid 30c: If the skin is waxy, you have stomachaches, and are very thirsty.
Apis 30c: If the skin is waxy, but transparent-looking, you have little urine output (the urine may contain dark deposits), and thirst is absent.

Apocynum can 30c: If you are very thirsty, but drinking upsets your stomach, have frequent indigestion, and feel pressure in the chest and abdomen.

Arsenicum 30c: If you are very thirsty, but only for frequent small amounts of liquid, and have shortness of breath with exertion and/or it wakes you up from sleep.

Take the appropriate remedy in the morning, as needed. Discontinue taking as soon as there is improvement in your symptoms.

Nutritional Supplements

The following supplements can help relieve water retention, according to naturopathic physician Linda Rector Page, N.D., Ph.D.:[5]

Vitamin C crystals with bioflavonoids and rutin (a citrus flavonoid): 1/2 teaspoon in water or juice every 2–3 hours until symptoms subside; take 3000–5000 mg daily to help prevent edema.

Vitamin B complex: 100 mg daily with additional vitamin B6 (250 mg 2 times daily).

Bromelain: 750 mg 2 times daily, with meals; an enzyme compound found in pineapple; aids digestion and facilitates nutrient absorption.

Betaine HCl: 3 times daily; hydrochloric acid (HCl) aids digestion and facilitates nutrient absorption.

Reflexology

Lymphatic system

Stone/Crystal Therapy

For edema, use moonstone, says Daya Sarai Chocron, a vibrational healer based in Northampton, Massachusetts. Hold the stone, wear it, carry it in your pocket, or lay it on the affected part for 15–20 minutes daily, as needed.

Eye Problems (Eyestrain, Bloodshot, Dry Eyes, Circles)

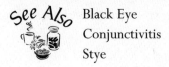

See Also Black Eye
Conjunctivitis
Stye

Common minor ailments associated with the eyes are eyestrain, bloodshot eyes, dry eyes, and dark circles under the eyes.

Eyestrain, or fatigue of the eyes, results from overuse, typically in reading, detail work, or computer work. The symptoms include aching, burning, and/or watering eyes, blurred vision, difficulty focusing, eyelid tics, light sensitivity, and headaches.

The red appearance of bloodshot eyes is produced by congestion and dilation of the small blood vessels in the eyes.

Dry eyes, an uncomfortable or even painful lack of lubrication by the tear ducts in the eyes, can be a function of vitamin A deficiency, age, the use of contact lenses, chronic conjunctivitis, or Sjögren's syndrome (an immunological disorder).

Aside from fatigue, dark circles under the eyes may be an indication of allergies, iron deficiency, or kidney or liver malfunction.[1]

Essential Oils

Essential oil should not be used in the eyes, states Kurt Schnaubelt, Ph.D., scientific director of the Pacific Institute of Aromatherapy in San Rafael, California. However, you can use a hydrosol—aromatic water that is a coproduct of the essential oil distillation process. Green Myrtle hydrosol can be effective for eyestrain, dry eyes, or bloodshot eyes. Spray it directly into the eyes up to 6 times per day to relieve these conditions, says Dr. Schnaubelt.

Flower Essences

Queen Anne's Lace and Harvest Brodiaea flower essences combined in a misting bottle are beneficial for fatigued, bloodshot, and/or dry eyes, states Richard Katz, founder of the Flower Essence Society.

Spray the mist around your face and eyes and in your immediate environment 2–4 times daily, or more often as needed. (For instructions on preparing a misting bottle, see part 3, "Flower Essences," "Directions for Use," p. 372.) The clearing that occurs with this remedy can result in a lessening of dark circles under the eyes as well.

Pretty Face and Crab Apple flower essences mixed in Self-Heal cream and applied topically can bring light into the face, which also lessens dark circles. Use 6–10 drops of each essence per 1 ounce of Self-Heal cream. Apply over the entire face, including the area under the eyes, 2–4 times daily, as needed. You can also use this mixture as a "mask." Instead of working the cream into the skin, apply a light layer and leave it on for 10–15 minutes. The slower absorption rate allows the ingredients to work more gradually into the skin on an energetic level. Either method is effective.

Food Therapy

Eat:

Protein (B vitamins), sunflower and sesame seeds, foods high in vitamins A, C, and E, selenium, and zinc. (For a list of foods containing these nutrients, see part 3, "Food Therapy," pp. 377, 378.)

Avoid:

Or limit sugar, caffeine, alcohol.

Herbal Medicine

Eyebright (*Euphrasia officinalis*) has been used for centuries as an herbal treatment for all manner of eye ailments, including eyestrain, bloodshot eyes, irritation, infection, and allergic symptoms. Herbalist Earl Mindell, R.Ph., Ph.D., recommends taking eyebright orally to promote eye health and good vision and using it in an eyewash to ease tired, irritated, or inflamed eyes. Take 1 capsule of eyebright 1–3 times daily or 15–40 drops of eyebright extract mixed in liquid every 3–4 hours. Eyewashes containing eyebright and other beneficial herbs are available commercially. Using an eyecup, rinse your eyes 3–4 times daily during an acute eye problem.[2]

Homeopathy

For eyestrain, Drs. Andrew Lockie and Nicola Geddes recommend the following homeopathic remedies:[3]

Nat mur: If there is dull, aching pain when you move your eyes, if it is worse with exertion, in a draft or in the hot sun, and with emotional stress or grief, and the symptoms are relieved by cold compresses and fresh air.

Ruta: If the eyes burn and feel strained and/or hot after a long period of study or reading, the eyes are red, the symptoms are worsened by rest or lying down or drinking alcohol, and improved by movement; you may also have a headache.

Take the appropriate remedy at a 6c potency 4 times daily for up to 7 days.

Homeopathic eyedrops, available in health food stores, can also alleviate eyestrain, and dry and bloodshot eyes as well.

Nutritional Supplements

Red, irritated eyes are one of the signs of vitamin B deficiency. Taking a vitamin B complex supplement daily can help prevent eyestrain. Research conducted in Japan demonstrated the efficacy of B vitamins, notably B12, in reducing eyestrain among computer workers.[4]

Dry eyes can be due to a vitamin A deficiency, as tears actually contain this nutrient. Take 25,000 IU daily as needed for dry, scratchy eyes.[5]

In addition to vitamin A and B complex, other nutrients essential to eye health are vitamins C, and E, selenium, and zinc. Make sure you are eating enough foods high in all of these nutrients and/or take a good supplement containing them.

Reflexology

Eyes, neck, cervical spine, head/brain, kidneys

Stone/Crystal Therapy

For eye problems, use yellow prenite, green apophylite, gem rhodochrosite, amethyst, or clear quartz, says Katrina Raphaell, crystal healing therapist and author of the crystal reference series *The Crystal Trilogy*. Place the stone on your closed eyes, or on the most distressed area near your eyes. Visualizing your health goal, leave the stone in place for 5 minutes. Do this 3 times daily. For ongoing healing, wear the stone, hold it, or carry it in your pocket.

Other Remedies

Half a fresh fig placed over each closed eye and left there for 20 minutes can help remove dark circles under the eyes, states nutritionist Ann Louise Gittleman, N.D., C.N.S., M.S.[6]

Dampen a cloth with witch hazel (available in drugstores and supermarkets) and lay it across your closed eyes to reduce bags under the eyes.[7] Witch hazel has astringent and anti-inflammatory properties, which help tighten eye tissues and reduce puffiness.

Fatigue

Fatigue has become a way of life in the United States. Workload, the pace many people keep, stress, poor diet, high caffeine consumption, and lack of sufficient sleep combine to keep many people in a constant low-grade state of fatigue. The remedies here are not intended to enable you to maintain your mad pace and fatiguing habits, but to support your body on an occasional basis. To prevent your body's breakdown into illness, you might want to examine the lifestyle factors that contribute to your fatigue and make changes where possible.

Eating healthfully, exercising regularly, getting enough sleep, and reducing/managing stress can go a long way toward preventing fatigue. Even those who follow healthy life practices succumb now and then to tiredness, however. Fatigue is difficult to avoid in modern life. The remedies here can give your body the support it needs at those times.

If you suffer from unusual tiredness that lasts longer than a few weeks, it is important to determine the cause, as fatigue is also a symptom of many illnesses.

Essential Oils

For a "fatigue-fighting" bath, aromatherapist Roberta Wilson recommends combining essential oils of Rosemary (3 drops), Orange (2 drops), Peppermint (1 drop), and Thyme (1 drop). Add the blend to a tub of warm water and immerse yourself in the water for 20–30 minutes, as needed. For an oil blend to inhale when you need energy, combine Rosemary (8 drops), Elemi (6 drops), Peppermint (4 drops), Basil (3 drops), and Ginger (1 drop), says Wilson. Keep the blend in an airtight bottle and take a whiff as needed for energy.[1]

Flower Essences

There are different flower essences for different types of fatigue. Patricia Kaminski, an herbalist and flower essence therapist from Nevada City, California, offers the following guidelines:

Echinacea: For fatigue with immune system depletion and "shattering" life events.

Aloe Vera: When an extreme work period or workaholic tendencies culminate in physical burnout.

Hornbeam: For fatigue related to activities or situations that the soul dislikes (Monday morning blues).

Olive: For exhaustion from overwhelming physical exertion or prolonged physical stress.

Take 4 drops of the appropriate flower essence for your fatigue, 2–4 times daily, as needed.

Food Therapy

Eat:

Lean protein, whole grains, small and frequent meals/snacks to stabilize blood sugar, foods high in potassium, magnesium, iron, and vitamin C. (For a list of foods containing these nutrients, see part 3, "Food Therapy," pp. 377, 378.)

Avoid:

Sugar, caffeine, soft drinks, alcohol, processed foods, fatty foods, limit dairy.

Herbal Medicine

For fatigue, Teresa Boardwine, an herbalist from Washington, Virginia, recommends adaptogenic herbs. These herbs support adrenal gland function, and by so doing, boost the immune system. Adaptogens activate the immune system at a deep level and ease wear and tear on the body. Unlike stimulants, they increase energy while nourishing and building up the body. Since they are tonics, they can be taken long-term. Boardwine recommends the following adaptogens:

American ginseng (*Panax quinquefolius*): This type of ginseng is more cooling than Oriental ginseng (*Panax ginseng*). It is especially useful for the fatigue that accompanies a stressful period and for convalescing after surgery (after the initial acute stage). Buy a root and nibble on it during the day, but avoid after 5 P.M. so its stimulating effects don't disrupt your sleep. Or you can take it in tincture form. To ensure quality, look for a tincture derived from plants grown in the United States (Vermont and Wisconsin are two states that produce American ginseng). During a stressful period, take 1 dropperful of the tincture twice daily. Again, do not take it in the evening. As maintenance, take 1/2 dropperful up to 3 times daily. Monitor your dosage to determine what works for you.

Siberian ginseng (eleuthero, *Eleutherococcus senticosus*): This type of ginseng is good for everyday life with its daily stressors. It is also helpful for those with tough schedules and when fatigue is accompanied by problems with mental clarity. In women whose hormones are out of balance and who suffer from premenstrual syndrome, Siberian ginseng can help restore equilibrium. Take 2 capsules twice daily.

Homeopathy

The following are common homeopathic remedies for simple fatigue, according to Drs. Andrew Lockie and Nicola Geddes:[2]

Arsenicum: Indicated for fatigue from overwork, accompanied by strong anxiety, inability to sleep, weakness after even slight exertion, and a feeling of not being able to function, with worry that other people will notice; worse in a draft and cool surroundings and from 2 to 3 A.M., and improved in the morning.

Calc carb: Indicated for fatigue produced by stress from worry, accompanied by restlessness, weakness, and dizziness after even slight exertion, faintness in the morning, and constantly feeling cold; worsened by cold drinks and food and the very smell or sight of food and from midnight to 2 A.M., and improved by warmth, hot drinks, and lying down with the head elevated.

Nux vom: Indicated for fatigue produced by stress, lack of sleep, and overwork, accompanied by irritability, severe chilliness, tense muscles, indigestion, early morning waking, and faintness on waking; worsened by stimulants, spices, and eating, and improved by warmth and sleep, and in the evening.

Take the appropriate remedy at a 30c potency 2 times daily for up to 14 days.

Nutritional Supplements

Natural medicine practitioner David Carroll cautions against indiscriminate supplementation in an attempt to combat fatigue. The following supplements are the ones you really need, he says; others are superfluous unless prescribed by a qualified practitioner to address a specific problem:[3]

High-potency vitamin B complex: Take as directed.
Vitamin C: 2,000–4,000 mg daily.
Vitamin E: 100 IU daily.
Brewer's yeast: 1 tablespoon with every meal.
Rutin: 100 mg daily; a citrus flavonoid antioxidant.
Optional: Kelp and natural cod-liver oil.

Reflexology

Adrenal glands, pituitary, thyroid, diaphragm, spine

Stone/Crystal Therapy

For fatigue, try citrine, red calcite, or green tourmaline, suggests Katrina Raphaell, crystal healing therapist and founder of the Crystal Academy of Advanced Healing Arts in Kapaa, Hawaii. Place the stone on the center of your body at the level of the heart or over your solar plexus (top of the abdomen, below the ribs). Leave it in place for 5 minutes while you visualize health. Do this 3 times daily, as needed. In addition, wear the stone, hold it, or carry it in your pocket for ongoing benefits.

Other Remedies

Michael Cottingham, a clinical herbalist from Silver City, New Mexico, notes that fatigue can be caused by not drinking enough water. He and many other health practitioners cite 8 glasses daily as the healthy minimum for water consumption. "Water can be one of the ultimate first aid remedies," says Cottingham.

Flu

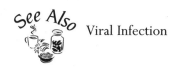 See Also Viral Infection

The many strains of influenza, or flu, manifest in the body in a variety of ways. Some affect primarily the respiratory system with a cold and cough, others the gastrointestinal tract with vomiting and diarrhea; and still others focus their attack on the muscular system, producing aches and pains. Generalized body ache, fever, chills, headache, sore throat, and fatigue are common to flu in general, with other symptoms occurring in combination.

Flu is a contagious viral infection. Though the symptoms resemble those of a cold, they are more severe and last longer. The remedies below can ease the severity, shorten the length of time a bout of flu lasts, and provide the immune system with important support to overcome the infection.

Essential Oils

For an antiviral diffusion, combine essential oils of:

Ravensare: 3 parts
Naiouli or Eucalyptus: 1 part

Lemon: 1 part
Rosewood: 1 part
Lavender: 1 part

Diffuse in the sickroom. You can also use this blend for steam inhalation 2–3 times daily, as needed. Put 6–8 drops in a bowl of boiled water, drape your head and the bowl with a towel, and inhale.[1]

To relieve the body aches of flu, use Juniper essential oil in massage or bath.[2]

Flower Essences

Self-Heal and Yarrow Special Formula can serve as the foundational healing agents for flu. Other flower essences to address the specific emotions, mental attitude, and environmental conditions of the individual are recommended, states Patricia Kaminski, a flower essence therapist and codirector of the Flower Essence Society. Self-Heal supports the body's innate healing ability. Yarrow Special Formula strengthens and protects against environmental toxicity and stress. Take 4 drops of each 2–4 times daily, or as needed.

Food Therapy

Eat:

Soup (especially miso), garlic, ginger. Drink plenty of fluids (soup, herbal tea, diluted vegetable juice).

Avoid:

Sugar, dairy, bread, meat, caffeine, alcohol.

Herbal Medicine

"Flu has a purpose," says Karen Vaughan, E.M.T, A.H.G, a clinical herbalist from Brooklyn, New York. "Upper respiratory infection helps us clean out debris in our intercellular spaces that didn't get eliminated on its own through the lymphatic system. If you suppress a cold, it can become flu. If you suppress flu, it may go deeper into the body and become a more serious illness." Taking aspirin to lower a fever means that you return the body to a temperature more hospitable to the virus; one of the functions of fever is to kill viruses. Vaughan's approach to flu treatment is to speed up the natural process rather than suppress it (provided that the fever is not too high and the patient is not an infant). Specific treatment for flu depends on the individual and the type of flu, but there are some measures that are helpful for all. Here is her general program for flu:

Tea: Use equal parts of boneset (also known as feverwort, *Eupatorium perfoliatum*), yarrow (*Achillea millefolium*), and elder (*Sambucus nigra*) berries. Put 1/2 cup of the herbal mix in 1 quart of boiled water, cover, and let steep for 15–25 minutes. Put in a thermos and drink as much as possible until the fever breaks (1–2 quarts daily for the first few days is usually what it takes). These herbs have a tradition of use in fever management. They are diaphoretics, meaning that they promote sweating, which speeds the process of elimination of toxins. Boneset is bitter, but when you're sick, often the taste won't bother you. When you start objecting to the taste, that's a sign that you are getting better and can cut down on the tea.

Bath: Run a hot bath and add 4–5 drops of Eucalyptus, Tea Tree (*Melaleuca alternifolia*), or Sage essential oil. These oils all help open up respiration. Stay in the bath until the body heats up as much as possible. Drink some of the above tea while you're in the bath. Immediately afterward, wrap yourself up and get into bed under comforters; don't cool off first. All of this encourages sweating out your illness. With this process, you're engaging the body's own immune response.

After the fever breaks: Make elderberry tea (infused) with decocted astragalus (*Astragalus membranaceus*) to aid the immune system. To make the decoction, put a few slices of fresh astragalus into a quart of boiling water, cover, and simmer for 15 minutes. Remove from the heat, add 1/2 cup of elderberries, cover, and let steep for 15–25 minutes. Strain and discard the astragalus, but you can eat the strained berries if you like. Drink 4 cups of the blend daily.

For immune support during flu season, use fresh astragalus slices in dishes such as rice and soup. Remove the slices after cooking; don't eat them. It is probably better to use these slices to prevent disease, but to withold them if you come down with an infection, says Vaughan, noting that in Chinese medicine it is believed that tonic herbs such as astragalus and ginseng can feed the pathogen.

Variations:

- If you have a dry, scratchy throat, add slippery elm (*Ulmus rubra, U. fulva*) bark to the boneset, yarrow, and elder tea; mix 1 teaspoon of slippery elm into the 1/2 cup of dried herbs. You can also suck on slippery elm lozenges as needed.

- If you are thin, frequently cold, and have chills and fever, put a few slices of fresh ginger into boiling water for 1–2 minutes. Strain and add the liquid to the boneset tea blend. You can also munch on ginger with meals, eat pickled sushi ginger, and/or suck on candied ginger (but don't overdo the sweets). The ginger is warming and can help with chills. Also take garlic, which is a strong antiviral. Mince a clove of garlic while holding it together, then let it sit for 10 minutes to oxidize into healthful compounds. Dip a spoon into honey, then touch it to the garlic so the whole minced clove sticks to the honey. Place the spoon upside down in your mouth and swallow the mixture. "For some reason, it goes down better when you do it upside down like this," notes Vaughan. Take up to 5 cloves daily.

- If you're a person who is frequently cold or you have more chills than fever during the flu, take 2–3 teaspoons daily of something that was used during the plague in Europe in the fourteenth century (reportedly by thieves who wanted to burglarize plague victims' houses without becoming ill) and is still a part of the French pharmacopeia. A warming formula called Seven Seas Vinegar, it is actually a blend of wormwood, rosemary, rue, sage, lavender, calamus, pepper, cinnamon, clove, nutmeg, garlic, and camphor. You can get it at health food stores or on herbal Web sites.

A note about echinacea and goldenseal: Although many people reach for these herbs when they feel a cold or flu coming on, Vaughan believes they should not be used prophylactically and should not be mixed (as they are in a number of commercial tinctures) because they are for different purposes. Echinacea (*E. spp.*) best addresses "bad blood and lymph," which may manifest as chronic inflammation, chronic infection, abscesses, skin ulcers, fever, eczema, foul discharges, or swollen glands. Echinacea can arrest early-stage flu, but is better combined with boneset or elder than with goldenseal. Goldenseal (*Hydrastis canadensis*) should be reserved for persistent upper respiratory infections that you just can't seem to shake, those with entrenched copious phlegm, or pneumonia. With goldenseal, there is an environmental issue involved as well. The herb is an endangered species, so if you're going to use it, make sure that you get cultivated goldenseal and not wild.

Vaughan recommends first giving your body a chance to fight the infection with its own immune reactions, aided by the methods above. If by the third day of your flu, there is no progress, then you can turn to echinacea. Consistency is more important than quantity when taking echinacea, she notes. Put 2 tablespoons of tincture in a liter bottle of water and sip it all day.

The boneset tea above doesn't work well for children because of its bitter taste, so for them Vaughan uses lemon balm (*Melissa officinalis*). Fevers can be dangerous for infants, and lemon balm can help bring the fever down. Put 1 cup of dried lemon balm leaves in 1 quart of boiled water, cover, and steep for 25 minutes. Strain and pour it in the baby's bath. When you put the baby in, the water should be the same temperature as the baby. Keep the baby in the bath while the water cools (toys to keep him or her entertained are a good idea). The infant's temperature should drop with that of the bath water.

For toddlers to adults, Vaughan makes lemon balm tea. Put 3 tablespoons of the dried leaf in 1 quart of boiled water, cover, and let steep for 15–25 minutes. Add stevia or honey for sweetening (only for children over 1 year old). You can also add dried peppermint (*Mentha piperata*) to the lemon balm to vary the taste. An adult should drink 2–4 cups per day; reduce the child's dose according to body weight. Drink until the feverishness abates.

Vaughan also keeps a lemon balm electuary (a sweet medicated paste) on hand during flu season. To make this, put several handfuls of fresh lemon balm in the blender and chop up fine. Add honey to make a paste. Vaughan recommends using local honey because it is from local pollen. Eating this honey can help protect you from developing allergies to the pollen in the area. Children love electuaries. Never give honey to a child who is less than a year old, however, because of the danger of infant botulinum. "Botulinum, which causes regular botulism, and infant botulinum are different," says Vaughan. "It is well-known that infants should not use honey because the spores are present. Older children and adults are not susceptible to infant botulinum."

Giving your kids an electuary "lollipop" (the paste on a spoon) is an easy way to administer a healing herb (fresh mint and dried ginger root powder also make good electuaries). Keep the electuary in a jar (it doesn't have to be refrigerated) and add water as needed. The honey tends to make it stiffen after a while. You can also freeze lemon balm or elderberry tea into popsicles to give a feverish child.

Homeopathy

The following homeopathic remedies are commonly indicated for flu, according to Stephen Cummings, M.D., and Dana Ullman, M.P.H.:[3]

Gelsemium: If your body feels tired, weak, and heavy, you just want to lie still and be left alone, and you have chills that run up and down the spine.

Bryonia: If motion worsens the symptoms, there is thirst for cold drinks, you are irritable and don't want people around, and you feel worse in warm rooms and better in cool air.

Rhus tox: If you have aches and pain when lying still, which get worse with movement but feel better if you continue moving, feel restless and chilly, and have a dry mouth and dry, sore throat.

Eupatorium: If you have such strong, aching pain that you feel as if your bones are breaking, chills (particularly in the morning), and a desire for ice cold drinks; if you had a runny nose, red eyes, and were sneezing before the achiness began.

Oscillococcinum: for the initial phase of flu, take during the first 48 hours of the onset of generalized fluish symptoms before the appearance of distinguishing symptoms as delineated above.

Take the appropriate remedy at a potency of 6c(x) or 12c(x) every 6 to 8 hours for 2–3 days. Discontinue when your symptoms improve.

Nutritional Supplements

For flu, naturopathic physician Bradley Bongiovanni, N.D., of Independence, Ohio, recommends the following combination of supplements and herbs:

Vitamin C: 1,000 mg 3 times daily for 10–14 days.
Zinc: 30 mg twice daily for 10–14 days.
Elderberry extract: 2 ml 3–4 times daily for 10–14 days.
Olive leaf extract: 1,000 mg 3 times daily for 10–14 days.
Feverwort: 2 ml 3–4 times daily for a week; also known as boneset, herb to relieve body/muscle aches.

Reflexology

Lungs, chest, diaphragm, lymphatic system, adrenal glands, pituitary, intestines

Stone/Crystal Therapy

When you have the flu, use jade, says Daya Sarai Chocron, a vibrational healer and author of *Healing with Crystals and Gemstones*. While in bed, hold the stone in your hand, place it near you or under your pillow, or lay it on your body for 15–20 minutes daily, as needed. If it is a child who has the flu, as a precaution make sure the gemstone is too large to be swallowed.

Food Poisoning

While true food poisoning arises from eating poisonous mushrooms or other poisonous food, the term generally refers to illness as a result of eating food contaminated by harmful bacteria. Such contamination occurs through faulty refrigeration, cooking, or handling.

The symptoms of food poisoning include nausea, abdominal cramps, vomiting, diarrhea, fever, and headache. Their onset may be soon after eating the contaminated food or as long as 48 hours later. The delayed onset and the fact that the symptoms resemble those of flu result in people mistakenly concluding that they are suffering from the flu.

The two most common types of bacteria involved in food poisoning are *Salmonella* and *Staphylococci,* in that order. Undercooked meats and eggs, raw fish and seafood, and food kept too long at room temperature are sources of *Salmonella* poisoning. *Staphylococci* are often present in the nose and throat, so coughing or sneezing by food handlers or others in the vicinity can easily infect food.

It is always a good idea to consult your doctor in a case of food poisoning. While the less serious varieties can often be home-treated, some kinds (such as botulism, caused by the bacteria *Clostridium botulinum*) are potentially life-threatening. If symptoms of any kind of food poisoning continue for more than 24 hours, seek medical assistance.

Essential Oils

For food poisoning, medical aromatherapist Julia Fischer of Northern California advises 1 teaspoon of green illite or montmorillonite clay (also known as bentonite clay) mixed in 6 ounces of Geranium hydrosol. Drink this every 20 minutes until the symptoms subside. In between drinking the clay mixture, put 1 drop of Peppermint and 1 drop of Anise essential oil (therapeutic quality only) on the back of your hand and lick the drops off.

Flower Essences

Self-Heal can serve as a foundational healing agent for food poisoning. Other flower essences to address the specific emotions, mental attitude, and environmental conditions of the individual are recommended, states Patricia Kaminski, a flower essence therapist and codirector of the Flower Essence Society. Self-Heal supports the body's innate healing ability. Take 4 drops 2–4 times daily, or as needed.

Food Therapy

Julia Fischer recommends that your food intake over the 24 hours following the food poisoning consist only of plain brown rice with salt, simple miso (with or without seaweed), carrot juice with ginger, and ginger tea.

Water, diluted juice, shakes (see "Diarrhea, Nutritional Supplements," p. 125), and electrolyte drinks are the best "food" remedies for food poisoning, notes Alan Christianson, N.M.D., a naturopathic physician from Scottsdale, Arizona. Here is his electrolyte replacement formula (makes 1 quart):

    1 cup white grape juice
    3 cups water
    1/2 teaspoon salt
    1 teaspoon baking soda
    1 teaspoon liquid magnesium citrate
    1/4 teaspoon Lite salt (potassium chloride)

Herbal Medicine

Ginger (*Zingiber officinale*) tea can help soothe the stomach in cases of food poisoning. Sage (*Salvia officinalis*) tea clears the body of toxins.[1] Add ginger powder or sage leaves to a cup of boiled water and let steep. Or you can boil slices of fresh ginger root for 10–15 minutes.

To assist the liver in getting rid of the toxins, use milk thistle (*Carduus marianus, Silybum marianum*) seed after contracting food poisoning, says herbalist Christopher Hobbs. Take 3–4 capsules daily for 3–5 days. Or you can take it in tincture form; on the first day, 2 droppersful every 3–4 hours, then for the next 3–4 days after that, 1 dropperful 3 times daily.[2]

Homeopathy

Maesimund B. Panos, M.D., has recommended Arsenicum album "countless times" for food poisoning. "Thus far, it has never failed me," she states. Take in a 6x potency every hour for 3–4 times. Take it after that only if vomiting and diarrhea continue, or if you feel weak.[3]

Nutritional Supplements

To aid the body in getting rid of the toxins of food poisoning and resolving the episode quickly, Dr. Christianson recommends the following supplements:

Activated charcoal: This binds with toxins and speeds their removal from the body. Take 30 capsules or 2 tablespoons of liquid in divided doses over the first day. If needed, continue taking for a second day.

Probiotics: It is important after the intense diarrhea that typically accompanies food poisoning to repopulate the intestines with the beneficial bacteria normally found there. Supplemental probiotics contain *Lactobacillus acidophilus* and *Bifidobacterium bifidum*, among other strains. There is an issue with the quality and purity of probiotic products. Be sure to get powder or capsules that require refrigeration. Take 5–10 billion organisms daily in 2–3 divided doses for a week. (The product will tell you how many organisms are in a specified amount.) Don't take long-term because it can disrupt the balance of other bacteria.

Colostrum: This is the initial mother's milk released to a nursing infant (or other mammal). It is highly antimicrobial and works to strengthen the infant's immune system. The supplement is a preparation derived from bovine colostrum. Take 1 teaspoon of the liquid with meals 3 times daily for 2 weeks. The colostrum helps restore the immune integrity of the gut, and its antimicrobial activity works against the bacteria involved in the food poisoning. Even after the diarrhea is gone, the harmful bacteria remain. To prevent a recurrence of the diarrhea or the development of a chronic condition, it is important to restore the intestinal environment and keep the bacteria from overgrowing again.

Reflexology

Stomach, intestines, kidneys, liver

Stone/Crystal Therapy

Carbon-C60 is a useful stone for food poisoning, states Melody, author of the crystal reference series *Love Is in the Earth*. Take 3–5 drops of elixir, no less than 5 times daily for 2 days. (For instructions on making an elixir, see part 3, "Stone/Crystal Therapy," p. 403.)

Other Remedies

Alkalinizing the body can alleviate the symptoms of food poisoning. Stir 1/2 teaspoon of cream of tartar into 1/2 cup of warmed water (not microwaved), says Sue Reynolds, M.S.W., L.M.T., a certified herbalist and aromatherapist from Goleta, California. Continue to stir as you drink. The strong alkalinizing effect will throw off your sodium-potassium balance, so half an hour after taking the cream of tartar, drink some water or juice with 1/2 teaspoon of salt dissolved in it. Sea salt is preferable, and vegetable juice masks the salt taste best. You can take this two-phased remedy 2–3 times in several hours if necessary.

Fungal Infection (Athlete's Foot, Jock Itch, Nails, Oral Thrush)

 See Also For vaginal fungal infection, see "Vaginal Yeast Infection."

Included in the category of fungus are yeasts, molds, and ringworm, in addition to other kinds of fungi.

Ringworm is a common fungus that causes infection (known as tinea) all over the body. Athlete's foot is ringworm of the feet (tinea pedis). Jock itch is ringworm of the groin area (tinea cruris). Ringworm of the nails is known as tinea unguium.

Athlete's foot is so named because the warmth and moisture of sweaty footwear and shower and locker rooms promotes the growth of ringworm. The symptoms are itching, burning, cracking, and soreness between and under the toes.

The symptoms of jock itch are redness and itching in the groin area. Like sweaty socks, the moisture of perspiration in tight clothes creates an ideal environment for the growth of ringworm.

A fungal nail infection can cause swelling and discoloration, and the nails may become brittle. The infection can raise the nail as the fungus grows in the nail bed, and ultimately destroy the nail if untreated.

Candida albicans is a yeast fungus. It normally inhabits the body and does not create a problem until an imbalance of some kind allows an overgrowth of the yeast. Oral thrush is an overgrowth of *Candida* in the mouth. It is characterized by white patches in the mouth and sometimes on the lips and in the throat as well. Oral thrush is a common affliction among infants (particularly those who have been given antibiotics) and people with lowered immunity.

Other forms of *Candida* overgrowth are vaginal yeast infection (see "Vaginal Yeast Infection") and candidiasis, a systemic overgrowth of the yeast (such a condition is beyond the scope of first aid; seek medical help).

Essential Oils

An essential oil blend can be used externally to treat fungal skin infections, says naturopathic physician Boyer B. Cole, N.M.D., of Cottonwood, Arizona. Combine equal parts of Tea Tree (*Melaleuca alternifolia*), Eucalyptus, Geranium, and Thyme Thujanol (a nonirritating and highly antimicrobial type of Thyme essential oil). Mix the essential oil blend with olive oil in a 1:1 ratio. For a fungal nail infection, athlete's foot, or jock itch, apply the mixture topically to the affected area 1–2 times daily. If it is irritating (this may be the case with jock itch), you can dilute the blend with more olive oil.

Your symptoms will likely subside relatively quickly, but to get rid of the fungus completely and prevent a recurrence, you should continue applying the treatment once daily for 3 months, notes Dr. Cole. "The problem with fungus is that people stop treating it. When fungus is attacked, it puts out spores deep in the skin," he explains. "The spore form can last in your skin for a long time. Then when the environment is right, the spores open up and put out fungus." If you keep up the bombardment for 3 months, you kill off the active fungus and give the skin a chance to shed out the spores.

To treat a fungal infection of the nails, medical herbalist Amanda McQuade Crawford, M.N.I.M.H., Dip.Phyto., recommends Thuja essential oil used externally and silica taken internally as a daily supplement (see "Nutritional Supplements," following). Put 1 drop of the Thuja oil in 1/4 ounce of vegetable oil. Massage this blend into the affected nail bed(s) daily. Let it soak in, or wipe away the excess. Avoid hand contact with detergents and harsh chemicals. Follow this program for 6 months, which is the time it takes for a new nail to grow out.

For oral thrush, herbalist Kathi Keville recommends Lavender and Tea Tree (*Melaleuca alternifolia*) essential oils. However, as these oils are too strong to use undiluted in the mouth, mix 8 drops each of Lavender and Tea Tree with 2 tablespoons of vegetable oil. Using a clean finger or a cotton swab, gently apply the mixture to the inside of the mouth, emphasizing the areas where there are patches of thrush. This is completely safe for infants, says Keville, noting that the mother must also treat her nipples with the mixture because *Candida* passes back and forth between a nursing baby's mouth and the mother's nipples.[1] Repeat the treatment daily until the thrush clears up.

Flower Essences

Self-Heal and Yarrow Special Formula can serve as the foundational healing agents for fungal infection. Other flower essences to address the specific emotions, mental attitude, and environmental conditions of the individual are recommended, states flower essence therapist Patricia Kaminski of Nevada City, California. Self-Heal supports the body's innate healing ability. Yarrow Special Formula strengthens and protects against environmental toxicity and stress. Take 4 drops of each 2–4 times daily, or as needed.

Food Therapy

Eat:

Garlic, chamomile, vegetables, olive oil, yogurt, foods high in B vitamins (see part 3, "Food Therapy," p. 378).

Avoid:

Sugar (all forms, including fruit and fruit juice), soft drinks, processed foods, yeast, certain fermented foods (see below).

"There is nothing like living sauerkraut for oral thrush," says David R. Field, N.D., L.Ac., a naturopathic physician from Santa Rosa, California. He has seen this work very well with his patients who have HIV infection and are prone to oral thrush. By "living," he means it contains live beneficial bacteria. Pasteurized sauerkraut in a can or jar is "dead," meaning it contains no live bacteria, and will not work, notes Dr. Field. Get the refrigerated variety. Eat 1 tablespoon 4–5 times daily, chewing it well. Drink the juice as well. "The tangy feeling you will get in your mouth is the bacteria in the sauerkraut killing the yeast," says Dr. Field. Although people with yeast infections are often told to avoid fermented foods, there are two types of fermentation, he explains. Foods fermented by bacteria, such as sauerkraut and yogurt, are actually beneficial. It is the foods that involve fungal fermentation that promote yeast overgrowth. These include miso, beer, wine, and bread (with the exception of pure sourdough, which involves bacterial fermentation).

Herbal Medicine

Medical herbalist Chanchal Cabrera, M.N.I.M.H., A.H.G., of Vancouver, British Columbia, recommends using the following herbal remedies for fungal infection as long as symptoms are present:

Garlic: Take fresh garlic orally. Odorless garlic pills are worthless, according to Cabrera, because the active ingredient in garlic is carried in its essential oil, which is what smells. To lessen the strong odor, chop up a clove of garlic, put it on a teaspoon, and swallow it like a pill, without chewing it. Take it at night before you go to bed to reduce the daytime smell.

Tea tree (*Melaleuca alternifolia*) oil: For athlete's foot, jock itch, or a fungal infection of the nails, apply undiluted tea tree oil to the affected area 2–3 times per day. In the groin area, it may sting or prickle for a minute or two, but it won't hurt you. For oral thrush, buy a diluted form of tea tree oil to use as an oral rinse. You can't really dilute it yourself because the oil doesn't mix with water. Follow the manufacturer's directions for use.

Pau d'arco (*Tabebuia avellanedae* or *T. ipe*): This herb is also known as lapacho or taheebo. You can use it internally and topically. Make a decoction from the bark by simmering 1 teaspoon of bark in 1 cup of water for 15 minutes. Drink a cup twice a day. Use the tea as a skin wash on the affected area or a foot soak for athlete's foot, 2–3 times daily.

Marigold (*Calendula officinalis*): Use a tincture; marigold doesn't taste good as a tea. Take 1 teaspoon twice a day.

You can use all of the above concurrently, especially if the infection is a bad one.

Homeopathy

For a topical fungal infection (feet, nails, jock itch) with itching and burning, take Sulphur 6c or 12c once a day until symptoms disappear, advises homeopathic physician Michael G. Carlston, M.D., of Santa Rosa, California. For oral thrush, take Antimonium crudum at the same dosage.

Nutritional Supplements

Take probiotics to help restore the proper balance of bacteria in the body and counteract fungal overgrowth, recommends Dr. Field. Live bacteria, or "live-bac," products are best; live-bac is a licensed process of bottling beneficial bacteria (such as acidiphilus and bifidus) that ensures the bacteria remain live. Take 2 capsules 3 times daily (take no more than 6 per day), as needed.

For infants, you should use pediatric probiotics because their balance of intestinal flora is slightly different from that of adults, says Dr. Field. *Bifido bacterium bifidus*, *Bifido bacterium infantus*, and *Lactobacillus acidophilus* are the most important beneficial bacteria for infants. Put a little of the powder in the infant's mouth daily until the thrush is gone. Nursing mothers can administer the powder by putting it on their nipples before nursing.

For a fungal infection of the nails, Amanda McQuade Crawford suggests taking the mineral silica, which helps build strong nails, along with applying her topical treatment above (see "Essential Oils"). Take the supplement according to the manufacturer's dosage.

Reflexology

Treat the area of the foot corresponding to the part of the body afflicted by fungal infection, other than athlete's foot. Do not use reflexology for that condition.

Stone/Crystal Therapy

For a fungal infection, use periclase and moss agate, recommends Melody, author of the crystal reference series *Love Is in the Earth*. Apply the periclase as an elixir on the site of infection 3 times daily for 3 days. Tape the moss agate on the affected area with hypoallergenic tape, and leave it on for 2–3 days. (For instructions on making an elixir, see part 3, "Stone/Crystal Therapy," p. 403.)

Other Remedies

Applying a selenium shampoo (certain dandruff shampoos are selenium based) to the affected area can knock out a fungal infection, says Dr. Field. At bedtime, apply the shampoo directly on the skin, without water, and let it dry. Leave it on overnight. Do this nightly for 2–4 weeks.

If you suffer from jock itch, wear boxers rather than briefs, advises Dr. Field. For athlete's foot, wear cotton socks or sandals with no socks when possible. Check your bathroom to see if conditions are promoting your athlete's foot. Make sure the shower and tub area are clean and free of mold, and avoid damp bath mats.

Getting sunshine directly on the area of fungal infection is also helpful, notes Dr. Field.

Dr. Carlston also stresses the importance of environmental management. Since it's the wet, warm condition that allows the fungus to grow, keep the area dry as much as possible. Putting cornstarch in your socks helps athlete's foot because it soaks up moisture. Using it as a powder in the groin area is helpful for jock itch for the same reason.

Gas (Flatulence)

Medically, flatulence is excessive gas in the intestines. A certain amount of gas is a normal aspect of digestion. Some of it is absorbed through the intestinal wall, while the remainder is released through the rectum as the smelly emission that makes flatulence a socially uncomfortable affliction.

It is the insufficient breakdown of food that, for the most part, creates flatulence. The problem begins when food enters the small intestine virtually intact. The intestines are unable to break it down and the food remains there until bacteria ferment it. Gas is released in the fermentation process.[1] Carbohydrates such as beans are known to be problematic in this regard.

Food allergies, enzyme deficiencies, intestinal disorders, poor diet, and antibiotics can all produce flatulence.

Essential Oils

Massaging the abdomen with essential oils can help alleviate gas, says aromatherapist Valerie Ann Worwood. Blend 2 drops of Cardamom and 3 drops of Peppermint in 1 teaspoon of vegetable oil. Massage in a clockwise direction. This blend is especially useful if the gas is painful. Other useful oils for flatulence include Coriander, Dill, and Spearmint.[2]

Flower Essences

When gas is accompanied by sensory overload or overexposure to stimuli, take Dill, recommends Richard Katz, naturalist and founder of the Flower Essence Society. When it is accompanied by moodiness or extreme emotional sensitivity, take Chamomile. For digestive disturbances related to travel, take Dill and Chamomile in combination or alternation with Yarrow Special Formula. The dosage for all is 4 drops under the tongue, no less than half an hour before eating, 2–4 times daily, as needed. During an acute attack, you can take the essence(s) as often as once per hour.

Food Therapy

Eat:

Ginger, yogurt.

Avoid:

Garlic, onions, broccoli and other *Brassica* vegetables (see part 3, "Food Therapy," p. 376), milk, food allergens.

Cook beans with kombu extract to reduce the flatulence factor, suggests naturopathic physician David R. Field, N.D., L.Ac., of Santa Rosa, California.

Herbal Medicine

Fennel (*Foeniculum vulgare*) seeds can help prevent gas, says Michael Cottingham, a clinical herbalist from Silver City, New Mexico. Fennel is a carminative, meaning that it has a soothing effect on the stomach and intestines. "It is a great circulatory herb," notes Cottingham, "and helps create circulation in the stomach." He suggests chewing on a pinch of fennel seeds after a meal.

Homeopathy

The following homeopathic remedies can help alleviate gas, states Maesimund B. Panos, M.D.:[3]

Carbo veg: If stomach gas results no matter what you eat, resulting in belching.

China (Cinchona): If your stomach fills with gas that won't go up or down, accompanied by bloating.

Lycopodium: If you feel full before you finish a meal or from even a light meal, your belt or waistband feels tight, and you have rumbling gas with farting.

Take the appropriate remedy in a 6x potency 3–4 times daily, or more often for acute symptoms. As symptoms improve, decrease the frequency. Stop taking the remedy when the improvement is well established. However, Dr. Panos cautions that the remedy should not be used on a regular basis to ease your gas. Rather, you need to address your eating habits and the underlying cause.

Nutritional Supplements

Dr. Field recommends probiotics and enzymes to improve digestion and ameliorate gas:

Probiotics: Live-bac products are best; live-bac is a licensed process of bottling beneficial bacteria (such as acidiphilus and bifidus) that ensures the bacteria remain live. Take 2 capsules twice daily for 3–4 weeks at least. This helps rebalance intestinal flora.

Digestive enzymes with HCl: Take 1–2 capsules of plant-based digestive enzymes with HCl (hydrochloric acid, a gastric digestive juice) midway through every meal. Taking the enzymes mid-meal prevents the body from relying on the supplement for its enzyme supply instead of producing its own. Take the supplement for 2–4 weeks.

Reflexology

Stomach, intestines, gallbladder, thyroid, liver, pancreas, solar plexus

Stone/Crystal Therapy

Citrine aids in digestion and can be helpful for gas. Place it over your solar plexus (top of the abdomen below the ribs) as needed or several times daily as prevention. You can also hold it, wear it, or put it in your pocket for ongoing benefits. Taking it as an essence is useful as well; drink a few sips 3 times daily. You can also charge massage oil with the stone's properties. Put the stone in a clear glass bottle of massage oil (such as sweet almond) and place the bottle on a sunny windowsill. Leave it there for a week, shaking it once a day. You can take the stone out of the bottle after a week or leave it in. Massage your abdomen and lower back with the oil, as desired.[4] (For instructions on making an essence, see part 3, "Stone/Crystal Therapy," p. 403.)

Other Remedies

A castor oil pack can help heal the gut, notes Dr. Field. Put castor oil on a hot towel and place it on the abdomen. Cover with plastic wrap to keep the heat in. Leave the pack in place until the heat is gone.

Gingivitis

Gingivitis is a common form of gum or periodontal disease (disease of the structures around the teeth). An inflammation of the gums (gingivae), it is marked by swelling, redness, and easy bleeding. If left untreated, it can advance into pyorrhea, in which pockets and pus develop in the gums, and the supporting structure of the teeth begins to disintegrate, leading to loss of teeth.

Allowing plaque (bacterial masses) to build up on the teeth is a major cause of gingivitis. If plaque is not removed, pockets that increase the likelihood of infection develop in the gums. Proper brushing and flossing are essential to gum health. In addition, there are a number of natural remedies that you can use as part of your oral hygiene program.

Denture problems, nutritional deficiencies, heavy metal toxicity, and mouth and upper respiratory infections can also contribute to gingivitis.

Essential Oils

Myrrh oil is an antiseptic, an astringent, and a healing agent. Apply 1 drop to the affected area of the gums 2 times daily, recommends Sue Reynolds, M.S.W., L.M.T., a certified herbalist and aromatherapist from Goleta, California.

Flower Essences

Self-Heal can serve as a foundational healing agent for gingivitis. Other flower essences to address the specific emotions, mental attitude, and environmental conditions of the individual are recommended, states Patricia Kaminski, a flower essence therapist and codirector of the Flower Essence Society. Self-Heal supports the body's innate healing ability. Take 4 drops 2–4 times daily, or as needed.

Food Therapy

Eat:

Fiber, buckwheat, foods high in bioflavonoids and vitamins A and C. (For a list of foods containing these nutrients, see part 3, "Food Therapy," pp. 377, 378.)

Avoid:

Sugar, soft drinks, fruit juice, caffeine, refined carbohydrates.

Herbal Medicine

Since dental problems can cause disease throughout the body, it is wise to take good care of your teeth and gums, notes Karen Vaughan, E.M.T, A.H.G, a clinical herbalist from Brooklyn, New York. To maintain healthy gums, strengthen gum tissues that are getting soft, and as a treatment for gingivitis, she recommends switching from toothpaste to a healing tooth powder. Here is her recipe. Combine equal parts of green clay, cultivated goldenseal (*Hydrastis canadensis*), and baking soda. Add 1/3 as much each of powdered calendula (*Calendula officinalis*, a tissue healer and anti-inflammatory) and myrrh (*Commiphora molmol*). Some people prefer to omit or reduce the amount of goldenseal in the tooth powder because it can color the teeth temporarily.

Brush with this powder each time you brush. After brushing, swish hydrogen peroxide around in your mouth for about a minute. Following this regimen for the rest of your life is a good way to help keep your teeth and gums healthy, says Vaughan. She notes that using this tooth powder can enable you to avoid the deep dental cleanings that gingivitis often necessitates. If your teeth are discolored from the goldenseal, brush for a few days with baking soda and hydrogen peroxide.

Note Goldenseal is an endangered plant. Use cultivated goldenseal rather than the wild variety.

Homeopathy

The following are among the numerous homeopathic remedies for gingivitis, as cited by Dr. Barry Rose of the Royal London Homeopathic Hospital:[1]

Ant crud: If the gums bleed easily and detach from the teeth.

Arg nit: If the gums bleed easily and the teeth hurt, but without tooth disease.

Carbo veg: If the teeth are sensitive, particularly when eating, and the gums bleed easily and retract during brushing.

Hepar sulph: If the gums bleed and both the gums and mouth are painful to touch.

Phos acid: If the gums bleed and retract from the teeth and the teeth feel cold.

Take the appropriate remedy in a 30c potency 4 times daily for 4 days.

Nutritional Supplements

The bioflavonoid quercetin can help reduce inflammation of the gums, says naturopathic physician Kathi Head, N.D., of Sandpoint, Idaho. Take 250 mg twice daily on an empty stomach. She also recommends an ongoing program to treat gingivitis and maintain the health of the gums thereafter:

Coenzyme Q10: Take 100 mg daily; co Q10 is an antioxidant and aids in energy production at the cellular level, which is especially beneficial for tissues where there is a rapid turnover of cells, as there is in gum and mouth tissue and skin.

Vitamin C: Take 500 mg twice daily; helps stablize the tissues and keep gums from bleeding.

Folic acid dental rinse: You can buy a folic acid dental rinse. Twice daily, swish it around in your mouth for one minute, then swallow it. As folic acid is vital for normal cell development and proliferation, it is especially necessary in tissue with rapid cell turnover.

Reflexology

Teeth

Stone/Crystal Therapy

Drusy botryoidal quartz is useful for gingivitis, notes Melody, author of the crystal reference series *Love Is in the Earth*. Take 3–5 drops of elixir 3 times daily for 11 days. Also use hypoallergenic tape to secure the quartz on the outside of the cheek over the problem area of the gums; leave it on for 11 days. As prevention, you can continue to take the elixir daily after symptoms are gone. (For instructions on making an elixir, see part III, "Stone/Crystal Therapy," p. 403.)

Gout

You may think that gout is an ailment of olden times, but it is still very much with us, as those who suffer from this painful condition can attest. Gout is actually a type of arthritis and a metabolic disorder, resulting from too much uric acid in the body. Uric acid is produced in the metabolism of purines, substances made in the body and found in certain foods, notably meats and organ meats. The uric acid crystallizes in the joints and other tissue, causing inflammation and severe pain.

In many cases, the first episode of gout affects only one joint, usually at the base of the big toe. Symptoms typically begin at night and occur in acute attacks, followed by remission. Of those afflicted by gout, 95 percent are men over the age of 30.[1]

Contributing factors to gout include heredity, overeating, obesity, a high-purine diet, and alcohol consumption.

Essential Oils

Benzoin essential oil is warming and has the ability to "melt away" blockages, according to aromatherapy authority Robert B. Tisserand. It is good for cold conditions of the joints such as gout. Rosemary, Fennel, and Juniper are also beneficial for gout, he says. Massage the affected area, as needed, using 5 drops of essential oil per 2 teaspoons of vegetable oil.[2]

Flower Essences

Self-Heal can serve as a foundational healing agent for gout. Other flower essences to address the specific emotions, mental attitude, and environmental conditions of the individual are recommended, states Patricia Kaminski, a flower essence therapist from Nevada City, California. Self-Heal supports the body's innate healing ability. Take 4 drops 2–4 times daily, or as needed.

Food Therapy

Eat:

Cherries, blueberries, leafy greens, complex carbohydrates, foods high in potassium, bioflavonoids, and vitamin C. (For a list of foods containing these nutrients, see part 3, "Food Therapy," pp. 376–378.) Drink plenty of water.

Eating a pound of Bing cherries daily can help prevent the formation of uric acid crystals, says naturopathic physician Alan Christianson, N.M.D., of Scottsdale, Arizona.

Eat celery and avocado to help lower uric acid levels in the body and use turmeric in your cooking for its anti-inflammatory properties, recommends herbal authority James A. Duke, Ph.D.

Avoid:

Refined sugar, refined carbohydrates, saturated fat, alcohol, high-purine food (meats, organ meats, shellfish, brewer's and baker's yeast, herring, sardines, mackerel, anchovies).

Herbal Medicine

Dr. Duke discovered the effectiveness of celery seed extract in relieving gout when he was suffering from the painful disorder himself. Celery (*Apium graveolens*) works for gout by helping to eliminate uric acid. Taking 2–4 tablets daily of the extract worked for him. Here are Dr. Duke's other herbal recommendations:[3]

Shiso zi su, (*Perilla frutescens*): A mint used widely as a food and medicine in Asia. Japanese research has identified compounds in shiso that inhibit the synthesis of uric acid. Add shiso to mint tea and drink a cup regularly.

Turmeric (*Curcuma longa*): Contains curcumin, an anti-inflammatory compound; take turmeric in capsules, as a tea, or spice your food with it.

Oat (*Avena sativa*): Tea made from the tops of this plant is a diuretic and helps lower uric acid levels

Willow (*Salix spp.*): The herbal aspirin; contains salicylates, which are what give aspirin its pain-relieving properties and which research has shown can reduce uric acid levels. Simmer 2 teaspoons of willow bark in a cup of boiling water for 20 minutes. Strain and drink as needed for pain and inflammation. Caution: If you are allergic to aspirin, don't use willow.

Homeopathy

The following are some of the remedies that may help alleviate gout, according to Dr. Barry Rose of the Royal London Homeopathic Hospital:[4]

Aconite: At acute onset of a swollen, red, shiny, very painful joint.

Ammon phos: For chronic, not acute gout.

Arnica: If the big toe joint is red and inflamed, the pain is worse at night, and the area is so sore that you are fearful of someone touching it.

Belladonna: If the acute symptoms are typical of gout and the slightest touch or jarring makes it worse.

Bryonia: If there is a large swelling.

Colchicum: If the smallest movement is agonizing, the area is extremely sensitive to touch, you feel weak, ill, and irritable, and all symptoms are worse at night.

Sabina: For acute and chronic gout if the symptoms are worse in a heated room and gouty nodes form in the affected area.

Urtica: For an acute attack that ends with urination in which there is a sand-like deposit.

Take the appropriate remedy in a 30c potency every hour for an acute attack; continue until your symptoms improve. For chronic gout, take the remedy 3 times daily for 1 day every 2 weeks.

Nutritional Supplements

The following supplement protocol can be effective for gout, according to Dr. Christianson:

Cherry extract: Cherries contain proanthocyanidins, substances in plants that inhibit the formation of uric acid crystals. Take 3 gel capsules 2 times daily.

Bromelain: This enzyme compound derived from pineapple acts as an anti-inflammatory when taken on an empty stomach. Take 250 mg twice daily without food.

Vitamin C: Take 500 mg twice daily.

EPA (eicosapentaenoic acid): This omega-3 essential fatty acid can help reduce inflammation, which leaves the pathways for uric acid less taxed so crystals are not as likely to form. Take 500 mg daily in any combination of oil, capsules, or food (cold-water fish are high in EPA, see above).

Take all of the above for as long as needed.

Reflexology
Kidneys

Stone/Crystal Therapy

The stone concretion, both as an elixir and placed on the problem area, can be helpful for gout, according to Melody, author of the crystal reference series *Love Is in the Earth*. For 2–1/2 days, take the elixir internally at a rate of 3–5 drops 3 times daily. Tape the stone on the affected site, using hypoallergenic tape, and leave it on for the same time period. You can also tape agatized limb cast on the affected area in the same manner. (For instructions on making an elixir, see part 3, "Stone/Crystal Therapy," p. 403.)

Hay Fever

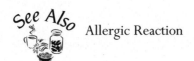 Allergic Reaction

Also known as allergic rhinitis, hay fever is an allergic reaction to airborne sustances, notably pollens, which results in inflammation of the mucous membrane lining the nasal passages. Hay fever tends to be a seasonal ailment, occurring when the offending plant is in bloom. Sneezing, headache, nasal discharge or congestion, and watery or streaming, itchy eyes are all part of the misery of hay fever. The throat and the roof of the mouth may be itchy as well. The histamines, which are released by the body as part of its immune response to what it regards as a foreign invader, are what produce these symptoms.

As with other allergies, it is not clear why certain people react allergically to pollen and other normal airborne substances. Heredity, food allergies, stress, *Candida* yeast overgrowth, intestinal parasites, excess mucus in the body (typically from a diet high in dairy and other mucus-forming foods), toxic buildup in the colon, nutritional deficiencies, and low thyroid function may be disposing factors in the development of hay fever and the severity of symptoms.[1]

Essential Oils

Lavender essential oil can ease a hay fever attack. Use 5 drops of essential oil per 2 teaspoons of carrier oil, and massage into the sinus area below the eyes, as needed. You can also sprinkle a few drops of Lavender, Lemon Balm, Eucalyptus, or German Chamomile on a tissue and simply inhale.[2] Note: Avoid German Chamomile if you are pregnant.

Flower Essences

Yarrow Special Formula can build up immune resistance to hay fever and help prevent attacks, says flower essence therapist Patricia Kaminski of Nevada City, California. Take 4 drops 2–4 times daily, beginning about 2 weeks before your hay fever season. Continue taking through the season, and as maintenance thereafter. During acute episodes, you can take the formula as often as hourly.

Food Therapy

Eat:

Garlic, onion, cold-water fish (salmon, mackerel).

Avoid:

Sugar, dairy, caffeine, alcohol, food additives and preservatives, food allergens.

Herbal Medicine

In treating hay fever, David Winston, A.H.G., a clinical herbalist and consultant from Washington, New Jersey, focuses first on normalizing the immune response, which is excessive with allergies. To that end, he recommends taking a formula comprising immune amphoterics, which are immune normalizers, meaning they increase immune activity if it is functioning below normal levels, and reduce it if the immune system is in overdrive. To make the formula, combine tinctures of the following:

Reishi mushroom (*Ganoderma*): 2 parts

Maitake mushroom (*Grifola*): 2 parts

Licorice (*Glycrrhiza glabra*): 1/2 part; if you suffer from hypertension, omit this herb.

Skullcap (Huang qin, *Scutellaria baicalensis*) root or dan shen (red sage, *Salvia miltiorrhiza*) root: 1 part of one or the other. (These herbs are not amphoterics, but work to reduce excessive immune response.)

Take 4–5 ml (roughly 4/5 to 1 teaspoon) of the blend 3 times daily. In addition, take 1 teaspoon daily of blueberry solid extract to increase your flavonoids. Flavonoids help to stabilize mast cells, which release histamine, thereby reducing the levels of histamine in the body.

It is best to begin this protocol 4–6 weeks before allergy season and continue throughout. Doing so may enable you to entirely avoid your usual hay fever. It can also work if you start in the middle of allergy season or an acute attack, but it may take a while for your body to respond.

If you still suffer hay fever attacks, despite following the program above, add the tincture formula below to the protocol, says Winston. It is designed for relief of symptoms and should only be used if the first formula was not sufficient on its own. Combine tinctures of these herbs:

Eyebright (*Euphrasia officinalis*): 1 part; use a tincture from the whole fresh plant, not a tincture made from the dried herb. (If your hay fever consists mainly of dry, red, itchy eyes, take this tincture alone instead of the blend; 20–30 drops 3–4 times daily.)

Echinacea (*E. spp.*): 1 part

Horseradish (*Armoracia rusticana*) root: 1 part

Bayberry (*Myrica cerifera*) root bark: 1 part

Yerba mansa (*Anemopsis californica*) root: 1 part

Take 4–6 ml (roughly 4/5 to 1–1/5 teaspoon) of this herbal tincture blend 3–4 times daily.

For relief of hay fever symptoms, medical herbalist Amanda McQuade Crawford, M.N.I.M.H., Dip.Phyto., of Ojai, California, cites the Ayurvedic herb albizzia as effective. Take 1/2 teaspoon of 1:2 strength tincture in water 2–3 times daily for 1 week. (The designation "1:2" refers to the ratio of the herb to its carrier liquid; you will find the ratio on the product label.) Albizzia can be used in combination with other natural treatments.

Homeopathy

Hay fever may best be treated with a constitutional remedy, so you may want to consult a homeopath for a deeper, comprehensive approach. The following are common remedies to provide relief from hay fever symptoms, according to London homeopath Miranda Castro:[3]

Allium cepa: If the hay fever produces typical cold symptoms and streaming eyes; the most common remedy.

Euphrasia: If the hay fever produces typical cold symptoms with inflamed eyes and a cough.

Sulphur: If the hay fever produces typical cold symptoms and inflamed eyes.

Take the appropriate remedy in a 6c or 12c potency every 4–8 hours, as needed. Discontinue the remedy when there is improvement. Repeat if necessary.

Nutritional Supplements

"Bee pollen works like a charm for hay fever," reports Joanne B. Mied, N.D., a naturopath and herbalist based in Novato, California. Start taking bee pollen 3–4 months before your allergy season begins. Take just a little at first to watch for an allergic reaction; some people are sensitive to bee pollen. If you develop any allergic symptoms, stop taking it. If not, build up to taking 3 capsules (450 mg each) daily. With this head start, you may not need to up the dosage during allergy season. But if you develop hay fever symptoms, take 6 capsules per day for the duration of the season. If you start taking the bee pollen when the allergy season is already upon you, build up to taking 6 capsules per day (as above) and continue at that dosage through the season. Be warned, says Dr. Mied, that quality makes all the difference. If you use a poor quality bee pollen, you may have to take twice as much to get the same effects as a better quality product.

Naturopathic physician Bradley Bongiovanni, N.D., of Independence, Ohio, recommends the following program for hay fever; take all until symptoms are resolved:

Bioflavonoids: 1,000 mg 2–3 times daily; antioxidant, anti-allergy, and anti-inflammatory.
Vitamin C: 1,000 mg 2–3 times daily; antioxidant.
Eyebright or nettle (*Urtica dioica*): 1,000 mg (capsules) or 2 ml (extract) 2–3 times daily; anti-inflammatory and anti-catarrhal (stopping flow of mucus and the runny, watery eyes of hay fever)
Flaxseed oil: 1,000 mg 2–3 times daily; anti-inflammatory.
Thymus gland extract: 500 mg 2–3 times daily; supports the immune system.

Reflexology

Sinuses, eyes, ears, face, head, neck, ileocecal valve (helps eliminate mucus), adrenal glands, pituitary

Stone/Crystal Therapy

Use roscherite to relieve and prevent hay fever, recommends Melody, author of the crystal reference series *Love Is in the Earth*. For acute symptoms, take 3–5 drops of elixir 4 times daily for 3 days. As maintenance, take the same dose 2 times daily throughout the allergy season. (For instructions on making an elixir, see part 3, "Stone/Crystal Therapy," p. 403.)

Headache

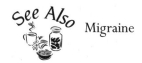

See Also Migraine

There are about as many variations on headaches as there are people who suffer from them. The pain can occur in different parts of the head; be acute or chronic; manifest as throbbing, stabbing, dull, penetrating, pressurized, or other equally descriptive kind of ache; and have any one or a combination of a vast array of causes as the source of the discomfort.

The great majority of headaches (some sources place it as high as 90 percent[1]) result from tension. The muscles of the scalp, neck, and/or shoulders tighten under stress. Muscle tension results not only in sore muscles, but also in decreased blood flow. Both of these factors can lead to a headache.

Other causes of headache include trauma to the head; eyestrain; food allergies; food reactions (the nightshade family—eggplant, potatoes, and tomatoes—produces headaches in some people); reactions to additives (MSG and aspartame are common culprits); too much caffeine, sugar, or salt; sinus infections; bacterial infections in other regions of the body; fever; flu; heatstroke; motion sickness; lack of sleep; toxic exposure or overload; constipation or other gastrointestinal disturbance; high blood pressure; hormonal imbalances; and anger, anxiety, or excitement.

Pain in the head is a sign that something is out of balance in the body. While it may be the result of a transient cause, it can indicate serious disease. If you suffer from recurrent or ongoing headaches, it is advisable to determine the underlying cause or causes of the pain and address healing on a deeper level. The following remedies can help relieve the occasional headache.

Essential Oils

There is a very simple and effective essential oil treatment for headaches, according to naturopathic physician Boyer B. Cole, N.M.D., of Cottonwood, Arizona. Rub 1–2 drops of Peppermint essential oil on the temples and the back of the head. "One to two doses usually knocks out a headache," notes Dr. Cole, "but you need to use a French or high-quality American oil. There is a lot of cheap Peppermint out there and it doesn't have the impact of the better oils."

Flower Essences

Lavender and Feverfew flower essences are beneficial in relieving a headache, notes naturalist Richard Katz of Nevada City, California. Take 4 drops under the tongue on a frequent basis until your symptoms subside. This can range from every hour to 4 times in a day.

Food Therapy

Eat:

Small and frequent meals/snacks for stable blood sugar, leafy vegetables, almonds, sardines, foods high in magnesium (see part 3, "Food Therapy," p. 377).

Avoid:

Sugar, greasy or fried foods, processed foods, red meat, dairy, food additives, aspartame, nitrite-cured meats (hot dogs, salami, bacon, sausage, bologna), chocolate (contains phenylethylamine, a headache-triggering amine), red wine and cheese (high in tyramine, another headache trigger), food allergens.

Herbal Medicine

For a headache, especially one caused by heat and sun, crush a fresh rosemary (*Rosmarinus officinalis*) sprig in your hand, take 5 deep breaths of the vapors while continuing to crush the sprig, suggests Michael Cottingham, a clinical herbalist from Silver City, New Mexico. "This can get rid of your headache in less than a minute," he notes. "It's a prime example of herbal first aid."

Naturopathic physician Jody E. Noé, M.S., N.D., of Brattleboro, Vermont, offers the following herbal headache formula. Combine equal parts of tinctures of skullcap (*Scutellaria laterifolia*), rosemary (*Rosmarinus officinalis*), woundwort (*Stachys palustris*), chamomile (*Matricaria recutita*), valerian (*Valeriana officinalis*), black cohosh (*Cimicifuga racemosa*), and lavender (*Lavandula officinalis*). Take 1 dropperful of tincture every hour as needed.

When a headache is not a migraine, poor circulation is usually the issue, notes Joanne B. Mied, N.D., a naturopath and herbalist based in Novato, California. Ginkgo (*Ginkgo biloba*), which promotes circulation, is therefore a good headache remedy. Take 120 mg of timed-release ginkgo once or twice in a day, 12 hours apart.

Homeopathy

Since pain in the head comes in many forms, there are numerous homeopathic remedies for headaches. The following are some of the most common, as outlined by Michael G. Carlston, M.D., of Santa Rosa, California:

Bryonia: If you want to hold your head still and not move to ease the headache, and are bothered by lights and noise.
Belladonna: For a right-sided headache with a hot flushed head and sensitivity to lights and noise.
Nux vom: If you have a stressed stomach disorder along with the headache and are chilly.

Take the remedy at a 30c potency 4 times a day. Pay attention to your symptoms. If your headache is gone, don't take the remedy.

Nutritional Supplements

The following supplements can help control and relieve headaches, according to natural healer Diane Stein:[2]

Multivitamin/mineral that contains 75 mg of vitamin B complex: Take as directed as a preventive measure.
Additional B complex: Take an additional 50–100 mg of B complex; this alone can be sufficient to stop headaches.
Vitamin B3 (niacin) and B12: When headaches are acute, take 500 mg daily of niacin and sublingual (under the tongue) B12 as directed by the manufacturer.
Vitamin C: 1,000 mg or more daily.
Calcium/magnesium: When you have a headache, take one pill of a combination supplement hourly, along with vitamin C, for a few doses; this can often stop a headache.

Vitamin E: Build up to taking 800 IU daily; antioxidant and an aid in circulation.

Coenzyme Q10: Take as directed; oxygenates the blood, relieves pain, and reduces stress.

Reflexology

Head/brain, neck, sinuses, spine (all), solar plexus

Stone/Crystal Therapy

Green and colorless tourmaline or amethyst can help resolve a headache, notes vibrational healer Daya Sarai Chocron, of Northampton, Massachusetts. Place the stone on the site of the headache for 15–20 minutes, as needed.

Other Remedies

Drink water. Dehydration is a common cause of headaches.

Pressing the acupressure point for headaches can alleviate head pain. The point (LI-4, which stands for the large intestine meridian, or energy pathway) is located in the web at the intersection of the thumb and index finger. Maintain moderate pressure on the point for 3 minutes on each hand.

Heartburn/Indigestion

Heartburn is a symptom of indigestion (dyspepsia), an umbrella term that means faulty or incomplete digestion of food, which can manifest in a variety of ways. Other symptoms of indigestion include stomachache, nausea, bloating, and excessive gas or burping.

In heartburn, digestive stomach acid (hydrochloric acid, or HCl) rises into the esophagus due to insufficient closure of the LES (lower esophageal sphincter), which normally blocks passage of the acids. The result is a burning sensation in the chest, thus the name "heartburn." This condition is also called acid reflux. Stomach acids may even rise into the mouth, as evidenced by a bitter taste.

Contributing factors in heartburn and indgestion include high intake of rich, spicy, fatty, or fried foods; deficiency of digestive enzymes; too much or not enough HCl; eating too fast or too much; stress; excess weight; pregnancy; and chronic constipation. It is important to note that not enough stomach acid rather than too much can cause heartburn and indigestion. In either case, antacids are not a proper treatment for the condition. They do not address the problem, and in fact, worsen it by throwing off the acid-alkaline balance of the stomach.

Indigestion can be an indication of a more serious disorder, such as an ulcer or intestinal or gallbladder disease. As with other conditions in this book, if your heartburn or other symptom of indigestion is chronic, it is a good idea to investigate the underlying cause(s) and get appropriate medical treatment.

Essential Oils

Eucalyptus and Peppermint can help prevent heartburn, notes aromatherapist Julie Oxendale, C.M.T., of San Francisco, California. Blend 2 drops of Eucalyptus and 3 drops of Peppermint essential oil in 1 teaspoon of vegetable oil. Using the blend, massage the chest, stomach, and lower back once daily for a week, as needed. Activating the lower back muscles and releasing the abdomen can alleviate constriction in the upper body. You can use Clove and Lavender instead, if you prefer. Follow the same procedure, using 2 drops of Clove and 3 drops of Lavender essential oil.

Flower Essences

Self-Heal can serve as a foundational healing agent for heartburn and indigestion. Other flower essences to address the specific emotions, mental attitude, and environmental conditions of the individual are recommended, states Patricia Kaminski, a flower essence therapist and codirector of the Flower Essence Society. Self-Heal supports the body's innate healing ability. Take 4 drops 2–4 times daily, or as needed.

Food Therapy

Eat:

Dinner emphasizing complex carbohydrates over protein; drink cabbage juice.

Avoid:

Heavy-protein dinner, fried and spicy foods, processed foods, soft drinks, iced drinks, alcohol, acidic foods (citrus, tomatoes, chocolate, coffee, black tea).

Herbal Medicine

DGL (deglycrrhizinated licorice) can be used preventively and also helps in an acute attack of heartburn, says Alan Christianson, N.M.D., a naturopathic physician from Scottsdale, Arizona. Take 1 teaspoon of powdered DGL (directly in the mouth rather than mixing it with water) 3 times daily for 2 weeks, then as needed. If you do not have high blood pressure or an ulcer, and are not taking oral steroids, you can use regular licorice (*Glycrrhiza glabra*) root powder.

Fennel (*Foeniculum vulgare*) seeds can help prevent heartburn and indigestion, says clinical herbalist Michael Cottingham of Silver City, New Mexico. Fennel is a carminative, meaning that it has a soothing effect on the stomach and intestines. "It is a great circulatory herb," notes Cottingham, "and helps create circulation in the stomach." He suggests chewing on a pinch of fennel seeds after a meal.

Ginger (*Zingiber officinale*) is also helpful in deterring heartburn and indigestion, according to Cottingham. He recommends chewing crystallized ginger after a meal. Make sure to buy a high-quality crystallized ginger, so you get the benefits of the ginger. You can tell it's good if you feel a warming on your tongue after you bite into a piece. To ensure quality, you can make your own crystallized ginger. Here is Cottingham's recipe:

Peel the outer bark from 2 pounds of fresh ginger root, cut the roots into slices the thickness of checkers, and boil in sugar syrup. To make the sugar syrup, bring 2 quarts of water to a boil, then add sugar, stirring until it is dissolved. Add as much sugar as the water can hold and still dissolve; about 5 cups of sugar. After boiling the ginger in the syrup for 30–40 minutes, remove the slices and lay them on a cookie sheet. Bake in the oven at 200 degrees for 5–6 hours.

Herbalist Penelope Ody points to slippery elm (*Ulmus rubra*) as a good herbal solution for heartburn.[1] It is well-known as a digestive aid that soothes the mucous membranes of the gastrointestinal tract. Take 2–4 capsules before every meal, or as needed, for heartburn.

Homeopathy

The following are homeopathic remedies commonly indicated for heartburn and indigestion:[2]

Arsenicum: If heartburn "creeps" up the chest and throat.
Carbo veg: If indigestion is accompanied by flatulence.
Kali mur: If indigestion is the result of eating fatty foods.

Take the appropriate remedy in a 6x or 6c potency 3 times daily, or more often as needed. Stop taking the remedy when your symptoms improve. The remedy should not be considered an ongoing solution for your digestive problems. If your heartburn is recurrent, you need to investigate and resolve the underlying causes.

Nutritional Supplements

Digestive enzymes with or without added betaine HCl (hydrochloric acid) can be useful in resolving heartburn, as they facilitate complete digestion of food. Before you take them, however, you need to know if you are deficient in HCl, so you can choose the correct supplement. Nutritional authorities James F. Balch, M.D., and Phyllis A. Balch, C.N.C., offer a simple test to determine your HCl status. Here's how it's done:

Next time you have heartburn, take 1 tablespoon of fresh lemon juice or apple cider vinegar. If it gets rid of your heartburn, you are deficient in stomach acid. If your heartburn gets worse, you already have too much HCl. If the latter is the case, do not supplement with HCl or digestive enzymes that contain it. If the former is the case, you could benefit from a combination product.[3] Take the appropriate enzyme product (at the dosage directed) in the middle of every meal. That will prevent your body from coming to rely on this outside supply of enzymes and cutting back on its own production.

Reflexology

Stomach, diaphragm, pancreas, gallbladder

Stone/Crystal Therapy

For heartburn, Matlockite and green fluorite are best used as elixirs, notes Melody, author of the crystal reference series *Love Is in the*

Earth. Take 3–5 drops of matlockite elixir 3 times daily for 3 days, or the same dosage of green fluorite elixir for 2–3 days. A maintenance dose of either elixir is 3–5 drops twice daily. You can also place red coral or pyrope garnet on the chest over the area of greatest discomfort. Keep the red coral in place with hypoallergenic tape for 6 hours or the pyrope garnet for 6–8 hours. Use as needed on an ongoing basis. (For instructions on making an elixir, see part 3, "Stone/Crystal Therapy," p. 403.)

Other Remedies

Chew your food slowly and well.

Raw potato juice can ease and help prevent acid reflux. Put a washed, unpeeled potato in a juicer, add an equal part of water to the resulting juice, and drink right away. Do this 3 times daily until your condition is resolved.[4]

Hemorrhoids

Hemorrhoids, or piles, are varicose veins of the anus. The veins may become swollen and inflamed as a result of straining during defecation (as in chronic constipation), prolonged sitting (especially on hard, cold surfaces) or standing, or pregnancy. Diarrhea and overuse of laxatives have also been implicated in the development of hemorrhoids.[1] Lack of exercise, food allergies, and excess weight may be contributing factors as well.

Symptoms include itching, pain, burning, and bleeding. Hemorrhoids on the outside of the anal opening are external hemorrhoids; these are generally painless. Internal hemorrhoids are enlarged veins in the anal canal, but can protrude and cause severe pain.

Essential Oils

For hemorrhoids, Jeanne Rose, an aromatherapist and herbalist based in San Francisco, California, recommends topical applications of MQV (*Melaleuca quinquenervia viridiflora*), also known as True Niaouli. It can be applied neat and has a more delicate scent than Tea Tree

(*Melaleuca alternifolia*) oil, whose properties are similar. Use as needed several times daily.[2]

Flower Essences

Self-Heal can serve as a foundational healing agent for hemorrhoids. Other flower essences to address the specific emotions, mental attitude, and environmental conditions of the individual are recommended, states Patricia Kaminski, a flower essence therapist and codirector of the Flower Essence Society. Self-Heal supports the body's innate healing ability. Take 4 drops 2–4 times daily, or as needed.

Food Therapy

Eat:

Fiber, complex carbohydrates, berries, onion, parsley, legumes, green tea, foods high in vitamin K (see part 3, "Food Therapy," p. 378).

Avoid:

Sugar, refined foods, caffeine, alcohol, dairy, red meat.

Herbal Medicine

For the acute stage of hemorrhoids, Michael Cottingham, a clinical herbalist from Silver City, New Mexico, cites oak (*Quercus robur*) bark tincture. Oak bark is a heavy astringent. One of the actions of astringent herbs is to tighten and shrink tissue. To shrink your hemorrhoids quickly, take 30–50 drops of oak bark tincture 3–4 times daily for 3 days. Do not take for longer than 3 days.

According to Cottingham, the main causes of hemorrhoids are too many fatty and oily foods, which have caused lymph congestion and a fat absorption problem in the small intestines; not drinking enough water; and not getting enough exercise. In most cases of chronic hemorrhoids, lymphatic congestion is a major factor, he says. (The lymph system is the body's filtering system. Lymph fluid flows between cells in the body, transporting beneficial substances between tissues and the bloodstream and also foreign substances for elimination from the body; lymph nodes filter the fluid.)

To help get the lymphatic system flowing freely again and thus prevent a recurrence of hemorrhoids, Cottingham recommends taking a combination of red root (*Ceanothus americanus*) and ocotillo (*Fouquieria splendens*) bark. Red root has a great ability to clear congestion in the lymph system and has a long history of use for that purpose. "Red root is one of the most important lymphatic plants," says Cottingham. Ocotillo can help the intestines absorb fat and works in the pelvic area as a lymphatic mover. Use equal parts of ocotillo bark and red root tinctures, and take 30 drops of the mix 3 times daily for a month. It is also important in conditions of lymph congestion to drink lots of water (at least 8 glasses daily) to aid the body in clearing the congestion. "Water can be one of the ultimate first aid remedies," observes Cottingham.

Homeopathy

The following are common homeopathic remedies for hemorrhoids, according to naturopathic physicians Robert Ullmann, N.D., and Judyth Reichenberg-Ullmann, N.D.:[3]

Aesculus: If the primary symptom is pain "like small sharp sticks in the rectum" and the pain lasts a long time after defecation; purple, painful, external hemorrhoids.

Collinsonia: If the primary symptom is pain "like small sharp sticks in the rectum" with painful, bleeding hemorrhoids and chronic constipation alternating with diarrhea.

Hamamelis: If the primary symptom is swelling and considerable bleeding, with throbbing in the rectum and pain lasting long after defecation; purple, swollen hemorrhoids.

Nux vom: If your hemorrhoids follow too much stress or overindulgence in rich food, stimulants, drugs, or alcohol, result from chronic constipation, and are itchy and painful.

Sulphur: If there is a lot of rectal itching and rectal spasms, the hemorrhoids are large and in bunches, both internal and external, and diarrhea drives you out of bed to the bathroom at 5 A.M.

Take the appropriate remedy in a 30c potency every 4 hours until your symptoms improve. Stop taking the remedy; take another dose if the symptoms recur. If there is no improvement with 3 doses, you probably are not using the correct remedy.

Nutritional Supplements

The following program of supplements can help relieve and prevent hemorrhoids, states Bradley Bongiovanni, N.D., a naturopathic physician from Independence, Ohio; take all on an ongoing basis:

Vitamin A: 10,000 IU 3 times daily; aids tissue healing.
Vitamin C: 1,000 mg 3 times daily; strengthens capillaries and veins.
Vitamin D: 200 IU 2 times daily; aids tissue healing.
Bioflavonoids: 1,000 mg 3 times daily; anti-inflammatory.
Glycosaminoglycans (GAGs): 50 mg 3 times daily; promote the production of mucin (a glycoprotein in mucus), which lubricates and soothes the tissues, allowing them to heal.
Flaxseeds (ground fresh): 1–2 tablespoons daily; grind in an herb or coffee grinder and sprinkle on food; source of fiber and anti-inflammatory essential fatty acids.

Reflexology

Hips/pelvis, lower spine, sigmoid colon, rectum, diaphragm, solar plexus, lymphatic system, adrenal glands

Stone/Crystal Therapy

Blue sodalite can reduce swelling and inflammation, and may be helpful for hemorrhoids. You need to use a stone equal in size to or larger than the affected area. Place the stone over your hemorrhoids and rest quietly several times a day for 10–15 minutes.[4]

Hiccups

Hiccups are caused by uncontrollable spasms of the diaphragm and glottis (sound-producing element of the larynx) that produce a kind of cough on the inhalation, thus the quirky disorder's alternative name—hiccough.

Indigestion, swallowed air, alcoholism, irritation of the diaphragm, and phrenic nerve (the nerve serving the diaphragm) disturbance are among the causes of hiccups.

Essential Oils

Natural healer Diane Stein cites Basil, Sandalwood, and Tarragon as essential oil remedies for hiccups. Sniff the oil directly from the bottle or put a few drops on a handkerchief or tissue and inhale the aroma that way, as needed for hiccups. You can use Basil and Sandalwood in a blend, if you desire.[1]

Flower Essences

Five Flower Formula (Rescue Remedy) can help ease hiccups by stabilizing breathing and instilling calm, according to Patricia Kaminski, a flower essence therapist and educator from Nevada City, California. Take 4 drops under the tongue as often as once every 5 minutes. Also rub drops over the stomach area, then lay your hands on your stomach, breathe deeply, and allow the flower essences to take hold. Continue treatment until the hiccups subside.

Food Therapy

To stop hiccups, eat a slice of hard, dry bread by breaking off small pieces and chewing each one slowly and thoroughly. Eat the whole slice in this manner.[2]

Herbal Medicine

Naturopathic physicians Mildred Jackson, N.D., and Terri Teague, N.D., D.C., recommend dill (*Anethum graveolens*) leaf tea to stop hiccups. Combine 1 teaspoon of dill leaf with 1 cup of boiled water. Strain and sip slowly. The herb helps equalize oxygen in the bloodstream and diaphragm.[3]

Homeopathy

Dr. Barry Rose of the Royal London Homeopathic Hospital cites the following remedies for hiccups:[4]

Cyclamen 12c: For hiccups during pregnancy; take up to 3 times daily, as needed.

Nux mosch 12c: For hiccups with gassy indigestion; take hourly until symptoms improve.

Wyethia 30c: For hiccups alternating with burping; take 3 times daily for 2–3 days.

Nutritional Supplements

While it is not a good idea to take any supplement while you have hiccups due to the danger of choking, taking digestive enzymes with your meals can help prevent the formation of gas and thus deter hiccups, says Diane Stein.[5] Take the enzymes in the middle of the meal. This prevents your body from developing a reliance on the supplements for its enzyme supply and consequently lowering its own production of digestive enzymes.

Reflexology

Diaphragm, stomach

Stone/Crystal Therapy

Diane Stein recommends golden or clear beryl held, worn, or carried in the pocket; and golden apatite in essence form. Drink the essence 3–4 times daily, as needed.[6] (For instructions on making an elixir, see part 3, "Stone/Crystal Therapy," p. 403.)

Other Remedies

Sometimes the old remedies are best. Clinical herbalist Karen Vaughan, E.M.T, A.H.G, of Brooklyn, New York, swears by the glass-of-water trick to put an end to hiccups. Fill a glass of water and drink the whole thing from the top (wrong) side of the glass. You need to bend over and drink "upside-down." "This works ninety percent of the time," says Vaughan. "Plus you're relaxing while you do it, and you get water, which is always a good thing."

"A tablespoon of [dry] sugar will usually stop hiccups," states herbalist Matthew Wood of Minnetrista, Minnesota, citing another folk remedy.

Hives (Urticaria)

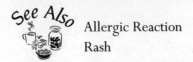

See Also

Allergic Reaction
Rash

Medically termed urticaria, hives are an allergic outbreak of itchy wheals (red bumps with white centers) on the skin in response to something ingested, inhaled, or contacted. The allergen (reaction-causing substance) can be almost anything: a food, a medication, a chemical, a plant, an insect bite, even cold or heat. In addition to these, food additives, the heat of physical exercise, emotional stress, certain bacterial and viral infections, and an overgrowth of *Candida albicans* (yeast-like fungus) have been implicated in hives.[1] Hives can come and go in a matter of hours or last for a day or more. In many cases, the cause of the hives remains a mystery.

As with the symptoms of other allergic responses, such as sneezing and runny nose and eyes, the skin rash of hives is a reaction to histamine, which the body releases in response to what it perceives as a foreign invader (the allergen). The rash is similar in appearance to that produced by stinging nettle; thus another name for hives is nettle rash. (In fact, the hairs of the stinging nettle plant inject histamine into you when you touch them.)

In some cases, the swelling of hives occurs in the respiratory tract and can be severe enough to block breathing. If your airways are involved in your allergic reaction, seek emergency medical care immediately. Further, as with other conditions in this book, if you suffer from chronic hives, it is an indication of an underlying imbalance. Rather than simply applying first aid to relieve the wheals and itching, you need to look into the deeper causes of your condition and get the appropriate therapy to redress your body's imbalance.

Essential Oils

Chamomile and Melissa essential oils "will quickly relieve most attacks of urticaria," states Patricia Davis, founder of the London School of Aromatherapy. Commonly used to relieve allergies, the oils work on the physical level for hives, she says, but also on the emotional aspect of the disorder, as they are de-stressing. Put 4 drops of Chamomile and 2 drops of Melissa in a lukewarm bath. Use no more than this, cautions Davis, or the bath could be irritating to the skin rather than soothing. Take the baths as needed, but if stress is a major factor in your case of hives, she advises continuing the baths for a time after the lesions have healed.[2]

Flower Essences

Self-Heal can serve as a foundational healing agent for hives. Other flower essences to address the specific emotions, mental attitude, and environmental conditions of the individual are recommended, states Patricia Kaminski, a flower essence therapist and codirector of the Flower Essence Society. Self-Heal supports the body's innate healing ability. Take 4 drops 2–4 times daily, or as needed.

Food Therapy

Eat lots of vegetables and dandelion, advises Karen Vaughan, E.M.T, A.H.G, a clinical herbalist from Brooklyn, New York. You can put dandelion (leaves and root) in salad or cook it like spinach. Eat as much of it as you can during a hives outbreak, says Vaughan, and include it in your regular diet thereafter. Violet leaves can also be cooked like spinach and are high in minerals and vitamins, she notes.

Avoid:

Dairy, eggs, chicken, shellfish, cured meat, food additives, alcohol, citrus fruit, chocolate, food allergens (often implicated in hives).

Go easy on animal products, grains (especially flour), fruits, and sugar, says Vaughan. These foods are harder to digest or tend to create allergic reactions, and the sugar from sweets and fruit can feed skin reactions.

Avoid spicy food because it causes vasodilation (opening of blood vessels), which can contribute to hives, notes naturopathic physician David R. Field, N.D., L.Ac., of Santa Rosa, California.

Herbal Medicine

First, try to identify the cause of your hives, advises Karen Vaughan. "In general, however, hives are an indication that the liver isn't detoxifying sufficiently," she notes. Hives are an attempt by the body to get rid of toxins. Treatment should support the liver and also relieve its toxic load by drawing out rather than suppressing the hives. Using cortisone, a common conventional treatment for hives, only drives the toxins back into the body.

Vaughan recommends the following protocol for hives:

Take liver-supporting herbs: In addition to eating fresh dandelion (see "Food Therapy" above), take 2 droppersful of dandelion (*Taraxacum officinalis*) tincture 3 times daily for as long as symptoms are present. Dandelion both supports the liver and helps draw toxins out through the skin. Grind milk thistle (*Carduus marianus, Silybum marianum*) seeds in a coffee or herb grinder and sprinkle them on salads and cereals. Milk thistle supports and protects the liver. You can take milk thistle tincture or powdered extract as well.

Apply poultices to draw out toxins. Mix green clay powder with water to make a paste and put it on the affected area. If your skin shows signs of infection, use echinacea (E. spp.) tincture instead of water to form the paste. Cover the poultice to keep it from drying too quickly. A cabbage leaf works well, as does plastic wrap. Tie or wrap a handkerchief or clothing around the site to keep the poultice in place. If you are treating your legs, you can put on leggings, for example. Leave the poultice on all day if the rash is bad. Apply a new poultice at night.

If your skin is dry, don't use the clay. Make a violet (*Viola odorata*) or comfrey (*Symphytum officinale*) leaf poultice instead. If there is an active infection, don't use the comfrey though, because it is a powerful skin healer and will close the infection over. Violet is high in salicylates (the active ingredient in aspirin is derived from salicylates) and other anti-inflammatories. To prepare the violet leaf poultice, put a handful of fresh leaves in the blender and chop up fine. Add just enough water to make a goop. Apply, cover, and wrap as with the clay poultice. For comfrey, combine comfrey leaf with enough water to make a goop and keep the hairs of the comfrey from irritating the skin. Follow the same procedure as with the other poultices.

Use a topical healing ointment if desired: Compound ointments of grindelia (*Grindelia camporum*) and sassafras (*Sassafras albidum*) can be helpful in resolving hives and are available in health food stores or on herbal product websites.

Herbalist Matthew Wood of Minnetrista, Minnesota, suggests treatments for different manifestations of hives:

Goldenrod (*Solidago vigaurea*) tincture: For hives with dry skin, fatigue, and exhaustion.
Agrimony (*Agrimonia eupatoria*) tincture: For hives with tension.
Nettle (*Urtica dioica*) tincture: For hives with edema, especially of the fingers; you can also take nettle as tea, as needed.

Take 3 drops of the appropriate tincture every hour when the hives are acute, 3 times daily thereafter until the condition is resolved.

Homeopathy

Apis mellifica is well known as a homeopathic remedy if the hive is large and swollen like a bee sting with burning and stinging, says Matthew Wood. Take any potency from 6c to 30c, once or twice daily. Discontinue taking when your symptoms improve.

Nutritional Supplements

For hives, Dr. Field recommends the bioflavonoid (an antioxidant plant substance) quercetin. It has significant anti-allergy activities, inhibiting both the production and release of histamine and other inflammatory substances.[3] Take 500 mg on an empty stomach 2 times daily for a week.

Reflexology

Treat the adrenal glands and the areas of the foot corresponding to the parts of the body where the hives erupted.

Stone/Crystal Therapy

Asphaltum, both placed on the rash and applied as an elixir, can bring relief in about 6 hours, states Melody, author of the crystal reference series *Love Is in the Earth*. Use hypoallergenic tape to keep the stone in place. Wet the area with the elixir 1–2 times in the initial 6 hours. You can apply it as needed for maintenance thereafter. (For instructions on making an elixir, see part 3, "Stone/Crystal Therapy," p. 403.)

Other Remedies

In the case of hives, "you *have* to do stress reduction," says Dr. Field. Whether it's meditation or exercise, it's important to find what works for you, since stress is typically a component of the condition, he explains.

Hot Flashes (Menopausal)

Menopausal hot flashes may begin with an uncomfortable feeling in the abdominal area, followed by a chill, then a rush of heat traveling upward to the head, accompanied by sweating and the face flushing red. Women experience hot flashes as they near menopause, typically between the ages of 45 and 55.

While conventional medicine holds that hot flashes are caused by estrogen deficiency, evidence suggests that the problem is more often estrogen dominance, or a skewed ratio between estrogen and progesterone. At menopause, estrogen levels drop only 40 percent to 60 percent, while progesterone levels can plummet to almost zero. In addition, women in industrialized countries ingest xenoestrogens (estrogen-mimicking chemicals) from our food supply and environmental pollutants, further skewing the balance.

The view that estrogen deficiency is not the problem is supported by the fact that many women on estrogen replacement therapy (ERT) and women with normal levels of estrogen still suffer hot flashes and that natural progesterone therapy often resolves the problem of hot flashes.[1] To ensure that you are addressing your specific hormonal imbalances, it is advisable to have your hormone levels checked, especially if you are considering hormone therapy.

The remedies here can help restore hormonal balance and ease the discomfort of hot flashes.

Essential Oils

Julie Oxendale, C.M.T., an aromatherapist based in San Francisco, California, recommends the following essential oil formula for hot flashes:

Clary Sage: 10 drops
Geranium: 11 drops
Sage: 2 drops
Lemon: 7 drops

Combine the oils in 2 tablespoons of vegetable oil. Use 5 drops of this mixture to 1 teaspoon of massage oil and massage all over the body once a week on an ongoing basis. Note that Clary Sage is a different plant from Sage. "Clary Sage is known as the female fixer," says Oxendale. "It's great for hormonal balancing."

Flower Essences

Tiger Lily, Sage, and Black Cohosh flower essences can help balance the hormones and alleviate hot flashes, states Patricia Kaminski, an herbalist and flower essence therapist from Nevada City, California. Take 4 drops of each, 2–4 times daily as maintenance. During a hot flash, increase the frequency of dosage as needed. "These are the baseline flower essences," notes Kaminski. "Others may be indicated, according to the specific emotional state."

Food Therapy

Eat:

Soy, kelp, fiber, foods high in vitamin E (sunflower seeds, almonds, wheat germ oil).

To help prevent hot flashes, the most important factors in diet are keeping blood sugar levels stabilized and getting a balance of protein and the right kinds of fats to support hormonal production, states Ann Louise Gittleman, N.D., C.N.S., M.S., nutritionist and author of *Super Nutrition for Menopause,* among other books. To that end, eat nuts between meals, sprinkle ground flaxseed on your food, and use dressing containing olive oil on salads daily.

Avoid:

Sugar, chocolate, alcohol, red meat.

Sugar depletes calcium and magnesium needed for bone building, says Dr. Gittleman. These minerals are also potent blood sugar stabilizers.

Herbal Medicine

For hot flashes, mix equal parts of chaste tree (*Vitex agnus-castus*) seed, sage (*Salvia officinalis*) leaf, and/or black cohosh (*Cimicifuga racemosa*) root, says Mindy Green, A.H.G., M.S., an herbalist from Boulder, Colorado. Use one teaspoon of the mix per cup of boiled water. Steep for 15 minutes, then strain. Drink a cup 1–4 times daily for 1–6 months or ongoing as needed.

Homeopathy

"Hot flashes are mostly the province of constitutional homeopathic treatment," according to Michael G. Carlston, M.D., of Santa Rosa, California. This means treatment involves a homeopath's determining the single remedy that is appropriate for your particular constitution and cluster of physical, emotional, and psychological symptoms or characteristics. However, in the absence of this deeper treatment, as a homeopathic first aid measure, you can take Belladonna or Glonoinum in a 12c or 30c potency when you are having a hot flash.

Nutritional Supplements

To help control hormonal fluctuations and the resulting hot flashes, Dr. Gittleman recommends essential fatty acids and vitamin E, along with natural progesterone.

Essential fatty acids: Take 2 tablespoons daily of a liquid combination of evening primrose and flaxseed oils.

Vitamin E: Take 400–1,200 IU daily. (Note: do not take vitamin E if you are on blood-thinning medication.)

Natural progesterone: Creams for this natural hormone treatment contain varying amounts of progesterone. Per application, you should get 20 mg of USP (U.S. Pharmacopeia, the standard for the preparation) natural progesterone. Rub the cream on your throat, instructs Dr. Gittleman. Do 1–2 applications per day, depending on your symptoms, for 25 days out of the month, with 5 days off, if you have stopped menstruating. If you are still menstruating, do not use the progesterone during your period. Progesterone cream has the advantage over oral progesterone of not having to pass through the liver, where a large portion of the hormone gets discarded. If you decide to take oral progesterone, however, you should do so only under the care of a doctor.

Reflexology

Diaphragm, ovaries, uterus, fallopian tubes, endocrine system

Stone/Crystal Therapy

Angelite, chrysocolla, and gem silica can be beneficial for hot flashes, according to Katrina Raphaell, crystal healing therapist and author of the crystal reference series *The Crystal Trilogy*. Place the stone directly on the body at the site or sites of distress. Keep it in place for 5 minutes while visualizing your health goal. Do this 3 times daily. As prevention and for ongoing healing effects, wear the stone, hold it, or carry it in your pocket.

Inflammation
(Natural Anti-Inflammatories)

Inflammation is the immune system's response to any injury to body tissue, whether the source of that injury is a bacterial or other microbial infection or a physical trauma. Inflammation can occur internally or externally, anywhere in the body.

The purpose of inflammation is protective: to destroy invading organisms or contain the damage. To this end, the body increases blood flow to the site of the injury, then renders the capillaries more permeable so white blood cells and other important components in the blood can move rapidly from the bloodstream to the injured tissue. Once the problem is overcome or contained, tissue healing can take place.

The cardinal signs of inflammation are heat, redness, swelling, and pain. Although it may be painful, inflammation is a normal mechanism of the immune system, unless it becomes chronic (as with weakened immunity) or is inappropriate (as in autoimmune disorders such as rheumatoid arthritis and multiple sclerosis).

The remedies here are natural anti-inflammatories that do not suppress the normal immune response, but ease the pain of inflammation, speed the inflammatory process, and support your body in its healing response to an injury or infection.

Essential Oils

"Everlasting (*Helichrysum italicum* var. *serotinum*) is, along with German Chamomile, one of the strongest anti-inflammatory oils in aromatherapy," states Kurt Schnaubelt, Ph.D., scientific director of the Pacific Institute of Aromatherapy in San Rafael, California. He also cites Moroccan Chamomile for its "spectacular anti-inflammatory properties," along with Lemon Verbena, Myrrh, and Yarrow.[1] Note: Do not use German chamomile if you are pregnant. Use the method of delivery that is appropriate for your inflammatory condition, as needed. (For instructions on using essential oils, see part 3, "Essential Oils," pp. 366–68.)

Flower Essences

Self-Heal and Yarrow Special Formula can serve as the foundational healing agents for inflammation. Other flower essences to address the specific emotions, mental attitude, and environmental conditions of the individual are recommended, states Patricia Kaminski, a flower essence therapist and codirector of the Flower Essence Society. Self-Heal supports the body's innate healing ability. Yarrow Special Formula strengthens and protects against environmental toxicity and stress. Take 4 drops of each 2–4 times daily, or as needed.

Food Therapy

Eat:

Apples, black currants, garlic, ginger, onion, sage, cayenne, turmeric, the tropical fruits pineapple, mango, kiwi, and papaya (these fruits contain enzymes that "digest" inflammatory products and thus speed the process). Drink plenty of water to help flush toxins and inflammatory products from the body.

Protein and dietary sources of essential fatty acids (EFAs) support the body in dealing with inflammation, says nutritionist Ann Louise

Gittleman, N.D., C.N.S., M.S. Flaxseed, pumpkin, walnuts, soybeans, canola oil, and fish (salmon, mackerel, and cod) are good sources of omega-3 EFAs. Safflower, corn, peanut, and sesame oils provide omega-6 EFAs, as do evening primrose, black currant, and borage oils.

Avoid:

Sugar, refined foods, soft drinks, alcohol, caffeine.

Herbal Medicine

It is actually more accurate to call anti-inflammatory herbs pro-inflammatory herbs, states medical herbalist Chanchal Cabrera, M.N.I.M.H., A.H.G., of Vancouver, British Columbia. Inflammation is "useful and necessary," she explains. "What we want to do is promote the inflammatory process in a controlled fashion such that we achieve resolution." Cabrerea adds that "the big problem with anti-inflammatories in the modern medical sense is that they inhibit the inflammatory response. That is not necessarily a useful thing."[2] (To avoid confusion, however, this discussion will stay with the term "anti-inflammatory.")

Cabrera cites licorice (*Glycrrhiza glabra*) root as an all-round, generic anti-inflammatory herb that can help resolve an inflammation quickly. It is useful for any kind of inflammation, she notes. Licorice supports the action of adrenal hormones, including cortisol (pharmaceutically known as hydrocortisone), one of the body's major anti-inflammatories.

Licorice root can be taken as a tincture or a tea (decoction), says Cabrera. To make the tea, simmer 1 teaspoon of shredded licorice root in 1 cup of water for 15 minutes. Drink a cup 2–3 times per day. If you prefer the tincture, take 1 teaspoon twice daily. Use the tea or tincture for as long as symptoms are present. You can also chew on licorice root to get its anti-inflammatory effects.

Caution:

People who suffer from high blood pressure or water retention should not use pure licorice root, which can aggravate these conditions. Use DGL (deglycrrhizinated licorice; licorice from which glycrrhizinic acid has been removed) instead; follow manufacturer's recommended dosage.

As a topical application for inflammation, Cabera recommends cayenne (*Capsicum spp.*), which as a rubefacient increases blood flow to the area, which in turn speeds the clearing process of inflammation. (See "Pain".)

A turmeric electuary (sweet medicated paste) is good for any kind of inflammatory condition, from hives to arthritis, says Karen Vaughan, E.M.T, A.H.G, a clinical herbalist from Brooklyn, New York. To make the electuary, mix powdered turmeric (*Curcuma longa*) with black pepper or ginger (90 percent turmeric and 10 percent pepper or ginger), which will help the turmeric penetrate. Mix the powders with honey to make a paste. Vaughan recommends using local honey because it is from local pollen. Eating this honey can help protect you from developing allergies to the pollen in the area. Eat 1–2 teaspoons of the electuary daily. Keep the electuary in a jar (it doesn't have to be refrigerated). The honey tends to make it stiffen after a while, so make a looser paste than you think necessary. If you have a tendency toward inflammatory conditions, take the electuary on an ongoing basis.

Homeopathy

See the particular type of inflammation.

Nutritional Supplements

To help reduce inflammation, take 400 mg of a combination of EPA (eicosapentaenoic acid) and DHA (docosahexaenoic acid) 3 times daily, says Dr. Gittleman. EPA and DHA are omega-3 essential fatty acids.

Bromelain, an enzyme compound found in pineapple, is another natural anti-inflammatory. Dr. Gittleman suggests taking 1,000 mg daily (ideally divided into 3 doses). Take on an empty stomach. Taken with food, the enzymes work on digesting the food rather than breaking down the inflammatory products. A number of supplement formulations combine bromelain with the flavonoid quercetin, which research has shown to be significantly anti-inflammatory as well.[3]

Reflexology

Treat the area of the foot corresponding to the part of the body where the inflammation is located.

Stone/Crystal Therapy

Green and colorless tourmaline are anti-inflammatory gemstones, according to Daya Sarai Chocron, a vibrational healer based in Northampton, Massachusetts. Lay the stone on the affected part of the body for 15–20 minutes daily, as needed, until the inflammation subsides.

Insect Bites and Stings

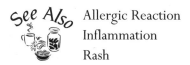 **See Also**   Allergic Reaction
Inflammation
Rash

Bites or stings by nonpoisonous insects such as mosquitoes, spiders, mites, ticks, and bees can produce annoying and uncomfortable itching and/or raise welts on the skin. Often it is the saliva of the insect that creates these problems. Your body's inflammatory response is its attempt to contain the invading substance. Applying natural remedies can help neutralize the effects of a bite or sting. There are also natural bug repellents that can help prevent insect bites and stings.

If you have been stung, check to see if there is a stinger left in the skin. If so, remove it with tweezers. Avoid squeezing it to prevent the contents of the stinger from expressing into your skin. If the problem is a tick, do not use the popularly advocated techniques of a lit cigarette, match, lighter, or gasoline to remove it. Do not touch the tick; ticks can carry disease, such as Lyme disease or Rocky Mountain spotted fever. Again, use tweezers, and grasp the head of the tick as close to the skin as possible. Exert slow backward pressure until the tick is removed.

In some cases, people respond allergically to the bite or sting of a nonpoisonous insect. Wasp and hornet stings are particularly problematic in this regard. If you know that you are highly allergic or if you feel any respiratory symptoms, such as tightness in the chest or wheezing, from a few minutes to several hours after an insect bite or sting, seek emergency medical care immediately. Also seek such care if you have been bitten by a poisonous or venomous insect, such as a black widow spider.

Essential Oils

Dab Lavender or Tea Tree (*Melaleuca alternifolia*) essential oil on bites or stings, says herbalist Mindy Green, A.H.G., M.S., of Boulder, Colorado. You can also mix Lavender oil with baking soda—the traditional remedy for stings—to make a paste; apply as needed.

Naturopathic physician Boyer B. Cole, N.M.D., of Cottonwood, Arizona, also recommends Lavender, but he blends it with Helichrysum. Combine 4 parts Lavender essential oil to 1 part Helichrysum essential oil. Dab 1 drop of the blend on the bite or sting 4 times daily. Keep applying it until the swelling and itching subside.

To make an "Insect Deterrent Synergistic Blend," combine essential oils of Lemongrass (8 drops), Thyme (4 drops), Lavender (4 drops), and Peppermint (4 drops), says aromatherapist Valerie Ann Worwood. To deter mosquitoes while you're sleeping, put 2 drops of the blend on a cotton ball and place it near your bed. To deter insects from feeding on you, mix 2 drops of the blend with 2 teaspoons of carrier oil and apply to your skin. You can also just add the blend to lotion you use. If you are particularly attractive to mosquitoes and other biting insects, Worwood recommends combining 30 drops of Lavender with 2 tablespoons vegetable oil and applying it as needed to protect you.[1]

Flower Essences

Topical applications of Self-Heal cream mixed with Five Flower Formula (Rescue Remedy) can relieve the itching and swelling of an insect bite or sting, says Richard Katz, naturalist and founder of the Flower Essence Society. Use 6–10 drops of Five Flower Formula per 1 ounce of cream, and apply topically 4–5 times daily for 1–3 days or until the skin returns to normal. You can also mix Five Flower Formula with clay powder (available in health food stores) and enough water to make a paste. Apply to the bite or sting and leave it on for 1–2 hours. This helps pull toxins out. Then apply the Self-Heal cream with formula added, as directed above.

Food Therapy

Drink plenty of fluids to flush the toxins from the bite or sting out of the body.

Avoid:

Sugar, alcohol, meat.

Sugar both suppresses the immune system and makes you more attractive as a feast for insects.

Herbal Medicine

Plantain (*Plantago major*) is helpful for bee stings and insect bites, says Chanchal Cabrera, M.N.I.M.H., A.H.G., a medical herbalist from Vancouver, British Columbia. Not only is it a powerful drawing agent, but it is also antimicrobial, has pain-relieving properties, and promotes healing. In addition, it grows everywhere, so is readily at hand when emergency first aid is needed.

As a drawing agent, plantain will pull out the venom and other substances introduced by the bite or sting. It contains vitamin A, zinc, and allantoin (found also in egg whites and the herb comfrey), all of which aid healing.

Pick fresh plantain leaves. Mash them into a pulp by chewing them, using a mortar and pestle, or putting them in a blender or herb grinder. Place the pulp over the bite or sting and wrap gauze around it. If you're in the woods, you can use a bandanna or other piece of clothing in place of the gauze. Leave the plantain on until the pain subsides. You can apply a fresh poultice if the pain persists.

Prickly pear cactus pads are another drawing agent and can pull the poison from an insect bite or sting, says clinical herbalist Michael Cottingham of Silver City, New Mexico. If you get bitten by a fire ant or other insect, or are stung by a wasp, and you're in a place where prickly pear cactus grows, use a stick to knock a pad off the cactus, brush off the prickles, and rub off the spine. Then cut the pad open and slap it on the bite or sting. "You will feel relief in seconds," states Cottingham. One pad for 20–30 minutes can eliminate ill effects. See "Boil" for more information on prickly pear cactus and how to use it at home.

Homeopathy

Take Ledum palustre 30c twice daily for 3 days as treatment for an insect bite or sting, suggests naturopathic physician David R. Field, N.D., L.Ac., of Santa Rosa, California. Apis mellifica 30c is indicated for bee stings or other insect bites charactized by red swelling and stinging pain. Take every 15 minutes for up to 6 doses.[2]

Nutritional Supplements

Vitamin E, vitamin C, or bromelain (derived from pineapple) can be applied topically to relieve the pain and inflammation of an insect bite or sting. Use liquid vitamin E or break open a capsule. In the case of vitamin C, use powder or crush a few tablets into powder and moisten with water to make a paste. For bromelain, crush tablets and prepare in the same way as the vitamin C. Apply any of the three remedies to the bite or sting as needed.[3]

Reflexology

If the insect bite or sting swells or becomes inflamed or infected, treat the area of the foot corresponding to the part of the body where the bite or sting occurred.

Stone/Crystal Therapy

Green obsidian with perlite, both placed on the bite and applied in elixir form, can bring relief from an insect bite in 1–2 hours, according to Melody, author of the crystal reference series *Love Is in the Earth*. Apply the elixir 1–2 times during that time period. Keep the stone in place with hypoallergenic tape. The stone also protects against infection from the bite. For an insect sting, apply moonstone in elixir form 2–4 times for 1 day, and also tape the stone on the sting site for the same period. Moonstone can help prevent an allergic reaction to a sting. (For instructions on making an elixir, see part 3, "Stone/Crystal Therapy," p. 403.)

Other Remedies

Ice the area for 20 minutes as soon after the bite or sting as possible, advises Dr. Field. Repeat as needed.

Lemon and apple cider vinegar are both useful antiseptic remedies, taken internally and applied topically to the bite or sting. Drink 1/2 teaspoon of fresh lemon juice in 1 cup of water every 1–2 hours and dab the juice on the bite or sting as needed. Alternatively, drink 1/4 teaspoon of apple cider vinegar in 1 cup of water every 1–2 hours, and dab vinegar on the bite or sting 2–3 times daily.[4]

Insomnia

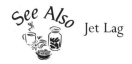 See Also Jet Lag

Insomnia is difficulty in falling and/or staying asleep. Nearly everyone experiences this problem at some point in life. The factors that contribute to sleeplessness are many, including stress, anxiety, depression, pain, magnesium deficiency, certain medications, recreational drugs, alcohol, caffeine, smoking, overeating, strenuous exercise too close to bedtime, lack of exercise, and fear of insomnia. Research has found that 50 percent of insomnia cases are due to psychological factors.[1]

A chronic sleep disorder is beyond the scope of household treatments for minor ailments. It indicates a deeper problem than the occasional inability to fall or stay asleep. It may be advisable to seek medical assistance to determine the causes of your chronic sleeplessness.

Essential Oils

Aromatherapist Valerie Ann Worwood designed a "General Synergistic Blend for Insomnia," using the following essential oils:

Clary Sage: 3 drops
Vetiver: 2 drops
Lavender: 2 drops
Valerian: 1 drop

Blend the oils and use 3 drops in a before-bedtime bath. You can also use the blend in a diffuser during the night, or put 2 drops in 1 teaspoon of vegetable oil and rub it on any part of your body you like.[2]

Flower Essences

For the various varieties of insomnia, flower essence therapist Patricia Kaminski of Nevada City, California, recommends the following flower essences:

Benediction flower oil: For insomina due to the stress of life transitions such as a new job, a move, or death of a loved one; use in a bath or massage before sleeping

St. John's Wort: For insomnia accompanied by disturbing dreams and general restlessness; take 4 drops 2–4 times daily, as needed.

White Chestnut: For insomnia accompanied by repetitive thoughts and intense mental activity; take 4 drops 2–4 times daily, as needed.

Red Chestnut: For insomnia accompanied by constant worry about another; take 4 drops 2–4 times daily, as needed.

With your bedtime dose of the oral remedies, it also helps to take a bath to which you've added St. John's Shield or Benediction. (For instructions on using flower essences in baths and massage oil, see part 3, "Flower Essences," "Directions for Use," p. 372.)

Food Therapy

Eat:

Complex carbohydrates for dinner rather than heavy protein, foods containing tryptophan (milk, cottage cheese, fish, dates, turkey, bananas).

A drop in blood sugar levels during the night is often an issue in not being able to stay asleep, says nutritionist Ann Louise Gittleman, N.D., C.N.S., M.S., of Bozeman, Montana. To counteract this problem, she recommends eating some avocado or some almond butter on toast one hour before going to bed. There is wisdom in the old remedy of a warm glass of milk as a sleep aid. Milk contains the amino acid tryptophan, which is a precursor to serotonin, a calming brain neurotransmitter (chemical messenger). If you employ the milk remedy, Dr. Gittleman advises that you use only milk that is organic and free of BGH (bovine growth hormone).

Avoid:

Sugar, alcohol, caffeine (all forms, including chocolate).

Dr. Gittleman recommends avoiding sweet foods before bed because such foods adversely affect blood sugar levels, which can disturb sleep.

Herbal Medicine

As magnesium deficiency is frequently implicated in insomnia, clinical herbalist Karen Vaughan, E.M.T, A.H.G, of Brooklyn, New York, suggests trying a magnesium supplement first (see "Nutritional Supplements" below). If that doesn't produce results, then you can turn to the herbs here. While valerian is a common herb recommended for insomnia, Vaughan considers oatstraw, kava-kava, or passionflower superior. If you prefer to take valerian, make sure you are using a tincture made from the fresh root rather than dried valerian. In a few people, valerian has the opposite effect of that intended. Instead of relaxing them, it makes them hyperactive. Dried valerian has more of a tendency than fresh to produce that effect, but the reaction depends on the person. Here are Vaughan's recommendations for the other herbs:

Oatstraw (*Avena sativa*): Oatstraw is a good nervine, or nervous system restorative. To make an infusion, pour 1 quart of boiled water over 1 ounce of dried oatstraw in a bottle. Cap the bottle and leave overnight. Strain it in the morning and drink 2–4 cups daily, with one of these cups taken before bed. The infusion doesn't keep longer than 2 days.

Kava-kava (*Piper methysticum*) or passionflower (*Passiflora incarnata*): Before bed, take 2 droppersful of one or the other tincture.

Homeopathy

The following are common homeopathic remedies for insomnia, say Stephen Cummings, M.D., and Dana Ullman, M.P.H.:[3]

Coffea: If an overactive mind (but not anxiety or irritability), caffeine, or a sudden emotion is keeping you awake.

Arsenicum: If you can't sleep due to anxiety and fears or you are "too tired" to sleep, as after heavy exertion.

Nux vom: If your insomnia is the result of coffee, alcohol, or drug use, mental strain, or too much studying, and you are irritable.

Pulsatilla: If one obsessive thought keeps you awake.

Ignatia: If your sleeplessness is due to grief.

Chamomilla: If your sleeplessness is due to irritability, physical pain, or sedative dependence.

Passiflora: For insomnia in children and the elderly, which is not particularly distinguished by symptoms; also indicated for an overactive mind.

Take the appropriate remedy at a potency of 6c(x) or 12c(x) up to every 30 minutes for as many as 3 doses. If you still can't fall asleep after 3 doses, try another remedy, but don't take more than 2 remedies in a night.

Nutritional Supplements

"We are getting one-third less minerals in our diet than thirty years ago," states Karen Vaughan. "People in the United States are not getting enough magnesium from their food." One of the symptoms of magnesium deficiency is insomnia. Simply taking a magnesium supplement can often resolve sleep problems. Vaughan recommends taking up to 2,000 mg of magnesium citrate or magnesium aspartate with 1,000 mg of calcium daily, divided into 3 doses. Magnesium citrate or aspartate is better absorbed and utilized by the body than magnesium oxide or magnesium sulfate.[4]

Dr. Gittleman concurs on the use of magnesium. In her experience, magnesium, inositol, and salt are the three remedies that work the best for occasional insomnia. Here are her recommendations:

Magnesium: Take 400 mg of magnesium before bed. If you wake up during the night and can't get back to sleep, take another 400 mg. A magnesium deficiency may be involved in difficulty in staying asleep.[5]

Inositol: Take 650 mg of inositol before bed. A member of the vitamin B family, inositol is necessary in the function of serotonin and other neurotransmitters.

Salt: If your system is too acidic, it may interfere with your sleep. Simply putting 1/4 teaspoon of sea salt under your tongue or dissolving it in warm water and drinking it at bedtime can neutralize the acidity and allow you to get a good night's rest.

 Note While melatonin has become a popular sleeping aid, it is a hormone and as such should be used carefully, not as a simple sleeping pill on an ongoing basis. If your melatonin levels are normal, you shouldn't be taking it. Unneeded supplementation could throw off your circadian rhythm (sleep-wake cycle).[6] Low melatonin levels are quite common among the elderly,[7] but regardless of your age, a low melatonin level may not be the problem behind your insomnia. You might want to try some of the remedies here before you consider melatonin, or have your melatonin level checked. If you do use melatonin, the recommended dosage is far higher than the amount your body produces daily, so you may want to start with half the dosage suggested by the manufacturer.

Reflexology

Adrenal glands, diaphragm, thyroid/parathyroid, pancreas, pituitary, ovaries/testes

Stone/Crystal Therapy

For insomnia, try hematite, celestite, labradorite, amethyst, or smoky quartz, recommends crystal healing therapist Katrina Raphaell of Kapaa, Hawaii. At bedtime, position the stone on your third eye (on the forehead, between the eyes), in your hand, or under your pillow. Count backwards from ten to zero, exhaling on each number. As you exhale, focus on your breath, and let go of all thoughts (aside from the countdown) and tension. During the day, wear the stone, hold it, or carry it in your pocket.

Other Remedies

Don't go right from watching television or using the computer to bed, advises Karen Vaughan. "We need a break from EMFs [electromagnetic fields]," she explains. It is difficult for the body to go right from EMF stimulation to sleep. Similarly, many practitioners have cited the presence of electrical devices such as digital alarm clocks in the bedroom as interfering with or deterring sleep.

Deep breathing or a differential relaxation exercise while lying in bed can aid sleep, says Vaughan. Differential relaxation is tightening and letting go of muscles, moving progressively through the body, beginning with the toes and ending with the scalp.

Jet Lag

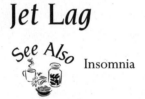 *See Also* Insomnia

The fuzzy-headedness, performance problems, fatigue, sluggishness, and sleep difficulties of jet lag (medically termed desynchronosis) are familiar to anyone who has flown from one time zone to a significantly different one. The greater the time difference between departure point and destination, the greater the jet lag.

The source of the symptoms is the disturbance of one's internal clock and its attendant biological rhythms, such as the sleep-wake cycle. The sooner you can reset your inner clock to the new time zone, the sooner you will be free of the discomfort of jet lag. Natural remedies can help speed this process and alleviate the symptoms.

Flying itself—especially the often low oxygen level in the pressurized cabin and the changes in altitude—is somewhat stressful on the body and contributes to the symptoms of jet lag. There are steps you can take to ease some of the stress of flying and prevent or at least lessen jet lag.

Essential Oils

Chanchal Cabrera, M.N.I.M.H., A.H.G., a medical herbalist from Vancouver, British Columbia, travels frequently, so has developed a good program for minimizing jet lag. She carries Lavender and

Peppermint essential oils whenever she flies. "Peppermint wakes you up and Lavender relaxes you. I often have to go right to a meeting or presentation when I get off the plane, so I either sniff peppermint out of the bottle or put some on a Kleenex or the cuff or collar of what I'm wearing to help me get rid of the grogginess of jet lag." At bedtime, you can take a bath with a few drops of Lavender essential oil in it, sniff it before you go to sleep, or put some on a Kleenex and tuck it into the pillowcase, says Cabrera. Peppermint and Lavender are also useful in relieving headaches, she notes.

As a complete program for jet lag, aromatherapist Julie Oxendale, C.M.T., of San Francisco, California, suggests the following:

- If you are flying at night and want to sleep on the flight, take a bath a few hours before you have to be at the airport. Put 1 drop each of Lavender and Roman Chamomile in the bath water. This is wild or fine Lavender, not Spike Lavender, which will not produce the same effects. During the flight, put 1 drop of each on a handkerchief and tuck it into your collar or pillow, so you can inhale it for relaxation.
- Walk as much as possible in between flights and after you arrive at your destination. Put 1 drop each of Lavender and Roman Chamomile on a handkerchief, carry it with you, and inhale frequently as you are walking.
- In the morning after you arrive at your destination, take a bath with 2 drops each of Peppermint and Eucalyptus in the water. If you are showering instead, put 1 drop of each oil on a shower sponge or loofah and wipe over your body after you have washed. Do this for 3 days.
- Before you go to sleep at night after arriving, take a bath with 1 drop each of Lavender and Geranium in the water. Or you can put 1 drop each in 1 ounce of a carrier oil (sweet almond, apricot kernel, avocado, or olive oil) and massage (or get a friend to massage) the blend into your shoulder blades, upper back, chest, and solar plexus. Inhale deeply during the massage. Do this for 3 days.
- To revive you during the day, use Grapefruit essential oil. Put 1 drop on a handkerchief and inhale the aroma. Or you can dilute the

Grapefruit (20 drops in 4 ounces of carrier oil) and put 1 drop of the blend on the pulse point of your wrist. Use as needed.

• To get you over the shock of the time change, to smooth a rough transition, put 1 drop each of Peppermint and Geranium on a shower sponge and wipe over your body after you have washed.

Flower Essences

For jet lag, take Yarrow Special Formula and Morning Glory in combination, recommends naturalist Richard Katz of Nevada City, California. On the day before and after your flight, take 4 drops of each flower essence at least 4 times during the day, but as often as once per hour. Base your dosage on the extent of jet lag you usually experience (slight, moderate, or severe symptoms) or, in the case of the day after your flight, the extent of jet lag you are experiencing on this trip. During the flight, take 4 drops every hour.

Food Therapy

Chanchal Cabrera suggests some dietary practices that can ease travel strain on your body and help prevent jet lag:

• Eat lightly the day before and the day after you travel. Your food intake should be low in carbohydrates and high in protein. Drink lots of water and avoid alcohol and stimulants such as coffee.
• Drinking lots of water during your flight—a big glass every hour—really helps for jet lag.
• Don't eat much while flying. Stay off the carbohydrates, and eat fruit, vegetables, and protein. You can order a fruit plate as a special meal beforehand, or bring appropriate food with you if you want more than fruit.

Herbal Medicine

Cabrera recommends ginger (*Zingiber officinale*) as a good remedy for several problems associated with air travel. Ginger can help settle your stomach if you suffer from air sickness. Since it also promotes peristalsis (contraction and relaxation of smooth muscle, which moves matter through the intestines), ginger can help prevent the constipation that sometimes occurs with a plane trip. Bring a tin of ginger candies, dissolve them in a cup of hot water, and sip as a tea. Or carry ginger tea bags or crystallized ginger. You can also make a pot of fresh ginger tea before you travel and bring it with you in a thermos, or water bottle if cool, suggests Cabrera. To make ginger tea, chop up a knob of fresh ginger (about the size of the end of your thumb, or a 1-inch length) in 2 cups of water, and simmer, covered, for 10 minutes. Drink the tea throughout the flight.

Homeopathy

Cocculus indicus is a homeopathic remedy that can alleviate jet lag, according to Stephen Messer, N.D. Take at a potency of 6c, 5–10 minutes before you get on the plane. Once you're at your destination, take the remedy up to 2 times daily for 2–3 days. Cocculus will help you adjust to the new time zone, says Dr. Messer.[1]

Nutritional Supplements

Of nutritional supplements, Chanchal Cabrera has found melatonin the most useful in reversing jet lag, but she urges people to remember that it is a hormone. (Melatonin is produced by the pineal gland and regulates the sleep-wake cycle.) Although melatonin is available over the counter, Cabrera advises using it conservatively. Your body naturally makes only 0.5 mg of melatonin daily, but the dosage range of most products starts at 1.5 mg, she notes. For jet lag, she recommends starting with only half a pill at bedtimes at the new location. That is all that many people require to help their body reset its internal clock. Adjust the dosage to your needs, however; 3 or even 6 mg is all right to take for a few days, says Cabrera. Take the melatonin nightly for 3–4 nights, until your sleep pattern is adjusted.

For those who don't want to use melatonin, an alternative is 5-HTP (5-hydroxy tryptophan), a plant extract that resembles the amino acid tryptophan in its effects. Tryptophan is a precursor to the neurotransmitter serotonin, which helps regulate sleep patterns. Follow the 5-HTP manufacturer's directions; dosage varies.

Taking extra antioxidants and vitamins and minerals that help protect against stress is also beneficial for jet lag. These nutrients include vitamins A, C, E, and B6, selenium, and zinc.[2]

Reflexology

Endocrine system, especially the pineal and pituitary glands

Stone/Crystal Therapy

Hematite is an excellent stone for jet lag, notes Katrina Raphaell, crystal healing therapist and founder of the Crystal Academy of Advanced Healing Arts in Kapaa, Hawaii. Before, during, and after flying, wear the stone, hold it, or carry it in your pocket. Some people find it effective to tape a piece of hematite to their solar plexus (at the top of the abdomen, below the ribs) when they fly, says Raphaell. She also recommends putting six pieces of hematite in your bath water at your destination.

Other Remedies

You can help your body reset its internal clock by mentally anticipating and adapting to the new time zone. Before arriving at your destination, set your wristwatch to the new time.

Jock Itch

See Fungal Infection.

Joint Soreness

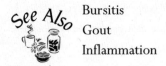

See Also
Bursitis
Gout
Inflammation

Painful or stiff joints can be caused by a multitude of factors. Overuse, injury, overexercise, and not stretching or warming up before exercise are common culprits. The remedies here can help alleviate occasional joint soreness. If you suffer from chronic joint soreness, you may have nutritional deficiencies or a joint condition such as arthritis. If the treatments below do not produce improvement and your joint soreness persists, seek medical help.

Essential Oils

For joints that feel hot and swollen, herbalist Penelope Ody recommends using an ice pack (a package of frozen peas also works) to cool the area, followed by a gentle massage with a blend of Lavender essential oil (20 drops) and infused St. John's wort oil (1 teaspoon). Repeat as needed.

For general joint stiffness, Ody suggests hot baths with 5 drops each of essential oils of Rosemary, Thyme, and Juniper.[1]

Flower Essences

Treat joint soreness internally and externally, says Patricia Kaminski, a flower essence therapist and educator from Nevada City, California. Take 4 drops of Dandelion flower essence under the tongue 2–4 times daily. Do Dandelion Dynamo flower oil baths and massages daily. Continue treatment until soreness subsides. (For instructions on using flower essences in baths and massage oil, see part 3, "Flower Essences," "Directions for Use," p. 372.)

Food Therapy

For their anti-inflammatory effects, use ginger and turmeric liberally in your diet, and eat foods rich in omega-3 and omega-6 essential fatty acids (EFAs), suggests Nick Buratovich, N.M.D., a naturopathic physician from Tempe, Arizona. In addition to giving your body the dietary support it needs for the current problem, these foods may prevent future episodes of joint soreness if you make them a regular part of your diet. (For a list of EFA-rich foods, see part 3, "Food Therapy," p. 376.)

Dr. Buratovich recommends avoiding coffee and other forms of caffeine (aside from green tea) because caffeine blocks endorphin receptors in the brain. As endorphins facilitate pain relief, people who consume a lot of caffeine tend to have a low threshold of pain. Avoid animal products because they contain arachidonic acid, which promotes inflammation. You may also want to avoid foods in the night-shade family (eggplant, tomato, green pepper, potato, paprika, and cayenne; tobacco is also a nightshade plant). In some people, night-shades increase inflammation as an allergic reaction.

Herbal Medicine

To ease aching joints, Jeanne Rose, an herbalist and aromathera-pist based in San Francisco, California, recommends an herbal bath. Simmer a handful each of chamomile (*Matricaria recutita*) flowers, sage (*Salvia officinalis*) leaves, comfrey (*Symphytum officinale*) root, tansy (*Tanacetum vulgare*), and myrtle (*Myrtis communis*) berries in 1 quart of water for 10–20 minutes. Strain into a warm bath and soak.

For a compress, pour 1 cup of boiled water over 1/4 ounce each of meadowsweet (queen of the meadow, *Filipendula ulmaria*), melilot (*Melilotus officinalis*), and wormwood (*Artemisia absinthum*), says Rose. Cool so it won't burn you, then dip a cotton cloth in the blend, wring out, and apply to the afflicted area. Repeat as needed.[2]

You can also take meadowsweet, which contains an aspirin-like substance, orally to help relieve joint soreness. Add 10–20 drops of the tincture to juice or water and drink 2–3 times daily, or take the herb in tea form.[3]

Homeopathy

There are a myriad of homeopathic remedies for joint pain and soreness, based on the specific characteristics of the pain. Here are a few, as cited by London homeopath Miranda Castro:[4]

Arnica: Indicated for joint pain and soreness made worse by touch.

Causticum: Indicated for joint pain with stiffness alleviated by heat and the warmth of bed and worse in dry cold and when rising from sitting; accompanied by restlessness at night.

Pulsatilla: Indicated for joint pain and soreness worsened by wet weather, heat, the warmth of bed, and the onset of movement, and after having a cold, and improved by cold compresses, fresh air, and walking.

Rhus tox: Indicated for joint pain and soreness that is worse after sitting, in damp weater, during a fever, at night, and when chilled, and improved by heat, warm compresses, the warmth of bed, and walking.

Take the appropriate remedy in a 6c or 12c potency every 4–8 hours, or more often during an acute episode. Discontinue the remedy when there is improvement. Repeat if necessary.

You can also apply arnica ointment to the affected area, as needed, to relieve soreness.

Nutritional Supplements

To help resolve joint soreness and ease the pain, the following supplements can be effective, according to Dr. Buratovich:

Glucosamine sulfate: 300 mg 3 times daily for 1–3 months; helps to rebuild cartilage.

Vitamin B3: 300–500 mg of niacinamide 3 times daily for 1–3 months. Niacin, the other form of vitamin B3, is biochemically different and does not produce the same effects of decreasing joint soreness and increasing range of motion that niacinamide does.

Vitamin B6: 100 mg 3 times daily for 1–3 months; helps reduce swelling.

DLPA (D,L-phenylalanine): 750 mg 3 times daily before meals for 1–3 weeks; a pain-relieving amino acid.

Tryptophan: 2–4 g 3 times daily for up to 1 month. This amino acid has been shown to reduce pain, perhaps by raising the pain threshold, although the exact mechanism is unknown.[5] To ensure uptake, avoid protein for 90 minutes before and after taking.

Reflexology

Treat the area of the foot corresponding to the part of the body where the sore joint is located.

Stone/Crystal Therapy

Place green calcite, hiddenite, green aventurine, or amethyst directly on the sore joint, recommends crystal healing therapist Katrina Raphaell of Kapaa, Hawaii. Keep it in place for 5 minutes while visualizing your health goal. Do this 3 times daily. In between treatments, wear the stone, hold it, or carry it in your pocket.

Kidney Stones

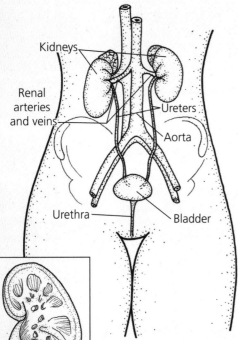

Kidneys

Renal
arteries
and veins

Ureters

Aorta

Urethra

Bladder

The pain of passing a kidney stone through the urinary tract is excruciating, as anyone who has experienced it can tell you. The stone is actually a sharp-edged crystal formed by an aggregation of mineral salts that normally float freely in kidney fluid. A minuscule kidney stone may pass through the tract without your even knowing it, but a larger stone causes great pain and can get stuck anywhere along the urinary passage, in the tubes (ureters) from the kidneys to the bladder, or in the urethra (tube from the bladder) before exiting the body.

Symptoms indicating the presence of a kidney stone include pain in the lower back, extreme radiating pain in the groin area, painful urination, chills and fever, and nausea progressing to vomiting in some cases.

While heredity may influence a tendency to form kidney stones, "The majority of kidney stones are entirely preventable," according to Michael Murry, N.D., and Joseph Pizzorno, N.D.[1] They point to diet as the main reason the incidence of kidney stones in the West has risen steadily over the past twenty years. The specific dietary factors are low intake of fiber and high intake of refined carbohydrates, animal protein, fat, salt, high-oxalate foods (peanuts and chard, among others), and calcium-containing and vitamin D-enriched foods, as well as high alcohol consumption.[2] Low water consumption can also be a contributing factor.

Although most kidney stones are calcium oxalate in composition, research suggests that natural dietary calcium is not the problem; rather, high calcium levels in the urine are the risk factor in the formation of stones.[3] If the body is absorbing the calcium from the food you eat, your urinary calcium levels won't be high. But if your body cannot absorb the calcium or other factors are causing it to be excreted in the urine, your risk of kidney stones may increase.

Poor absorption of calcium can be due to digestive problems or deficiencies in the substances required for calcium absorption (vitamin D and hydrochloric [stomach] acid). Overconsumption of milk and antacids (many people are now taking antacids as calcium supplements) can raise urinary calcium levels.[4] Caffeine, animal protein, and salt have also been linked to higher levels of calcium in the urine.[5] In addition, research has found that carbonated soft drinks may contribute to the formation of kidney stones.[6]

Kidney stones are a serious occurrence. Consult your doctor. The remedies here can help in passing a stone and/or preventing future stones, but should not be considered a substitute for medical care.

Essential Oils

Fennel is a diuretic (increases the flow of urine) and can help dissolve kidney stones, states aromatherapy authority Robert B. Tisserand. For general support of the kidneys, he cites Cedarwood, Clary, Eucalyptus, Juniper, and Sandalwood. Use in baths, or massage the painful area with a blend of 5 drops of essential oil per 2 teaspoons of vegetable oil.[7]

Flower Essences

Self-Heal can serve as a foundational healing agent for kidney stones. Other flower essences to address the specific emotions, mental attitude, and environmental conditions of the individual are recommended, states Patricia Kaminski, a flower essence therapist and codirector of the Flower Essence Society. Self-Heal supports the body's innate healing ability. Take 4 drops 2–4 times daily, or as needed.

Food Therapy

Eat:

Fiber, complex carbohydrates, green leafy and yellow vegetables (aside from high-oxalate greens), almonds, sardines, urinary tract cleansers (asparagus, celery, watermelon), foods high in magnesium, potassium, and vitamin B6. (For a list of foods containing these nutrients, see part 3, "Food Therapy," pp. 377, 378.) Drink plenty of water.

Avoid:

Excess sugar and salt, simple carbohydrates, high-fat foods, dairy foods, alcohol, rich and spicy foods, high-purine foods, high-oxalate foods. (For a list of foods containing these substances, see part 3, "Food Therapy," p. 377.)

Herbal Medicine

Hydrangea (*Hydrangea arborescens*) root capsules are excellent for kidney stones, states Joanne B. Mied, N.D., a naturopath, herbalist, and iridologist from Novato, California. (Note that hydrangea leaves are poisonous, but the root is not.) Take 9 capsules (325 mg each) daily until the pain is gone. Then cut back to 6 capsules daily. If the pain returns, go back up to 9. Drink lots of water, at least 8 glasses (8 ounces each) a day. Add a squeeze of fresh lemon to the water for an extra cleansing benefit.

Homeopathy

The following remedies are indicated for kidney stones, according to Dr. Barry Rose of the Royal London Homeopathic Hospital:[8]

Berberis: For usually left-sided kidney pain that is worse when standing, extends down to the bladder and down the back, is stabbing and tearing in nature, and accompanied by the constant desire to urinate.

Lycopodium: For usually right-sided kidney pain with painful urination, and a severe backache alleviated by the excretion of urine that contains a lot of red "sand."

Ocimum can: For right-sided pain with pain in the ureter, nausea, and frequent, painful urination in which there is red or yellow "gravel."

Sepia: When there is a "dragging sensation" in the bladder, a continual urge to urinate, and foul-smelling urine containing a reddish, clay-colored sediment.

Take the appropriate remedy in the highest potency available every 10 minutes until your symptoms improve, says Dr. Rose. Thereafter, take it periodically until the improvement holds.

Nutritional Supplements

If your kidney stones are the calcium oxalate type, as most are, supplementing with magnesium and vitamin B6 can effectively prevent a recurrence.[9] Naturopathic physician Alan Christianson, N.M.D., of Scottsdale, Arizona, recommends taking 400–600 mg of magnesium daily in 2–3 doses and 50 mg of vitamin B6 daily in one dose. You can take the magnesium on a long-term basis (for several years), but should take B6 only for 1 month. (Although it is extremely unlikely, vitamin B6 may cause neuralgia at doses over 100 mg taken daily for 3 months, notes Dr. Christianson.)

Reflexology

Kidney, bladder, ureters

Stone/Crystal Therapy

As an ongoing preventive measure, use nebula stone, which helps cleanse the kidneys, states Melody, author of the crystal reference series *Love Is in the Earth*. Take 3–5 drops of elixir 2–3 times daily. Also secure the stone over the kidneys (the lower back on each side) using hypoallergenic tape, and leave it on until you get relief. (For detailed instructions, see part 3, "Stone/Crystal Therapy," p. 403.)

Laryngitis

 See Also
Bacterial Infection
Sore Throat
Viral Infection

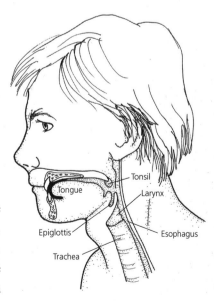

Laryngitis is inflammation of the larynx, or voice box, in the throat. Common symptoms are hoarseness, loss of the voice, a barking cough, and pain upon speaking. Laryngitis can be caused by a viral infection, overuse of the voice, loud shouting, exposure to cold or wet, or irritation from inhalants such as smoke, dust, or noxious vapors. If your laryngitis has not improved after a few days of treatment and resting your voice, seek medical assistance.

Essential Oils

In the middle of giving a lecture, herbalist Kathi Keville often demonstrates a simple essential oil remedy for laryngitis. "The students think I've taken the treatment for their benefit, but sometimes the therapy is all that allows me to complete the lecture," she comments. For this simple remedy, put 2 drops of Lavender essential oil in a bowl of steaming-hot water and inhale the steam. You can also do a steam with Eucalyptus or Peppermint essential oil; use 1/4 teaspoon of the oil to 3 cups boiled water. Drape a towel over your head and the bowl and inhale. Come out for fresh air as needed, but do at least 3 rounds of inhaling. Do this 2–3 times daily until your symptoms resolve.[1]

Flower Essences

Self-Heal and Yarrow Special Formula can serve as the foundational healing agents for laryngitis. Other flower essences to address the specific emotions, mental attitude, and environmental conditions of the individual are recommended, states Patricia Kaminski, a flower essence therapist and codirector of the Flower Essence Society. Self-Heal supports the body's innate healing ability. Yarrow Special Formula strengthens and protects against environmental toxicity and stress. Take 4 drops of each 2–4 times daily, or as needed.

Food Therapy

Eat:
Ginger, garlic.
Avoid:
Sugar, dairy, chocolate.

Herbal Medicine

Joanne B. Mied, N.D., a naturopath and herbalist based in Novato, California, recommends slippery elm (*Ulmus rubra, U. fulva*) bark tea for laryngitis. Open a capsule into a cup of boiled water and stir. Drink 1 cup at least 3 times daily, but you can drink it all day long if you like. Make sure to ingest the residue at the bottom of the cup as well.

A sage (*Salvia officinalis*) tea gargle is also useful for laryngitis, says herbalist David Hoffmann, M.N.I.M.H. Add 2 tablespoons of sage leaves to 1 pint of cold water, bring to boil, remove from heat, and let stand for 10 minutes. Strain the tea, and use it to gargle frequently throughout the day, reheating it as needed.[2]

Homeopathy

For laryngitis, Drs. Andrew Lockie and Nicola Geddes recommend the following homeopathic remedies:[3]

Aconite: If laryngitis is accompanied by a high fever; take 30c 4 times daily for up to 7 days.

Arg nit: If you lost your voice as a result of overuse in singing or shouting; take 6c 4 times daily for up to 6 days.

Phosphorus: If laryngitis is accompanied by a tickly, dry cough; take 6c 4 times daily for up to 7 days.

Nutritional Supplements

Propolis, zinc, and vitamins C and E are indicated for laryngitis, according to naturopathic physician Linda Rector Page, N.D., Ph.D. When the laryngitis is acute, take 500 mg of chewable vitamin C every hour. Suck on zinc gluconate or propolis lozenges every 2–3 hours as needed (do not exceed 30 mg of zinc in a day). Propolis, a plant resin collected by bees, is antibacterial and helps soothe inflamed mucous membranes. Take 400 IU of vitamin E daily as a preventive measure.[4]

Reflexology

Throat, sinuses (if involved)

Stone/Crystal Therapy

To alleviate laryngitis, place blue tourmaline at the throat for 8 hours, recommends Melody, author of the crystal reference series *Love Is in the Earth*. You can speed its effects if you also take it as an elixir (3–5 drops, 2–3 times or more daily). Stillbite placed at the throat for 8 hours is helpful, too. You can attach either stone with hypoallergenic tape or wear as a choker-type necklace. (For instructions on making an elixir, see part 3, "Stone/Crystal Therapy," p. 403.)

Other Remedies

Gargling alternately with lemon juice and black tea can help resolve laryngitis, say naturopathic physicians Mildred Jackson, N.D., and Terri Teague, N.D., D.C. Start with a lemon juice diluted in lukewarm water, then 1 hour later gargle with lukewarm black tea. Alternate every hour throughout the day. Do not drink the caffeine tea. Drs. Jackson and Teague note that the tannic acid in the black tea is soothing to the throat when alternated with the lemon.[5]

Memory Problems

Although less than optimal memory is generally associated with aging, memory lapses can occur at any age. In addition, a fading memory is not the inevitable consequence of growing older it was previously thought to be. Since factors that contribute to fuzziness in memory include poor diet, stress, overwork, some medications, and recreational drugs, there are obvious steps you can take to promote the longevity of your memory.

Poor circulation is another factor that can affect memory. Reduced blood flow (and the attendant reduction in oxygen, which is carried in the blood) to the brain compromises mental function. By improving your circulation through exercise and diet, you can help your mind, and your memory.

As neurotransmitters (the chemical messengers of the brain) are vital to the memory process, making sure that you are getting enough of the nutrients required in the production of neurotransmitters is another way to support optimal function of your brain and memory.

Note: Serious impairment of memory function is an indication of injury or disease and beyond the scope of this book.

Essential Oils

Rosemary is highly useful for memory improvement, notes herbalist Teresa Boardwine of Washington, Virginia. (See "Herbal Medicine" below.) It can also help with the brain drain of mental fatigue (what Boardwine calls "synapsus collapsus") and keep you awake when you have to drive or do mental work such as studying late at night.

There are numerous ways you can use Rosemary. Sniff Rosemary essential oil right from the bottle or put a few drops of it on a handkerchief and inhale. When you're driving or studying, tuck the handkerchief into your collar or apply the drops directly on the collar (oil can leave spots). At home or at work, you can put a few drops in water in an aromatherapy burner for diffusion in the air around you. Or use Rosemary oil in your bath. Add 10 drops of Rosemary oil to a tub of warm water, or "innoculate" your bath salts (5 drops of rosemary oil to 1 cup of bath salts).

You can even put Rosemary essential oil in your shampoo. The active constituents of the essential oil will be absorbed through your skin, enter the bloodstream, and increase oxygen flow to your brain. Cineole, an antioxidant constituent of rosemary, is able to pass through the blood-brain barrier, and has shown promise in protecting against Alzheimer's, notes Boardwine. To a 16-ounce bottle of shampoo, add 10–20 drops of Rosemary essential oil. You can use rosemary tincture instead of the essential oil; 1/2 ounce to 16 ounces of shampoo.

Flower Essences

Rosemary flower essence can help improve memory, states Richard Katz, founder of the Flower Essence Society. Take 4 drops under the tongue 2–4 times daily, as needed or on a maintenance basis.

Food Therapy

Eat:

Foods that contain the nutritional building blocks for neuotransmitters—kelp, wheat germ, tofu, salmon, foods high in choline and vitamins B1 and B12. (For a list of foods containing these nutrients, see part 3, "Food Therapy," pp. 376, 378.)

Avoid:

Refined sugar, processed foods, saturated fats, alcohol.

Herbal Medicine

To help improve the memory, herbalist Teresa Boardwine of Washington, Virginia, cites the oxygen-carrying plants rosemary and ginkgo. Increasing oxygen to the brain aids memory. (For rosemary, see "Essential Oils" above.) *Ginkgo biloba* has become popular and there are a lot of products to choose from. Not all are good quality. Look for tinctures derived from the whole plant. Take 1 dropperful 3 times daily. It is relatively slow-acting, so you need to take it for 4–6 weeks before you will notice results. Once you see improvement, you can switch to a maintenance dose of 1/2 dropperful twice daily.

Note: If you are on blood-thinning medication, you shouldn't use ginkgo. Active consituents in the herb called ginkgosides can act as blood thinners. Rosemary does not have blood-thinning properties, so use that herb instead.

Research has shown that ginkgo is one of the "four Gs" that enhance mental abilities, says herbalist Kathi Keville. The other three herbs in the quartet are gotu kola (*Centella asiatica*), ginseng (*Panax ginseng*), and Siberian ginseng (*Eleutherococcus senticosus*). Keville suggests the following formula to improve and preserve the memory: combine 1 teaspoon each of tinctures of ginkgo leaves and Siberian ginseng root with 1/2 teaspoon each of tinctures of gotu kola leaves and ginseng (*Panax*) root. Take half a dropperful 2–3 times daily. When an impending event or activity is going to require particular focus, take extra tincture an hour beforehand.[1]

Homeopathy

The following remedies are commonly indicated for memory problems, according to Dr. Barry Rose of the Royal London Homeopathic Hospital:[2]

Arg nit 12c: For poor memory in general.

Lycopodium 12c: If your memory is weak and your thoughts confused, and you make spelling errors.

Oleander 12c: If your memory is weak and your perception slow.

Take the appropriate remedy 2 times daily until your memory improves.

Nutritional Supplements

The following supplements can be beneficial in improving memory and preventing memory loss:[3]

Antioxidants: To neutralize free radicals that can damage brain cells, supplement daily with 1,000 mg of vitamin C, up to 10,000 IU of beta-carotene, and 100 mcg of selenium; antioxidants are more powerful when taken in combination rather than used singly.

Choline: Take 200–350 mg 2–3 times daily; necessary for the manufacture of acetylcholine (low levels of this neurotransmitter have been implicated in Alzheimer's disease[4]).

Lecithin: Take 1,200 mg with meals 2–3 times daily; found in soybeans, brewer's yeast, and wheat germ, lecithin is rich in choline and the B vitamins, which aid brain function.

Tyrosine: Take 500 mg on getting up in the morning, for 1–2 months; this amino acid is a precursor to the neurotransmitter norepinephrine, which influences memory. (Caution: do not take tyrosine if you are taking an MAO inhibitor drug.)

A beneficial commercial product aimed at improving memory is one that combines choline, vitamin B12, ginkgo, and gotu kola (see "Herbal Medicine" above).

Reflexology

Brain

Stone/Crystal Therapy

Fluorite, elestials, pyrite, calcite, and green tourmaline are useful stones for enhancing the memory, notes Katrina Raphaell, crystal healing therapist and author of the crystal reference series *The Crystal Trilogy*. Place three stones on your head, one over each eyebrow and one at the third eye (on the forehead, between the eyes). Leave the stones in place for 5 minutes while visualizing the health/memory benefits you desire. Do this 3 times daily. For ongoing benefits, wear the stone, hold it, or carry it in your pocket.

Other Remedies

Don't use aluminum cookware or deodorants or antacids that contain aluminum. Reseach suggests that higher than normal levels of aluminum in the body are a contributing factor in the development of Alzheimer's disease.[5]

Menstrual Cramps

Menstrual cramps, or spasms of pain in the lower abdominal region, typically begin just before or with the onset of menstruation, and may be accompanied by back pain. The medical term for menstrual cramps is "dysmenorrhea."

Pain associated with menstruation is considered by many to be a normal aspect of the menstrual cycle. This view is supported by the numbers: approximately 50 percent of menstruating women suffer menstrual cramps, and 10 percent of this group experience such severe cramps that they are incapacitated for several days of each period.[1]

The view of many alternative medicine practitioners, however, is that dysmenorrhea signals an imbalance of some kind. One form of implicated imbalance is an excess of estrogen in relation to progesterone (estrogen dominance).[2] An excess production of prostaglandins, hormone-like substances that regulate the contraction of the smooth muscle of the uterus, among other functions, has also been linked to painful menstruation. A high level of prostaglandins promotes uterine cramping.[3]

Other factors that may contribute to menstrual cramps are lack of exercise, fatigue, obesity, diet, smoking, and perhaps heredity. Serious medical conditions such as endometriosis can underlie dysmenorrhea. If the remedies below do not alleviate your cramps or you are one of those women who are incapacitated each month, you may want to get medical help to determine the cause of your menstrual problem.

Essential Oils

Medical aromatherapist Julia Fischer of Northern California offers an essential oil blend to ease menstrual cramps. Combine:

Lemon: 2 drops
Geranium: 2 drops
Clary Sage: 1 drop
Sage: 2 drops
Anise: 2 drops

Apply the undiluted blend to your lower abdomen and back as needed for cramps.

Flower Essences

For menstrual cramps, it works well to use flower essences internally and topically, says Patricia Kaminski, an herbalist and flower essence therapist from Nevada City, California. Take 4 drops each of Tiger Lily and Alpine Lily flower essences 2–4 times daily, or more often as needed. Some women do this as a maintenance dose for 6 months or longer to normalize conditions. Others have occasional flare-ups of cramping and begin this combination when premenstrual symptoms occur the week before their period. Still others take it only during menstruation. For a topical treatment, gently rub 1–2 tablespoons of Mugwort Moon Magic flower oil on the pelvic/abdominal area and cover with a hot compress. You can do this as often as needed to ease cramps.

Food Therapy

Eat:
Fiber, green vegetables, fish, tofu, eggs.
Emphasize warm foods over cold foods and make sure you are getting adequate protein in your diet (3–4 ounces per meal), adequate salt (miso soup can help with that), and enough fluids, says Paul Reilly,

N.D., L.Ac., a naturopathic physician and acupuncturist from Seattle, Washington.

Avoid:

Sugar, red meat, alcohol, coffee, saturated fats, gas-inducing foods, excess salt.

Avoid dairy unless you use products that are completely free of hormones, notes Dr. Reilly. Avoid sugar because, by increasing insulin, it increases the prostaglandins that promote cramping.

Herbal Medicine

To help relax your muscles and relieve pain, take either Jamaican dogwood (*Piscidia erythrina*), cramp bark (*Viburnum opulus*), or dong quai (*Angelica sinensis*), suggests Dr. Reilly. Take 2 capsules 3 times daily of one of these herbs, starting a day before your period and continuing during the days of cramping.

Menstrual cramps can arise from poor movement of the blood in the reproductive organs as a result of lymphatic congestion, says Michael Cottingham, a clinical herbalist from Silver City, New Mexico. (The lymph system is the body's filtering system. Lymph fluid flows between cells in the body, transporting beneficial substances between tissues and the bloodstream and also foreign substances for elimination from the body; lymph nodes filter the fluid.) Signs that chronic lymphatic backup may be the problem underlying your cramps include chronic constipation, varicose veins, feeling bloated or swollen throughout the month, not just during your period, and catching colds and flu often (due to the weakened immunity that accompanies lymphatic congestion).

Taking ocotillo (*Fouquieria splendens*) bark and red root (*Ceanothus americanus*) can help clear lymph congestion and reduce or eliminate the menstrual cramps, says Cottingham. Red root is well known for its ability to clear the lymphatic system. Ocotillo can help the intestines absorb fat, which is important in cases of lymph congestion, because the congestion is often the result of a high intake of fats or malabsorption of fats. Use equal parts of ocotillo bark and red root tinctures, and take 30 drops of the mix 3 times daily for a month. It is also important in lymph conditions to drink lots of water (at least 8 glasses daily) to aid the body in moving the congestion. "Water can be one of the ultimate first aid remedies," observes Cottingham. In addition, you may want to consider your diet and reduce your intake of saturated fats.

Julia Fischer recommends drinking herbal teas: peppermint, ginger, dandelion, red clover, and nettles.

Homeopathy

Naturopathic physicians Robert Ullmann, N.D., and Judyth Reichenberg-Ullmann, N.D., cite the following remedies for menstrual cramps:[4]

Belladonna: If there is throbbing pain and heavy, even gushing, bright red bleeding.

Mag phos: If the pain is alleviated by pressure and heat and you feel better after a hot bath.

Chamomilla: If the pain is very intense, the bleeding is profuse, dark, and clotted, and you are angry and highly irritable.

Take the appropriate remedy in a 30c potency every 15 minutes to 1 hour until your symptoms improve. Stop taking the remedy, repeat if the symptoms return. If there is no improvement with 3 doses, try a different remedy.

Nutritional Supplements

For treatment and prevention of cramps, Dr. Reilly recommends the following supplements in addition to a regular multivitamin/mineral:

Magnesium: "The first thing I think about for cramps is magnesium. It's a smooth muscle relaxant. Most Americans are deficient in it. They don't even consume the RDA [recommended daily allowance] for magnesium." Take 300–500 mg daily, Dr. Reilly suggests. In some people, magnesium excess can cause diarrhea, so you may need a lower dose. Sensitive people sometimes can take only 100 mg daily. Take as much within the dosage range as you can without diarrhea. Use magnesium aspartate or magnesium glyccinate. These forms are much less likely to produce loose stools.

Magnesium needs to be taken in balance with calcium, but between diet and a multivitamin/mineral, most of us get plenty of calcium, so there is no need to add more. If you consume less than 1,000 mg of calcium daily, between your diet and regular supplement, take or eat enough calcium to bring your total daily intake up to 1000 mg. (Note: 3 ounces of cheddar cheese has around 600 mg of calcium.)

Vitamin B6: 100 mg daily; helps the body utilize magnesium.

Cod liver oil: 1 tablespoon daily; provides EPA (eicosapentaenoic acid, an omega-3 essential fatty acid) and vitamin D, which are necessary for the absorption of calcium and magnesium. Take this supplement on an ongoing basis, not just for relief of cramps.

Bromelain: 300–500 mg on an empty stomach 3 times daily; a smooth muscle relaxant derived from pineapple enzymes.

Start taking all of the above—with the exception of cod liver oil, which you should take all the time—the day before your period and continue until your cramps typically subside.

Additionally, supplementing with omega-6 essential fatty acids, notably gamma-linolenic acid (GLA), found in evening primrose, black currant, and borage oils, can help counteract the excess prostaglandins that contribute to menstrual cramping. Take 500–1,000 mg of one of the oils 2 times a day for 3 months.[5]

Reflexology

Uterus, ovaries, fallopian tubes, pituitary gland, thyroid, pancreas, lumbar spine, intestines, lymphatic system

Stone/Crystal Therapy

To ease menstrual cramps, use gem silica, amethyst, smoky quartz, larimar/cuprite, or chrysoprase, states crystal healing therapist Katrina Raphaell of Kapaa, Hawaii. Place the stone directly on your lower abdomen over the site of the cramping. Leave the stone there for 5 minutes while visualizing your health goal. Do this 3 times daily. In between treatments, wear the stone, hold it, or carry it in your pocket for continual healing effects.

Other Remedies

Hot packs and sitz baths can help with cramps, says Dr. Reilly. Use a hot water bottle, a gel pack, or even rock salt heated in the oven and put in a pillowcase. A sitz bath (a special tub that allows you to immerse your pelvic region in water with your legs out of the tub; you can use a washtub big enough for you to sit in) with hot water up to your navel focuses heat on the uterus and helps relieve cramping.

Migraine

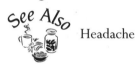 Headache

A migraine is a particularly excruciating type of headache. The pain can be disabling and is often accompanied by visual disturbances (spots, flashes, zigzags of light, and blurring), sensitivity to light, nausea, and vomiting. An "aura" of visual symptoms, along with numbness or tingling in the limbs, may forewarn the sufferer of an impending attack. The pain begins on one side of the head, often behind or above one eye, may or may not expand to a larger area, and lasts for hours or even days.

Until recently, science and medicine pointed to the cause of migraines as a vascular dysfunction; specifically, abnormal dilation of arteries in the brain. New findings, however, indicate that blood vessels are not the initial problem. Rather, it is abnormally excitable brain nerve cells (neurons) that, when triggered, fire off electrical pulses that, in turn, activate pain centers in the brain stem, resulting in a migraine headache. Changes in blood flow may occur in response to the electrical signals, but the blood vessels are not the instigators.[1]

Migraine triggers include food allergies, food additives, caffeine, stress, hormonal changes, and certain medications. As 80 percent to 90 percent of those afflicted with migraines have food allergies and research has demonstrated that eliminating the problem foods from the diet reduces or eradicates the symptoms of migraine,[2] it may be advisable for you to determine if you suffer from food allergies as well.

Preventing a full-blown migraine is easier than trying to get rid of the pain once it starts. Knowing the substances or conditions that trigger your migraine enables you to take steps toward avoiding them. The warning of the aura, which many migraine sufferers experience, makes that possible as well. Implementing the remedies here at the first sign of an impending migraine can help stop its progression.

Essential Oils

Coriander, Ginger, and Marjoram essential oils can help alleviate a migraine, says Jeanne Rose, an aromatherapist and herbalist based in San Francisco, California. Rub the chosen oil on the temples or other painful area of the head, or inhale via another essential oil delivery method, as needed.[3]

Flower Essences

The flower essence remedies cited for headache will probably be helpful for a migraine as well, says Richard Katz, founder of the Flower Essence Society, but he notes that the research compiled by the Flower Essence Society and on which they base their recommendations for flower essence treatment involved cases of headache, not necessarily of the migraine type. (See "Headache.")

Food Therapy

Eat:

Garlic, onion, flaxseed oil, cold-water fish, foods high in magnesium (see part 3, "Food Therapy," p. 376, 377).

Avoid:

Sugar, processed foods, fried foods, red meat, dairy, food additives (especially MSG), aspartame, nitrite-cured meats (hot dogs, salami, bacon, sausage, bologna), citrus, chocolate (contains phenylethylamine, a headache-triggering amine), red wine and cheese (high in tyramine, another headache trigger), food allergens, nightshade vegetables, food salicylates. (For a list of foods containing these substances, see part 3, "Food Therapy," p. 377.)

Herbal Medicine

Feverfew (*Tanacetum parthenium*) has a long tradition of use in treating and preventing migraines. Research has shown that the herb can reduce both the frequency and severity of the attack.[4] The herb is an anti-inflammatory and a vasodilator (helps to relax blood vessels). Sue Reynolds, M.S.W., L.M.T., a certified herbalist and aromatherapist from Goleta, California, recommends taking 2–4 capsules of high-parthenolide feverfew at the onset of a migraine, and 1–6 capsules daily as prevention. (Parthenolides are the active components of the herb.)

Homeopathy

Homeopathic physician Michael G. Carlston, M.D., of Santa Rosa, California, recommends the following:

Sanguinaria: For sharp, intense right-sided pain.
Spigelia: For sharp, intense left-sided pain accompanied by pounding of the heart.

In both cases, take a 12c or 30c potency of the remedy, every 1–2 hours for the duration of the migraine.

Nutritional Supplements

Joanne B. Mied, N.D., a naturopath, herbalist, and iridologist from Novato, California, suffered from regular migraines for years. She tried everything, but what finally resolved the problem was black currant oil, an essential fatty acid (EFA) supplement. After 3 months of taking it, Dr. Mied's headaches were gone. As migraines are an inflammatory problem, and in women often involve hormonal imbalance, EFAs are useful because they can help redress both issues, Dr. Mied explains. Take 9 capsules (250 mg each) of black currant oil daily. After you get results, you can reduce the amount according to your symptoms and find the maintenance dose that works for you.

As a supplemental protocol to prevent and relieve migraines, naturopathic physician Bradley Bongiovanni, N.D., of Independence, Ohio, recommends the following, which can all be taken on an ongoing basis:

Magnesium citrate: 800–1,000 mg, divided through the day.
Vitamin D: 200 IU 2–3 times daily.
Vitamin B2 (riboflavin): 100 mg 2–3 times daily; research has shown
    vitamin B2 to be useful in reducing migraines.[5]
Flaxseed oil: 1,000 mg 3 times daily; anti-inflammatory.

Reflexology

Head/brain, neck, sinuses, spine (all), solar plexus, liver

Stone/Crystal Therapy

Green fluorite and blue smithsonite are useful stones for migraine, according to Katrina Raphaell, crystal healing therapist and founder of the Crystal Academy of Advanced Healing Arts in Kapaa, Hawaii. Place the stone directly on the site of the pain in your head. Leave the stone in place for 5 minutes while visualizing your health goal. Do this 3 times daily. For ongoing healing benefits, wear the stone, hold it, or carry it in your pocket.

Other Remedies

In the years of pain before Dr. Mied finally found the solution to her migraines, the only thing that brought relief was to sit with her feet in hot water until the sweat came out on her forehead. It could knock out the migraine if she caught it early, Dr. Mied reports, but could also ease the severity if the migraine was already under way. When she was at work or traveling, running her hands under hot water or immersing them in a sink of hot water also helped, although it was not as effective as the foot soak.

Motion Sickness

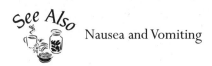

See Also — Nausea and Vomiting

Symptoms of nausea, dizziness, headache, and sleepiness characterize motion sickness, which is induced by the movements of a vehicle in which one is riding. Seasickness, airsickness, and carsickness are all forms of this malady, which can progress to vomiting.

Inner ear imbalance created by the overstimulation of travel motion and contradictory sensory signals (sitting in one place while the world moves by) produces motion sickness. Hunger, anxiety, and odors such as cigarette smoke can exacerbate the problem.[1]

As motion sickness usually does not end with the cessation of motion, it is best to practice prevention rather than treatment. If you know you are prone to motion sickness, using the remedies here can help you stop it before it starts.

Essential Oils

Lavender and Peppermint essential oils can provide relief from motion sickness, says Kurt Schnaubelt, Ph.D., scientific director of the Pacific Institute of Aromatherapy in San Rafael, California. Topically, apply the oil once at the acute stage; massage 1 drop of each on your temples. After an hour, apply again, if needed. Or you can blend 10 parts Lavender with 1 part Peppermint and rub some of the blend on your temples, the soles of your feet, and your solar plexus (below the ribs, a few inches above the navel). Do this as a preventive measure before embarking on your motion excursion, and repeat if symptoms develop.

You can also smell the oil instead. Simply put a few drops of either oil on a hankerchief, hold it under your nose, and inhale. Finally, instead of as a topical or inhaled application, you can take 1 drop of Peppermint essential oil internally, provided it is a therapeutic quality oil. One drop is sufficient.

Flower Essences

Self-Heal can serve as a foundational healing agent for motion sickness. Other flower essences to address the specific emotions, mental attitude, and environmental conditions of the individual are recommended, states Patricia Kaminski, a flower essence therapist and codirector of the Flower Essence Society. Self-Heal supports the body's innate healing ability. Take 4 drops 2–4 times daily, or as needed.

Food Therapy

Eat:

Easily digested food before your trip, ginger.

Avoid:

Fried or fatty foods before your trip; reduce sugar and simple carbohydrates to prevent blood sugar fluctuations.

Herbal Medicine

Ginger (*Zingiber officinale*) is widely known as a remedy for motion sickness. Clinical herbalist Michael Cottingham, of Silver City, New Mexico, recommends chewing crystallized ginger to promote circulation and relieve motion sickness. Eat a few pieces during your trip. This is a great remedy for children who get carsick. Children 8 years and older can nibble on 1–2 pieces over the space of a 4-hour drive; give younger children less.

Make sure to buy a high-quality crystallized ginger, so you get the benefits of the ginger. You can tell it's good if you feel a warming on your tongue after you bite into a piece. To ensure quality, you can make your own crystallized ginger. Here is Cottingham's recipe. Peel the outer bark from 2 pounds of fresh ginger root, cut the roots into slices the thickness of checkers, and boil in sugar syrup. To make the sugar syrup, bring 2 quarts of water to a boil, then add sugar, stirring until it is dissolved. Add as much sugar as the water can hold and still dissolve; about 5 cups of sugar. After boiling the ginger in the syrup for 30–40 minutes, remove the slices and lay them on a cookie sheet. Bake in the oven at 200 degrees for 5–6 hours.

If you prefer to take ginger in capsule form, take 3 capsules (500 mg each) with meals before traveling, recommends Joanne B. Mied,

N.D., a naturopath and herbalist based in Novato, California. While traveling on a boat or ship, take 3 capsules 3 times daily.

Homeopathy

For motion sickness, Michael G. Carlston, M.D., a homeopathic physician from Santa Rosa, California, suggests Tabacum when nausea predominates and Cocculus indicus when dizziness is predominant. Take the appropriate remedy in a 12c or 30c potency every 1–2 hours when motion sickness is acute. Pay attention to your symptoms. When you are no longer experiencing motion sickness, don't continue to take the remedy.

Nutritional Supplements

The following supplements can help prevent motion sickness, say James F. Balch, M.D., and Phyllis A. Balch, C.N.C.:[2]

Magnesium: Take 500 mg 1 hour before your trip.
Vitamin B6 (pyridoxine): Take 100 mg 1 hour before your trip, and another 100 mg 2 hours later.
Charcoal tablets: Take 5 tablets 1 hour before your trip.

Reflexology

Ear, diaphragm, pituitary gland, neck, spine

Stone/Crystal Therapy

For motion sickness, Melody, author of the crystal reference series *Love Is in the Earth*, recommends aurora borealis stone or brunckite placed at both wrists and taken as an elixir (3–5 drops 3 times daily). Implement both 3 days prior to the expected motion. (For instructions on making an elixir, see part 3, "Stone/Crystal Therapy," p. 403.)

Other Remedies

Massaging the acupressure point PC-6 (the inside of the wrist, two thumb widths above the wrist crease and between the tendons) is a traditional treatment for motion sickness. Wristbands with a bead that can be positioned to apply proper pressure to that point are available at drugstores, with instructions for placing the bead.

Muscle Aches and Pains

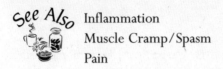

See Also   Inflammation
Muscle Cramp/Spasm
Pain

Sore muscles can result from overuse, injury or impact, unaccustomed activity or movement, more intense exercise than usual, maintaining one position for a prolonged period, and psychological/emotional stress. Muscle pain and aching is the result of stretching or overworking the fibers of the muscle. Swelling and inflammation can be involved if the muscle has been seriously overworked. Stressing the muscle fibers too much leads to a pulled or strained muscle.

The remedies here can help alleviate the minor aches and pains that we all experience at some point in our lives. Chronic pain signals a serious disorder and is beyond the purview of this book.

Essential Oils

To ease sore and overworked muscles, herbalist Colleen K. Dodt recommends massage with Lavender and Peppermint essential oils. Add 5 drops of each essential oil to 4 teaspoons (20 ml) of almond base oil. Use for massage as needed for muscle aches and pains.[1]

Flower Essences

Take Dandelion flower essence at a dosage of 4 drops under the tongue 2–4 times daily, or more frequently if needed, says Richard Katz, naturalist and founder of the Flower Essence Society. Also, use Dandelion Dynamo flower oil for daily baths and massages until soreness subsides. (For instructions on using flower essences in baths and massage oil, see part 3, "Flower Essences," "Directions for Use," p. 372.)

Food Therapy

Eat pineapple and papaya by themselves, not with other foods, to get the anti-inflammatory effect of the enzymes these fruits contain, suggests Nick Buratovich, N.M.D., a naturopathic physician from Tempe, Arizona. Foods rich in vitamins B3 and B6 are also indicated. (For a list of foods containing these nutrients, see part 3, "Food Therapy," p. 378.)

Dr. Buratovich recommends avoiding coffee and other forms of caffeine (aside from green tea) because caffeine blocks endorphin receptors in the brain. As endorphins facilitate pain relief, people who consume a lot of caffeine tend to have a low threshold of pain. Avoid animal products because they contain arachidonic acid, which promotes inflammation, says Dr. Buratovich, and you may also want to avoid foods in the nightshade family (see part 3, "Food Therapy," p. 377). In some people, nightshades increase inflammation via an allergic reaction.

Herbal Medicine

For muscle aches and pains, herbalist Earl Mindell, R.Ph., Ph.D., recommends eucalyptus (*Eucalyptus spp.*) ointment, which is warming and penetrating. Apply the ointment (available commercially) to the affected area, as needed. As a natural pain reliever to take internally, Dr. Mindell cites white willow (*Salix alba*) bark. White willow contains salicylates, the plant precursors of salicylic acid, the active ingredient in aspirin. While aspirin can irritate the stomach, however, white willow is beneficial to the digestive system. Take 2 tablets every 3–4 hours, as needed for pain.[2]

The traditional Chinese medicine Tiger Balm is another ointment for sore muscles containing warming, penetrating oils: in this case, camphor, menthol, cajeput, and clove. Use as directed. Tiger Balm is widely available in health food and other stores.

Homeopathy

Arnica montana, taken internally and applied topically, is the remedy of choice for muscle aches and pains. Maesimund B. Panos, M.D., recommends massaging the affected area with homeopathic arnica oil or ointment several times daily, as needed. Take the oral Arnica remedy in a 6x potency 3–4 times daily, or as needed. Decrease the frequency as symptoms improve. Stop taking the remedy when the improvement is well established.[3]

Nutritional Supplements

To relieve muscle aches and pains, Dr. Buratovich has found the following supplements useful:

DLPA (D,L-phenylalanine): 750 mg 3 times daily before meals for 1–3 weeks; a pain-relieving amino acid.

Bromelain: 2 capsules on an empty stomach 3 times daily until the pain is resolved; an anti-inflammatory enzyme compound found in pineapple.

Reflexology

Treat the area of the foot corresponding to the part of the body where your muscles are sore.

Stone/Crystal Therapy

Use green aventurine, green calcite, or black tourmaline, recommends crystal healing therapist Katrina Raphaell of Kapaa, Hawaii. Place the stone directly on the site of the muscle ache or pain. Visualizing your health goal, leave the stone in place for 5 minutes. Do this 3 times daily. Wear the stone, hold it, or carry it in your pocket for ongoing healing.

Muscle Cramp/Spasm

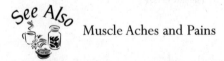 Muscle Aches and Pains

A muscle spasm is a sudden and involuntary movement or muscle contraction caused by tissue trauma or irritation. A spasm can be intermittent or sustained. Strong, painful, and sustained spasms are termed muscle cramps. Excessive sweating, as in exercise or heat, can produce a muscle cramp, as dehydration, a low salt level in the body, and electrolyte imbalance are all causes of cramping. Moving the involved muscle in a gentle stretch or flex can usually alleviate an exercise-induced cramp.

Nutritional deficiencies, particularly a skewed ratio of calcium to magnesium or a deficiency in vitamin E, also play a role in a tendency to cramp. Poor circulation is another cause, and may be a factor in the common phenomenon of night cramps, although the precise cause is unknown. Night cramps typically affect the legs and the feet.

Essential Oils

An essential oil massage can alleviate a muscle cramp or spasm and can be used preventively for nighttime cramping, says herbalist Penelope Ody. Combine 5 drops each of Ginger, Thyme, and Lavender essential oils in 1 tablespoon of almond oil. Massage the afflicted muscle, as needed. If you are prone to leg cramps during the night, massage your legs with this blend before going to sleep.[1]

Flower Essences

To relieve muscle cramps or spasms, apply Arnica Alleve flower oil on the affected area 2–4 times daily, recommends flower essence therapist Patricia Kaminski of Nevada City, California.

Food Therapy

Eat:

Foods high in vitamin E, potassium, and magnesium. (For a list of foods containing these nutrients, see part 3, "Food Therapy," pp. 377, 378.) Drink plenty of water.

Avoid:

Refined sugar, processed foods, soft drinks, food preservatives.

Herbal Medicine

Cramp bark (*Viburnum opulus*) and black haw (*Viburnum prunifolium*) are antispasmodic and can ease muscle cramps and spasms. Take one of these herbs as a tincture during an acute episode, says herbalist Teresa Boardwine of Washington, Virginia. Her recommended dosage is 1 dropperful every hour (but not more than 5 times) until cramps diminish. You should take the tincture with a little food, such as saltine crackers.

Homeopathy

For relief from a muscle cramp, take Magnesia phosphorica 6c at 5-minute intervals until there is a marked improvement. One dose may be sufficient. This remedy is particularly helpful for writer's cramp and cramping due to heavy exercise.[2]

Nutritional Supplements

Magnesium is a smooth muscle tranquilizer and can help prevent cramps and spasms, says Teresa Boardwine. If you are prone to these painful muscle contractions, add 500 mg, taken in one dose, to your regular multivitamin/mineral regimen. Do this for a month and see if it reduces the number of cramping episodes you experience. If it does, you can continue taking it as maintenance. Reduce the dosage gradually, first cutting down to taking 500 mg 5 times a week, then 3 times per week.

Naturopathic physician Nick Buratovich, N.M.D, of Tempe, Arizona, notes that magnesium can also produce rapid results for acute muscle cramp or spasm. He suggests taking calcium, another antispasmodic supplement, as well, along with vitamin E to increase circulation, as contracted muscles have a reduced blood supply. Here are his recommended doses:

Calcium lactate or calcium citrate: These chelated forms of calcium are the most easily absorbed. Take 500 mg 2–4 times daily until you get relief. Calcium both decreases muscular contraction and is a nervous system relaxant.

Magnesium glycinate: This form of magnesium is most easily absorbed and less likely to cause the diarrhea some people get when they take magnesium. Take 500 mg 1–3 times daily until you get relief. Magnesium can work surprisingly quickly to ease a muscle cramp or spasm. Note that muscle cramps are one of the signs of magnesium deficiency.

Vitamin E: 200 IU 4 times daily after meals for 1 month.

Reflexology

Treat the area of the foot corresponding to the part of the body where your spasm is located. You can also treat the solar plexus area on the foot to promote relaxation.

Stone/Crystal Therapy

Place holmquistite or stellerite on the site of the cramp or spasm for 4–6 hours or 8–10 hours, respectively, suggests Melody, author of the crystal reference series *Love Is in the Earth*. Use hypoallergenic tape to attach the stone. Alternate this treatment with taking 3–5 drops on an elixir of either stone 3 times daily. Due to possible lead content of these particular stones, prepare the elixir by placing the stone in a glass container, and put that container in the distilled water, rather than immersing the stone directly. Proceed with the elixir preparation as detailed in part 3, "Stone/Crystal Therapy," p. 403.

Nail Problems (Brittle, Ingrown)

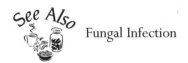 Fungal Infection

Brittle nails (nails that break, split, or chip easily) can be a sign of various nutritional deficiencies—iron, calcium, vitamin D, vitamin A, or protein (the B vitamins)—as well as a deficit of hydrochloric acid (HCl), the acid in the stomach that aids in digestion. A fungal infection can also cause nails to become brittle.

As outposts in the supply of nutrients by the blood, nails are good indicators of potential problems in the body. Deficiencies will affect the nails before they begin to have an impact on tissues that are better "fed" by the blood. Therefore, it is a good idea to keep an eye on your nails and keep them in good health.

When the edge on one or both sides of the nail grows into the soft tissue, it is known as an ingrown nail. Typically occurring on the big toe, it can become inflamed, quite painful, and susceptible to bacterial infection. An ingrown nail can be caused by improper nail trimming and/or ill-fitting shoes.

Essential Oils

To prevent infection in an ingrowing toenail, aromatherapist Valerie Ann Worwood recommends massaging the area daily with a blend of 10 drops each of Lavender and Tea Tree (*Melaleuca alternifolia*) essential oils in 1 tablespoon of vegetable oil.[1]

To strengthen brittle nails, blend 6 drops each of Lavender, Bay, and Sandalwood essential oils in 6 ounces of warm sesame or soy oil. Soak your nails for 15 minutes 1–2 times per week as long as needed.[2]

Flower Essences

Self-Heal can serve as a foundational healing agent for nail problems. Other flower essences to address the specific emotions, mental attitude, and environmental conditions of the individual are recommended, states Patricia Kaminski, a flower essence therapist and codirector of the Flower Essence Society. Self-Heal supports the body's innate healing ability. Take 4 drops 2–4 times daily, or as needed.

Food Therapy

Eat:

Eggs, more protein and fewer carbohydrates, cold-water fish, foods high in biotin, sulphur, and silica (For a list of foods containing these nutrients, see part 3, "Food Therapy," pp. 376, 378.)

Avoid:

Refined sugar, alcohol.

Herbal Medicine

"In general, the best remedy for nail problems is homeopathic Silica [see below] or one of the herbs containing high levels of silica," says Matthew Wood, an herbalist from Minnetrista, Minnesota. Herbs rich in silica, which helps build strong nails, include horsetail (*Equisetum arvense*), oatseed, and oatstraw (both *Avena sativa*). These herbs and homeopathic Silica are beneficial for splitting nails, hangnails, irritation in the bed of the nail, and ridged nails. They can also alleviate nail biting. Take 3–5 drops of tincture of horsetail, oatseed, or oatstraw, singly or in combination, 1–3 times daily for 6 weeks.

Homeopathy

Silica is an excellent homeopathic remedy for nail problems, as noted by Matthew Wood above. Take in a 6c potency once daily for a week, then once weekly for about 6 weeks. Discontinue taking when your symptoms improve.

For brittle nails, ingrown toenails, and when the ends of the toes and fingers are red, swollen, and dead-feeling, Dr. Barry Rose of the Royal London Homeopathic Hospital points to Thuja occidentalis 6c as the remedy. For brittle nails that grow out of shape, Dr. Rose suggests Antimonium crudum 6c. The dosage for either remedy is 3 times a day until your symptoms begin to subside; restart the remedy if the condition relapses.[3]

Nutritional Supplements

For brittle nails, take the mineral silica, says Amanda McQuade Crawford, M.N.I.M.H., Dip.Phyto., a medical herbalist from Ojai, California. Silica helps build strong nails. Take the supplement according to the manufacturer's dosage.

Nutritionist Ann Louise Gittleman, N.D., C.N.S., M.S., recommends the following supplements to restore health to brittle nails:[4]

MSM (methylsulfonylmethane): Take 500 mg 3 times daily; a source of sulfur, a necessary nutrient for healthy nails, hair, and skin.
Essential fatty acids: Take 1–2 tablespoons of flaxseed oil or flaxseed with evening primrose oil. Or you can take GLA (gamma-linolenic acid), the essential fatty acid found in evening primrose oil, in capsule form; take 2,000 mg of GLA daily.
Vitamin B complex: Take 100 mg 2 times daily for at least 2 months.
Biotin: Take extra biotin, 2.5–5 mg daily until your nails are healthy again; biotin is a member of the vitamin B family.

Stone/Crystal Therapy

Apatite is a good stone for nail problems, states crystal healing therapist Katrina Raphaell of Kapaa, Hawaii. Place the stone directly on the affected nail or nails. Keep it in place for 5 minutes while visualizing your health goal. Do this 3 times daily. Wear the stone, hold it, or carry it in your pocket for continual healing benefits.

Other Remedies

Apply lemon juice to your nails in the morning and again at night for a week.[5]

Putting apple cider vinegar on the nails can also strengthen them, according to Dr. Gittleman.

Nausea and Vomiting

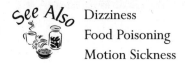 **See Also** Dizziness
Food Poisoning
Motion Sickness

Nausea is feeling queasy or sick to one's stomach. It may or may not lead to vomiting, the ejection of the stomach's contents through the mouth. Both have numerous causes, including food or other poisoning, bacterial or viral infections, inner ear problems, intestinal parasites, morning sickness in pregnancy, motion sickness, migraine headache, intoxication, overeating, certain medications, and stress, anxiety, or shock.

Nausea and/or vomiting can also signal a serious illness or disease. If you cannot determine a reasonable cause for your nausea or your nausea and vomiting persist, seek medical attention.

Essential Oils

Inhaling Cardamon, Lavender, or Peppermint is a quick remedy for nausea, according to aromatherapy authority Robert B. Tisserand. Peppermint "relieves nausea almost instantaneously," he says.[1] Sprinkle a few drops on a handkerchief or tissue and inhale the aroma, as needed.

Gently massaging the abdomen with Chamomile, Lavender, Lemon, or Peppermint essential oils, or putting a few drops on a hot compress placed over the stomach, can ease vomiting, according to Patricia Davis, founder of the London School of Aromatherapy. Repeat as needed.[2]

Flower Essences

Self-Heal can serve as a foundational healing agent for nausea and vomiting. Other flower essences to address the specific emotions, mental attitude, and environmental conditions of the individual are recommended, states Patricia Kaminski, a flower essence therapist and codirector of the Flower Essence Society. Self-Heal supports the body's innate healing ability. Take 4 drops 2–4 times daily, or as needed.

Food Therapy

Eat:

Bland, low-fat food, white basmati rice, miso soup; drink clear liquids to avoid dehydration if possible.

Avoid:

Soft drinks, spicy foods.

Herbal Medicine

Jody E. Noé, M.S., N.D., a naturopathic physician from Brattleboro, Vermont, recommends an herbal tea formula. Combine equal parts of catnip (*Nepeta cataria*), chamomile (*Matricaria recutita*), and a mint herb of your choice. Catnip is best fresh and is safe for all ages. Adjust the mint to taste if you find it too strong. Use 1 tablespoon of the mixture per 1–1/2 to 2 cups of boiled water. Let steep for 15 minutes and strain. Drink as needed for nausea or vomiting. You can also add a decoction of ginger (*Zingiber officinale*) or ginger syrup to the tea, or chew ginger candy. Note that ginger can be too stimulating for children and elders. Adjust as needed. To make the decoction, boil sliced ginger in water for 15 minutes.

Naturopathic physician David R. Field, N.D., L.Ac., of Santa Rosa, California, recommends the following herbs to calm the stomach:

DGL (deglycrrhizinated licorice): This is licorice root from which the potentially irritating glycyrrhizinic acid has been removed; DGL is soothing to the lining of the stomach. Open 1–2 capsules into 1/2 cup of cool water. Let it sit for 5–10 minutes. Drink this amount 2–3 times daily.

Slippery elm (*Ulmus rubra, U. fulva*): Take in the same way as DGL. This herb has a soothing effect on mucous membranes such as the stomach lining.

Ginger: Take 2 capsules 3–4 times daily as needed. Or drink ginger tea. Put 1 tablespoon of freshly grated ginger in 2 cups of boiled water, steep for 3 minutes, and then strain. Drink as needed for an upset stomach.

Homeopathy

The following are a few of the many homeopathic remedies indicated for nausea and vomiting:[3]

Ipecac: Indicated for terrible nausea or a "hanging down" sensation in the stomach such that nothing gives relief, even vomiting; a clean, red tongue

Nux vom: Indicated for nausea usually accompanied by cramps and painful vomiting or unproductive attempts to vomit, worsened by anger and alcohol.

Phosphorus: Indicated for nausea and vomiting accompanied by burning in the stomach and a craving for cold drinks to soothe it, but inability to hold the liquid down once it becomes warm in the stomach; worsened by warm drinks and putting hands in warm water.

Sepia: Indicated for terrible nausea with an empty feeling in the stomach, worse in the morning, and with motion, post-nasal drip, odors, and the thought of food; indicated for motion sickness.

Veratrum: Indicated for severe vomiting, sometimes projectile in nature, often accompanied by diarrhea, chills, and cold perspiration, particularly on the forehead; may be the result of vertigo.

Take the appropriate remedy at a 30c potency after vomiting or when nauseous, up to 6 times in a day.

Nutritional Supplements

To ameliorate nausea, naturopathic physician Linda Rector Page, N.D., Ph.D., recommends vitamin B6 (shown in studies to relieve nausea) and activated charcoal. The dosage for vitamin B6 is 50–100 mg; for charcoal, 500–1,000 mg.[4] Activated charcoal absorbs toxins and removes them from the body.

Reflexology

Stomach, diaphragm, solar plexus

Stone/Crystal Therapy

Green calcite, gold calcite, or peridot (green garnet) can help ease nausea and vomiting, says Katrina Raphaell, crystal healing therapist and founder of the Crystal Academy of Advanced Healing Arts in Kapaa, Hawaii. Place the stone directly on your abdomen over the area where your stomach distress is greatest. Leave the stone there for 5 minutes while visualizing your health goal. Do this 3 times daily. In between treatments, wear the stone, hold it, or carry it in your pocket for continued effect.

Other Remedies

Apple cider vinegar or fresh lemon juice can ease nausea. Put 1/2 to 1 teaspoon of vinegar and a bit of honey in 1 cup of warm water. For the lemon remedy, use the juice of half a lemon (it only works with fresh lemon juice) instead of the vinegar; the honey is optional. In either case, sip the mixture slowly.[5]

Nosebleed

Hemorrhage from the nose, known medically as epistaxis, can be caused by something as simple as strong blowing of the nose. This is because the lining of the nose is quite thin and it doesn't take much to break a capillary. A blow to the head, very dry air, atmospheric pressure change, infections affecting the nasal passages or sinuses, and nose-picking can also cause nose bleeding. Vitamin C deficiency and aspirin use may make you more prone to nosebleeds.[1]

The majority of nosebleeds involve capillary rupture in and blood flow from the front part of the nose. Although it may look gruesome, this type of hemorrhage is relatively easy to stop. Contrary to conventional wisdom, do not tilt your head back. Rather, sit down, lean forward slightly, and use your thumb and index finger to pinch your nostrils closed at the top (where the bone ends) for a few minutes, until the bleeding stops.

As with many other conditions in this book, nosebleeds can be an indication of a serious underlying disorder. If you suffer from recurrent nosebleeds or your nosebleed is in the rear of your nose (the blood runs into your throat), get medical care.

Essential Oils

Lemon is haemostatic, meaning it stops bleeding. Put a few drops of Lemon essential oil on a cotton swab and gently dab in the nostril(s).[2]

Flower Essences

To help calm the body or ease panic during a nosebleed, take Five Flower Formula, says naturalist Richard Katz of Nevada City, California. Take 4 drops hourly, or more often as needed. Yarrow and Pink Yarrow flower essences can be helpful in cases of nosebleed as a longer-term treatment for those who tend to bleed easily. Take 4 drops of each 2–4 times daily for several months.

Food Therapy

Eat:

Citrus fruit, dark green, leafy vegetables, other foods high in vitamins C and K. (For a list of foods containing these nutrients, see part 3, "Food Therapy," p. 378.)

Avoid:

Refined sugar.

Herbal Medicine

For nosebleed, Amanda McQuade Crawford, M.N.I.M.H., Dip. Phyto., a medical herbalist from Ojai, California, suggests plantain (*Plantago major*) or yarrow (*Achillea millefolium*) leaf. Yarrow is an astringent, which means it exerts a binding action on mucous membranes, tightening the tissue. Plantain has both astringent and soothing effects. Chop the fresh leaves of either herb and press out the juice. Holding the head back, rather than forward, use a cotton swab to dab up to 1/4 teaspoon of the juice gently in the affected nostril(s). You can repeat this 2–3 times if the bleeding continues for more than 5–7 minutes.

Homeopathy

Homeopathic physician Michael G. Carlston, M.D., of Santa Rosa, California, recommends the following remedies for nosebleed:

Phosphorus: When the blood is bright red and flowing, and you are thirsty for cool drinks.
Hamamelis: If the nosebleed is a dripping one.

Take the appropriate remedy in a 12c or 30c potency, followed by another dose after 10–15 minutes.

Nutritional Supplements

Make sure your diet is providing you with enough vitamin K, which is needed for proper blood clotting.

You can use vitamin E to help heal the nasal lining once the bleeding is under control. Use the liquid form or break open a capsule and gently dab the contents on the inside of the nose.[3]

Reflexology

Nose

Other Remedies

Apply ice or a cold compress to the nose.

Soak a cotton ball with lemon juice and gently place it in the affected nostril to stop a nosebleed.[4]

Pain (Natural Pain Relievers)

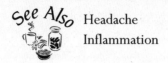 See Also Headache

Inflammation

It is somewhat antithetical to the tenets of alternative medicine to propose remedies for pain in general, rather than tailor the remedy to the specific nature of the individual's pain. This section is included because it is helpful to know the natural substances you can use when you want something to ease the hurt. With natural pain relievers, you can avoid the side effects of conventional medications.

Pain is actually a protective mechanism—the body's way of alerting you to a problem. Acute pain has a sudden onset, as with a headache or injury, and typically responds to pain relievers. Chronic pain, which may begin as acute pain, is an indication of a more deep-seated problem. While the remedies here might provide relief in cases of chronic pain, it is important to discover the cause of your chronic pain and seek appropriate medical treatment. In any case, pain relievers are not a substitute for necessary medical care.

Pain is like many other conditions in that there are factors that can heighten or lessen it. For example, stress and anxiety tend to worsen pain. It is impossible to say how much of this is physical (tight muscles make muscle pain worse) and how much emotional, because pain is a combination of sensory perception and emotional response. In other words, you might feel less pain from hitting your shin when you are in a calm state than when you are feeling tense and worried, even when the intensity of impact is the same.

In addition to emotional and psychological factors that influence the degree of pain you feel, what you eat (or don't eat) and drink can make you more susceptible to pain. Copper deficiency can lower the level of enkephalins, substances produced in the brain that act as natural pain relievers in your body.[1] Drinking coffee and other forms of caffeine may make pain worse because caffeine blocks the body's natural pain relievers from binding to necessary receptor sites.[2]

Essential Oils

Kurt Schnaubelt, Ph.D., scientific director of the Pacific Institute of Aromatherapy in San Rafael, California, cites Everlasting, Lavender, and Yarrow as pain-relieving essential oils.[3] (For instructions on using essential oils, see part 3, "Essential Oils," pp. 366–68.)

Flower Essences

Arnica Alleve flower oil and Love Lies Bleeding flower essence are natural pain relievers, states Patricia Kaminski, a flower essence therapist and educator from Nevada City, California. Use Arnica Alleve on the affected area 2–4 times daily, and take Love Lies Bleeding internally, 4 drops 2–4 times daily, as needed. During acute pain, you can take Love Lies Bleeding hourly or even more often. Alternate it with Five Flower Formula at the same dosage, as needed.

Food Therapy

Eat:

For their anti-inflammatory and pain-relieving effects, eat ginger, turmeric, and foods rich in omega-3 and omega-6 essential fatty acids, advises Nick Buratovich, N.M.D., a naturopathic physician from Tempe, Arizona. These foods can give your body the dietary support it needs for the current problem, and if you make them a regular part of your diet, they better equip your body to deal with pain in the future, thus minimizing its effects. (For a list of foods containing these nutrients, see part 3, "Food Therapy," p. 376.)

Given the link between copper deficiency and pain, making sure you are getting enough copper in your diet may raise your threshold of pain. Food sources of copper are nuts, legumes, buckwheat, and oysters and other shellfish.

Avoid:

Coffee and other forms of caffeine (aside from green tea).

Herbal Medicine

While many herbs can be used for specific conditions that produce pain, there are well-known herbal pain relievers, or analgesics. Chanchal Cabrera, M.N.I.M.H., A.H.G., a medical herbalist from

Vancouver, British Columbia, cites kava, valerian, California poppy, wild lettuce, and Jamaican dogwood. All should be taken according to your symptoms; the amount that provides pain relief differs with individuals.

Kava or kava-kava (*Piper methysticum*): Kava is a muscle relaxant. With pain, muscle tension impairs the blood supply to the area, which makes the pain worse. You can take kava as a tincture or in capsules. Take as much as you need to provide pain relief, but don't go beyond the upper limit of the dosage range suggested on the product. If you've never used kava before, start with a dosage below the lowest suggested dose, wait an hour, and see what happens. This is advisable because, though the vast majority of people have no problem with kava, a very few people can't take it. For them, kava is a stimulant rather than a relaxant. It's not harmful to these people; it just feels unpleasant.

Valerian (*Valeriana officinalis*): This herb works by acting on the brain to dull the sensation of pain. Dose according to your symptoms. If you take a lot, however, you may get a headache. Start with 1/2 teaspoon of tincture and gradually increase to up to 2 teaspoons daily, spread throughout the day.

California poppy (*Eschscholzia californica*) and wild lettuce (*Lactuca spp.*): These are very good, safe, natural painkillers, though not as well known as kava and valerian. Both contain opiates, but not the kind you can get hooked on. In addition to easing pain, they can suppress a cough, and since they are sedatives, they help you sleep. Take 1/2 to 2 teaspoons of California poppy or wild lettuce over a 24-hour period.

Jamaican dogwood (*Piscidia erythrina*): This analgesic herb is stronger and more effective than all of the above. Start with 1/4 teaspoon of tincture, and take up to 2 teaspoons over several hours, but definitely spread the doses out. Jamaican dogwood can give you a headache and produce grogginess.

Research has demonstrated that capsaicin and curcumin creams applied topically can be effective in reducing pain.[4] Capsaicin is the active component of cayenne pepper (*Capsicum spp.*) and curcumin is the active component of turmeric (*Curcuma longa*). Both work by depleting skin cells of substance P, a primary chemical messenger for pain impulses and an activator of inflammation. Capsaicin ointments are available commercially; follow the manufacturer's instructions for use.

Cabrera prefers using cayenne directly, noting that, as a rubefacient (increasing blood flow), cayenne opens up your blood vessels, which means the other ingredients in the commercial ointment, notably the carrier materials, get into your bloodstream more easily than they would otherwise. These other materials may contain chemicals. Some people have reactions to the ointments and think it's the cayenne, when it is actually the other substances in the preparation that are irritating.

You can mix cayenne with a little olive oil and rub it into the inflamed area (but not on an open wound), says Cabrera. Be careful in using it, she cautions. Don't use much cayenne, and test the mixture on a small area first, because it can burn the skin; very fair-haired and light-skinned people need to be particularly careful.[5] You can adjust the amount you use according to the results.

Homeopathy

There are myriad homeopathic remedies for pain, depending on the characteristics of the pain and the individual suffering it. Here are a few of the many possible selections, as cited by London homeopath Miranda Castro:[6]

Chamomilla: Indicated for people who are extremely sensitive to pain.

Opium: Indicated for people who don't feel pain when they should.

Arg nit, Hepar sulph, or Nitric acid: If the pain is needle-like.

Belladonna: If the pain is throbbing or shooting and appears and disappears suddenly; indicated for painful glands.

Hypericium or Rhus tox: If the pain is shooting.

Apis, Arsenicum, Phosphorus, Rhus tox, or Sulphur: If the pain is burning.

Apis or Silica: If the pain is stinging.

Take the appropriate remedy in a 6c or 12c potency every 1–2 hours, as needed. Discontinue the remedy when there is improvement. Repeat if necessary.

Nutritional Supplements

"Pain and inflammation feed off each other," notes Dr. Buratovich. "It's like the chicken and the egg. You don't know if you're hurting because you're inflamed or you're inflamed because you're hurting." Therefore, natural anti-inflamatories are useful for pain, along with supplements known for their pain-relieving properties (see "Inflammation").

As natural pain relievers, Dr. Buratovich cites the amino acids DLPA and tryptophan:

DLPA (D,L-phenylalanine): 750 mg 3 times daily before meals for as long as pain persists, but not exceeding 3 weeks.

Tryptophan: 2–4 g 3 times daily for up to 1 month. This amino acid has been shown to reduce pain, perhaps by raising the pain threshold, although the exact mechanism is unknown.[7] To ensure uptake, avoid protein for 90 minutes before and after taking.

Reflexology

Treat the pituitary area and the region of the foot corresponding to the afflicted part of the body.

Stone/Crystal Therapy

Stones that can help ease pain include malachite, chrysocolla, amethyst, green aventurine, and dow master quartz, notes crystal healing therapist Katrina Raphaell of Kapaa, Hawaii. Place the stone directly on the body at the site of distress. Visualizing your health goal, leave the stone in place for 5 minutes. Do this 3 times daily. You may also want to wear the stone, hold it, or carry it in your pocket for added benefit.

Poison Ivy/Oak Rash

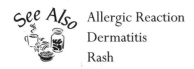 **See Also** Allergic Reaction
Dermatitis
Rash

As with other kinds of contact dermatitis, some people react strongly to exposure to the oily resin of poison ivy or poison oak, while others have no reaction after the same degree of exposure. Those who are sensitive to either plant break out in a red rash where contact occurred, from a few hours to as long as a week later. The rash is extremely itchy and blisters develop. Scratching the rash spreads it.

Reaction can occur at any time of the year, but most cases arise in the spring when the sap is running and the plants are plentiful. Smoke can carry the resin as well, to exposed skin and, more dangerously, to the lungs. Some people are so sensitive that petting a dog who has run through poison ivy/oak is enough to raise a rash.

Severe cases can result in fever, inflammation, headache, and swollen glands. If you develop these symptoms or if you have inhaled the smoke of burning poison ivy/oak and know that you are prone to reaction, seek medical care immediately.

Prevention is the best policy. Avoid contact with the plant and wear long pants and long sleeves when going into areas where poison ivy or poison oak is likely to be growing. If you have come in contact with either plant, wash with soap and water as soon as possible. Launder your clothes as well; as with pets, clothing can retain the resin.

Essential Oils

Lavender and Patchouli essential oils can help resolve a poison ivy/oak rash. Lavender is antiseptic and facilitates skin healing. Patchouli is also antiseptic and astringent as well, which aids in drying up weepy sores. Use in daily baths or with compresses as needed.[1] (For instructions on using essential oils, see part 3, "Essential Oils," p. 366–68.)

Flower Essences

Poison Oak flower essence taken before exposure can build up immunity and prevent a reaction to the plant, says Richard Katz, founder of the Flower Essence Society. Take 4 drops 2–4 times daily, beginning 1 month prior to anticipated exposure.

Food Therapy

Eat:

Fresh foods.

Avoid:

Fried and processed foods.

Herbal Medicine

For a poison ivy or oak rash, Joanne B. Mied, N.D., a naturopath and herbalist practicing in Novato, California, recommends black walnut (*Juglans nigra*). As the alcohol-based tincture tends to dry out the skin, break open black walnut hull capsules and add enough olive oil to the powder to moisten. Apply to the affected area twice daily or as needed for itching. As black walnut stains, you can cover it with gauze or a bandage.

As an internal remedy to clear the rash by purifying the blood, herbalist Michael Tierra, L.Ac., OMD, recommends the following formula: combine 1 part chaparral (*Larrea tridentata*) powder, 2 parts yellow dock (*Rumex crispus*) powder, and 2 parts echinacea (*E. spp.*) powder. Put the mixture in gelatin capsules and take 2 capsules every 2 hours.[2]

Homeopathy

The following are common homeopathic remedies for a poison ivy/oak rash:[3]

Anacardium: If there is intense itching that is worse with scratching and warmth and better with rubbing and eating; especially when the rash is on the left side, the neck, torso, armpits, scrotum, and/or inner thighs.

Apis: If there is itching, burning, stinging, heat, and great swelling, made worse by heat and better with cold; especially when the rash is on the face (notably around the eyes), forearms, and hands.

Rhus tox: If there are severely itchy eruptions making you nervous and restless, and characterized by prickling, burning, and tingling and red, angry skin worse in the morning, made worse by cold, wet, and scratching, and improved by scalding hot bathing; especially when the rash is on fingers, hands, face, groin, and folds of skin.

Sulphur: If there is a severely itchy, moist, dusky red rash with burning, prone to secondary infection, worse at night, worsened by warmth in bed, heat, perspiration, and washing, improved by cool air and icy applications, and characterized by scratching the skin for relief until it is raw and bloody; especially when the rash is on the left side, folds of skin, face, and palms.

Take the appropriate remedy in a 30c potency 3–4 times daily for 2–3 days.

Nutritional Supplements

For a poison ivy/oak rash, Susan Roberts, N.D., a naturopathic physician from Portland, Oregon, recommends vitamins C and E to speed skin healing. With the onset of the rash, take 2–3 grams of vitamin C daily at least until the rash is resolved; longer is fine. After the oozing sores of the rash have closed, apply vitamin E oil (you can break open gel capsules if you don't have the bottled liquid form) directly on them 2–3 times daily until the skin is healed.

Reflexology

Treat the adrenal glands, kidneys, liver, and the areas of the foot corresponding to the parts of the body where the poison ivy/oak rash is.

Stone/Crystal Therapy

To help heal a poison ivy/oak rash, use serpentine, suggests crystal healing therapist Katrina Raphaell of Kapaa, Hawaii. Place the stone directly on the affected area. Leave the stone in place for 5 minutes while visualizing your health goal. Do this 3 times daily. Wear the stone, hold it, or carry it in your pocket for ongoing healing.

Other Remedies

Dr. Roberts cites three easy household remedies for a rash from poison ivy/oak. Stir 2–3 tablespoons of salt into 1/4 cup of apple cider vinegar. The salt won't dissolve completely. Dip a cloth into the mixture (it's fine to have undissolved salt stick to the cloth), and then rub the cloth back and forth over the rash. The salt feels good on the itchy rash. Do 2 times daily, or as needed. You can do this even where there are open, oozing sores. It will sting, but the vinegar helps dry out the rash.

Because heat breaks down histamines (the inflammatory substances involved in allergic reactions), blowing a hot hair dryer over the area can also ease the itching and help resolve the rash, states Dr. Roberts. This works for bug bites as well, she notes.

Taking an oat bath can alleviate the itching, Dr. Roberts says. Put 1 cup of oats in a knee-high stocking or in one foot of a pair of old pantyhose and tie off the top. This acts as a kind of tea bag. Immerse it and yourself in a tub of water. Do this 1–2 times daily, as needed for itching.

Psoriasis

Psoriasis is a complex skin disorder, the cause of which is unknown. While deeper treatment may be advisable if you suffer from psoriasis, the remedies here can give you relief from the itching and help clear up the scaly patches of the condition.

The red patches, covered with the characteristic silvery scales, most often develop on the scalp, elbows, wrists, knees, and back. They form when skin cells multiply out of control. The new cells pile up under the dead outer skin cells, which cannot be shed fast enough to keep up with the accelerated cell production. The fingernails frequently show signs of the disorder as well, becoming pitted and thick.

The mechanism behind the excessive production of cells is an imbalance between two regulating substances found in skin cells: cyclic GMP and cyclic AMP. A higher level of GMP than normal is associated with more rapid cell proliferation, while a higher level of AMP than normal is associated with a decrease in cell proliferation. Paul Reilly, N.D., L.Ac., refers to them as the gas and brake pedals of the cell. Research has uncovered increased GMP and decreased AMP in people with psoriasis.[1] Some of the treatment below is focused on bringing this ratio back into balance.

Psoriasis tends to run in families, and most often affects those between the ages of fifteen and twenty-five. Although the cause of the GMP-AMP imbalance and its attendant accelerated skin cell production has not yet been determined, faulty protein digestion, high intake of animal fats, essential fatty acid deficiency, toxic buildup in the intestines, liver toxicity, and weak immunity may play a role in psoriasis.[2]

Certain triggers are associated with outbreaks of psoriasis. These include infection, a stressful event, smoking, damage to skin, sunburn, certain medications, and excess alcohol consumption.

Essential Oils

Dr. Jean Valnet, regarded as the father of essential oil therapy, recommends Cajeput for psoriasis. Use in an ointment applied to the affected area at a ratio of 1 part Cajeput essential oil to 5–10 parts ointment. Apply as needed to alleviate your symptoms.[3] As an ointment, you can buy an unperfumed cream base, designed for use with essential oils, but be sure that it contains only pure natural ingredients and is free of chemicals. Or you can make your own ointment by combining 4 tablespoons of anhydrous lanolin with 2 tablespoons of almond oil, which produces 3 ounces of ointment.[4]

Flower Essences

Use flower essences internally and externally as treatment for psoriasis, recommends Patricia Kaminski, an herbalist and flower essence therapist from Nevada City, California. Take 4 drops of St. John's Wort flower essence 2–4 times daily; during an acute episode, you should take it at least 4 times daily, and more often if needed. Alternate topical applications of St. John's Shield flower oil and Self-Heal cream, 2–4 times daily. Continue treatment until your symptoms are resolved.

Food Therapy

Eat:

Fiber, red grapes, garlic, ground flaxseed (sprinkle on salads, cereal, and other food), cold-water fish, turkey, psoralen-rich foods (carrots, celery, parsnips, citrus fruit, figs, fennel), foods high in lecithin (see part 3, "Food Therapy," p. 377).

"Diet is really important in psoriasis," says naturopathic physician and acupuncturist Paul Reilly, N.D., L.Ac., of Seattle, Washington. "Dietary modifications alone may be enough to clear up your psoriasis."

Eating foods that contain psoralens can be therapeutic for psoriasis, says herbalist James A Duke, Ph.D., among other authorities. These plant compounds inhibit cell division and have been used traditionally in combination with sunshine (ultraviolet rays) to treat psoriasis. Go out in the sun immediately after eating high-psoralen foods to get the full benefits of PUVA (the relatively new name for the treatment—psoralens and one type of ultraviolet light), says Dr. Duke.[5]

Avoid:

Sugar, red meat, pork, and other animal fats, dairy, caffeine, alcohol, soft drinks, gluten, acidic foods (tomatoes, pineapple), allergenic foods.

Herbal Medicine

If attention to diet alone does not resolve your psoriasis, combine dietary practice with supplements and the following herbal remedies as a treatment program, says Dr. Reilly:

Sarsaparilla (*Smilax spp.*): 1/4 teaspoon of the molasses-like solid extract 3 times daily; or 2 capsules 3 times daily. This herb helps stimulate circulation and restore balance to out-of-balance systems.

Milk thistle (*Carduus marianus, Silybum marianum*): 1 capsule (containing 200 mg of standardized solid extract) 2 times daily; supports and protects the liver.

Boswellia: 500 mg in capsule or tablet 3 times daily; this Ayurvedic herb is anti-inflammatory and can help control proliferating tissue.

Neem oil: Apply this Ayurvedic herb oil with a cotton ball 1–2 times daily. Derived from a tropical tree, the oil has a long tradition of use in skin ailments.

David Winston, A.H.G., a clinical herbalist and consultant from Washington, New Jersey, offers some herbal guidelines for specific manifestations of psoriasis. These treatments can be used on a long-term basis, but he recommends working with a qualified herbalist to tailor treatment more closely to your individual needs:

For red, hot, inflamed skin: Combine equal parts of tinctures of gotu kola (*Centella asiatica*) and sarsaparilla. Take 4 ml (roughly 4/5 teaspoon) of the blend 3 times daily.

For dry, itchy, scratchy, scaly skin: Use 2 parts of burdock (*Arctium lappa*) seed tincture to 1 part of nonstandardized milk thistle tincture. Take 4 ml (roughly 4/5 teaspoon) of the blend 3 times daily.

For red, hot, scaly skin: Combine equal parts of tinctures of gotu kola, sarsaparilla, and burdock seed. Take 5 ml (roughly 1 teaspoon) of the blend 3 times daily.

For weepy, oozing skin: Take 3 ml (roughly 3/5 teaspoon) of yellow dock (*Rumex crispus*) tincture 3 times daily.

For weepy, oozing, red, inflamed skin: Combine tinctures of gotu kola (1–1/2 parts), sarsaparilla (1–1/2 parts), and yellow dock (1 part). Take 5 ml (roughly 1 teaspoon) of the blend 3 times daily.

There is also evidence that topical application of Oregon grape (*Berberis aquifolium*) root can have benefits for psoriasis, Winston adds. You can purchase a cream containing the herb or you can make your own poultices. Prepare a decoction by putting 2 teaspoons of Oregon grape root in 1 cup of boiling water. Cover, simmer for 15–20 minutes, and steep for another 20 minutes. Soak a cloth with the decoction, lay it on the affected area, and leave it on for an hour. Alternately, you can "paint" the affected area with the decoction and leave it on your skin to dry. In either case, do this twice a day if possible. Note that Oregon grape root stains clothing.

Finally, research has demonstrated the effectiveness of capsaicin, the active component of cayenne pepper (*Capsicum spp.*), applied as a cream in reducing the scaling, redness, and itching of psoriasis.[6]

Capsaicin works by depleting skin cells of substance P, a primary chemical messenger for pain impulses and an activator of inflammation. Studies have found higher than normal levels of substance P in the skin of psoriasis sufferers.[7] Capsaicin ointments are available commercially; follow the manufacturer's instructions for use.

Homeopathy

The following are homeopathic remedies commonly indicated for acute psoriasis:[8]

Arsenicum: For psoriasis in the elderly, debilitated, or emaciated, located on knees, upper limbs, and back of hand, and characterized by severe itching, burning and bleeding with scratching, improvement with warmth, and parchment-like, dry skin with large, greyish-white scales.

Graphites: For psoriasis in children, located behind ears and on head, genitals, and back of hand and characterized by hard skin and thick, whitish lesions that may ooze; itching or no itching, and worsening at night and with heat.

Petroleum: For psoriasis with severe dryness of the entire skin, located on hands, between fingers, on heels, and scrotum, and characterized by thick, white scaly lesions and cracks in folds, worsening with cold, dry weather.

Sepia: According to homeopath Roger Morrison, "The most common remedy across the board for psoriasis." Located on the eyelids, chin, limbs, and particularly genitals or around rectum; and characterized by thickening of the skin, shiny or fatty-looking white scales, no itching mostly, but times of severe itching, as with heat of bed, and worsened by winter.

Sulphur: For psoriasis with strong itching, located in the folds of skin, on the scalp, genitals, and soles of feet, and characterized by moist lesions and worsening at night, with the heat of bed, and with washing.

Take a single dose of the appropriate remedy at a 30c potency.

Nutritional Supplements

The first supplement practice Dr. Reilly implements with his patients with psoriasis is reducing their vitamin C intake. He recommends taking no more than 1,000 mg daily, and that includes the amount that is in your multivitamin/mineral. The reason for this is that vitamin C can stimulate cyclic GMP, which is already overstimulated in psoriasis, he explains.

As a supplement program for psoriasis, Dr. Reilly suggests the following in addition to a regular multivitamin/mineral:

Forskolin: Derived from *Coleus Forskohlii,* an herb used in Ayurvedic medicine, this substance can stimulate cyclic AMP, which can help counterbalance the excess cyclic GMP. Use a standarized product and take 2 capsules twice daily as a starting dose. Adjust that dose up or down as needed.

EPA (eicosapentaenoic acid): 4–6 g daily of this omega-3 essential fatty acid; that is usually 8–10 capsules, depending on the product.

Vitamin E: 1,200 IU daily.

Vitamin A: 10,000–25,000 IU daily.

Lactobacillus acidophilus and *Bifidobacterium bifidum*: These beneficial bacteria normally found in the intestines help prevent the formation of polyamines, compounds formed by putrefaction of protein in the digestive system. (Research indicates that polyamines trigger rapid cell division, not only in psoriasis, but also in cancer.) Use a powder that requires refrigeration. Take 1 teaspoon twice daily for the first month, 1/2 teaspoon twice daily for the second month, and 1/4 teaspoon twice daily thereafter.

HCl (hydrochloric acid): Taking HCl (digestive acid of the stomach) can aid weak or faulty digestion. Take 2–3 capsules in the middle of every meal. Taking this supplement before or after a meal can produce heartburn.

Vitamin D: 1,000 IU daily. Vitamin D cream applied topically is also useful.

Take all of the above supplements in tandem with the herbal program and dietary recommendations above. When your symptoms have begun to improve, usually in 4–8 weeks, you can begin to cut the dosages to find your maintenance level—the amounts you need to take to keep your psoriasis from returning. Cut the dosages by 25 percent the first month. If you don't have a flare-up of your skin condition, reduce the dosages by another 25 percent the following month. You can expect that a maintenance dosage will be 25 to 50 percent of the starting dosages.

Reflexology

Kidneys, adrenal glands, thyroid, pituitary

Stone/Crystal Therapy

Beneficial stones for psoriasis are sulphur, rose quartz, green tourmaline, and rhodachrosite, according to Katrina Raphaell, crystal healing therapist and founder of the Crystal Academy of Advanced Healing Arts in Kapaa, Hawaii. Place the stone directly on the affected area. Keep it in place for 5 minutes while visualizing your health goal. Do this 3 times daily. In between treatments, wear the stone, hold it, or carry it in your pocket for continual healing.

Other Remedies

Psoriasis is often responsive to sunlight. "Try to get thirty to forty-five minutes of sunlight several times a week," advises Dr. Reilly. He notes that some patients find brief tanning sessions helpful as well. Be careful to avoid burning or excessive tanning, however, as premature wrinkling and skin cancer are a concern with too much sun exposure. (See "Food Therapy" above.)

Puncture Wound

A minor puncture wound, piercing by a sharp, pointed object, is a special kind of injury because the opening of the wound is small relative to the depth, so the techniques of cleansing and disinfecting used on regular cuts and scrapes are not effective. A typical example of a puncture wound is stepping on a nail. The nail may be rusty and/or coated with all manner of dirt and bacteria, but you can't see what's left behind in your foot when you pull the nail out. The problem with puncture wounds is that the skin, with its miraculous ability to heal itself, will close over quickly. But if the wound has not been properly cleaned, infection may be festering deep within your foot or other injury site, unseen beneath the healing surface until it worsens and spreads upward.

In the case of puncture wounds, bleeding helps clean out the germs and debris. Don't try to stop the bleeding unless it is spurting or severe. Washing the wound with water is often not sufficient to flush out a deep puncture. The remedies here can aid in the process of cleaning and disinfecting a puncture type of injury. Obviously, if you step on a nail or other metal object, it is advisable to talk to your doctor about whether you need a tetanus shot.

Essential Oils

If the puncture wound is on the foot or hand, soak the wound in water to which you've added Lavender or Tea Tree (*Melaleuca alternifolia*) essential oil. These antibacterial oils can help disinfect the wound; immersion allows them to penetrate into the wound. Use 6–8 drops of either oil per cup of warm water, blending the mixture well to ensure dispersion. After the soak, dry the area and put 1–2 drops of either oil on the wound, or on gauze if you are bandaging it.[1]

Flower Essences

Self-Heal and Five Flower Formula can serve as the foundational healing agents for a puncture wound. Other flower essences to address the specific emotions, mental attitude, and environmental conditions of the individual are recommended, states Patricia Kaminski, a flower essence therapist and codirector of the Flower Essence Society. Self-Heal supports the body's innate healing ability. Five Flower Formula, which brings immediate calm and emotional neutralizing, is indicated for physical and/or emotional trauma. Take 4 drops of each 4 times daily, or more frequently if needed.

Food Therapy

Eat:

Protein, foods high in vitamin C and zinc (see part 3, "Food Therapy," p. 378).

Avoid:

Sugar and dairy.

Herbal Medicine

For a puncture wound, plantain (*Plantago major, P. lanceolata*) is excellent, says Chanchal Cabrera, M.N.I.M.H., A.H.G., a medical herbalist from Vancouver, British Columbia. Not only is it a powerful drawing agent, but it is also antimicrobial, has pain-relieving properties, and promotes healing. In addition, it grows everywhere, so is readily at hand when emergency first aid is needed.

As a drawing agent, plantain will pull out dirt, slivers, or other debris in the wound. It contains vitamin A and zinc, both of which aid healing, plus allantoin, a wound-healing substance that promotes cell proliferation and is also found in the herb comfrey, placental fluid, and egg whites. You can't use comfrey for a puncture wound because it is such a potent wound healer that it will seal the surface before whatever foreign matter is in the wound has had a chance to emerge. You need to draw out that matter before you heal the wound.

To that end, pick fresh plantain leaves. Mash them into a pulp by chewing them, using a mortar and pestle, or putting them in a blender or herb grinder. Place the pulp over the puncture wound and wrap gauze around it. If you're in the woods, you can use a bandanna or other piece of clothing in place of gauze. Leave the plantain on the wound for an hour, then check to see if it has pulled matter out of the wound. If you don't see anything, apply fresh plantain.

Leave the poultice on day and night, changing it daily, until the wound has sufficiently healed, which means it is closed over and looks clean.

Plantain is good for puncture wounds caused by a nail, notes Cabrera, but you should also talk to your doctor about whether you need a tetanus shot.

Prickly pear cactus pads can also clean a puncture wound by drawing out dirt and other foreign matter, according to Michael

Cottingham, a clinical herbalist from Silver City, New Mexico. After squeezing the puncture wound to expel debris and bleeding to aid in cleansing, apply a prickly pear cactus pad. If you are outside in a place where prickly pear cactus grows, use a stick to knock a pad off the cactus, brush off the prickles, and rub off the spine. Then cut the pad open and place it, gooey side down, on the wound. Leave the pad in place for 15–30 minutes. Usually, 1–2 applications are sufficient. Do one right after the other. In addition to aiding in cleaning the wound, the prickly pear increases circulation in the area, which helps reduce swelling. See "Boil" for more information on prickly pear cactus and how to use it at home.

Homeopathy

"Ledum is the best remedy for puncture wounds," states Maesimund B. Panos, M.D. "It prevents sepsis (disease germs in the blood and tissues) and promotes healing." Use Ledum lotion to wash the puncture wound, advises Dr. Panos, then soak the affected part in a basin of water with a few drops of Ledum added. Use a compress with Ledum lotion on it for body parts that can't be soaked in a basin. Repeat as needed.[2]

Nutritional Supplements

Taking the following antioxidants and vitamins essential to skin health may be beneficial after receiving a puncture wound:[3]

Beta-carotene: 25,000 IU.
Vitamin C with bioflavonoids: 2–5 g in divided doses, or to bowel tolerance (the dosage just below the amount that produces diarrhea).
Zinc: 25–50 mg.
Selenium: 100–200 mcg.
Vitamin B complex: 50–100 mg.
Silica: 1–2 mg.

Stone/Crystal Therapy

For a puncture wound, lay carnelian near the wound for 15–20 minutes daily, as needed, and/or hold the stone, wear it, or carry it in your pocket until the wound is healed, recommends vibrational healer Daya Sarai Chocron of Northampton, Massachusetts.

Rash

See Also
Allergic Reaction
Dermatitis
Diaper Rash
Hives
Insect Bites and Stings
Poison Ivy/Oak Rash

A rash is a general term for any eruption on the skin, often red in color and involving small bumps. The exact appearance and nature of the rash depend upon the cause. A temporary condition, a rash is a common symptom of an allergic reaction, whether to a food, an inhaled substance, or something touched, as in contact dermatitis. A rash can also be a sign of viral or bacterial infection, a skin disorder or other disease, or kidney overload. Heat can bring on a rash (prickly heat), as can certain medications (known as a drug rash).

The remedies here can alleviate the itching and redness of a rash, but it is advisable to determine the cause of the rash, if possible, and treat that problem specifically. If you know the source of your skin outbreak, refer to the appropriate section of the book for more focused treatment.

Essential Oils

Medical aromatherapist Julia Fischer of Northern California suggests an essential oil and clay application to remedy a rash. Combine essential oils of Geranium (3 drops), German Chamomile (2 drops), and Lavender (3 drops). Make a clay paste by combining this formula with 1–2 teaspoons of green or yellow clay powder. Add water as needed to thin the paste. Apply the paste to the affected area and leave it on until it is dry. Do this 2–3 times daily, for as long as needed. Or you can add the essential oil formula to a base of calendula fatty oil and/or St. John's wort fatty oil (3 teaspoons, or 15 ml, total of one or a combination of these fatty oils). Apply topically 2–3 times daily. An herbal fatty oil is a carrier oil that has been infused with a given herb, in this case calendula or St. John's wort.

For a rash caused by contact with stinging nettle, dab Lavender or Tea Tree (*Melaleuca alternifolia*) essential oil on the affected area. This is quite effective, according to herbalist Mindy Green, A.H.G., M.S., of Boulder, Colorado.

Flower Essences

As with other conditions of multiple causes, there are numerous flower essences indicated for a rash. Richard Katz, naturalist and founder of the Flower Essence Society, cites some common protocols:

For a rash accompanied by symptoms of anger: Scarlet Monkeyflower.
When discharging toxins: take both Crab Apple and Self-Heal.
For a rash located near the sexual organs or connected to emotional issues of shame and low-self esteem: take both Pink Monkeyflower and Sticky Monkeyflower.

Take 4 drops of the appropriate flower essence for your rash, at least 4 times daily. If taking 2 essences, take 4 drops of each. During the acute stage, you can take the essences more frequently, as often as hourly. Continue taking the essence(s) until the rash goes away.

Food Therapy

Eat:
Fresh foods, seaweed, miso soup, whole grains.
Drink vegetable juices, green drinks (chlorella, spirulina), and plenty of water to flush the toxins out of the body.
Avoid:
Sugar, processed and fried foods, refined carbohydrates, caffeine, meat, dairy.

Herbal Medicine

As topical treatment for an itchy rash, herbalist Penelope Ody recommends aloe vera gel, chickweed (*Stellaria media*), or plantain

(*Plantago major, P. lanceolata*). Simply apply the aloe vera gel as needed. Use a food processor or blender to make a pulp of the chickweed or plantain, and use it as a lotion on the rash.[1]

Sage (*Salvia officinalis*) tea is also useful for rashes, both as a topical treatment and taken internally, says herbalist and naturopathic health consultant James Kusick. "Sage helps to fight the toxins in the body and soothes the nerves," he explains. Add 1 teaspoon or more of sage per 1 cup of boiled water, let stand for 10–15 minutes, then strain. Drink as a tea and apply to the rash when cool enough. Combine powdered sage with enough water or vegetable oil to make a paste and gently spread the mixture on the worst areas of outbreak. Repeat all as needed.[2]

Homeopathy

For an allergic rash, Dr. Barry Rose of the Royal London Homeopathic Hospital cites the following remedies:[3]

Anacardium 6c: For a very itchy nettle rash, with high irritability

Arsenicum 30c: For a burning rash accompanied by restlessness, from eating shellfish.

Terebinth 30c: For a rash from eating shellfish.

Fragaria 30c: For a rash from eating strawberries.

Kali brom 30c: For a nervous rash, due to stress and anxiety.

Nat mur 30c: For a rash that itches more following exertion.

Rhus tox 30c: For a red, swollen, and very itchy rash that is better with warmth.

Sepia 30c: For a rash from dairy products that worsens in the warmth of bed.

Take the appropriate remedy every 3 hours until there is improvement.

Nutritional Supplements

Taking zinc and vitamins A and C, which are essential nutrients for the skin, can often ameloriate a rash, says Elson Haas, M.D., director of the Preventive Medical Center of Marin in San Rafael, California. His recommended daily dosages are:[4]

Vitamin A: 5,000 IU.
Vitamin C: 5,000 mg.
Zinc: Up to 30 mg.

Continue taking until your rash disappears.

Reflexology

Treat the adrenal glands and the areas of the foot corresponding to the parts of the body where the rash is.

Stone/Crystal Therapy

Use larimar, blue calcite, blue lace agate, or angelite as crystal therapy for a rash, recommends crystal healing therapist Katrina Raphaell of Kapaa, Hawaii. Place the stone directly on the affected area. Visualizing your health goal, leave the stone in place for 5 minutes. Do this 3 times daily. In between treatments, wear the stone, hold it, or carry it in your pocket for continual healing.

Other Remedies

James Kusick cites a useful kitchen remedy to neutralize the toxins in a rash and ease itching. Cook 2 cups of oatmeal in a cloth bag in 2 quarts of water for about 15 minutes. Remove the bag from the water, cool enough to use safely, then squeeze to expel the liquid over the rash. If you don't have a cloth bag, use a thin dish towel and strain after cooking to obtain the liquid to apply to the rash.[5]

Ringworm

See Fungal Infection

Sciatica

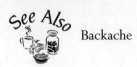 Backache

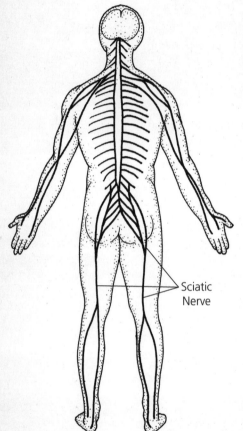

Sciatic Nerve

The sciatic nerve is the largest nerve in the body, running from the bottom of the spinal cord down the back of each leg. Sciatica is a painful condition, usually affecting one side or worse on one side.

A bulging or herniated (slipped) disk between the vertebrae in the lumbar (lower) portion of the spine can pinch the sciatic nerve and cause lower back pain, as well as mild to severe pain, tingling, and/or numbness radiating across the buttocks and down the back and/or outer side of the leg, sometimes all the way to the foot. Compression of the nerve can also occur in the buttocks or pelvis; prolonged sitting on a hard surface or pressure on the buttocks (wallet sciatica) can produce compression. Sciatica can stem from inflammation of the sciatic nerve as a result of infection, arthritis, or a toxic condition.

The remedies here can help relieve the pain of sciatica, but it is advisable to determine the cause of your sciatica and address that problem with the appropriate treatment. Vertebral involvement, for example, is a structural condition and needs the attention of an osteopath or other doctor specializing in musculoskeletal therapies.

Essential Oils

When the pain of sciatica is intense, massage is not advisable as a delivery method for essential oils, notes Julie Oxendale, C.M.T., an aromatherapist based in San Francisco, California. She suggests cold compresses instead. The oils that are effective for sciatica are Ginger,

Lavender, Nutmeg, Peppermint, and Rosemary. You can use one alone or combine several (don't use more than three). For a compress, soak a washcloth in icy water, squeeze it out, and put 1 drop of each of your desired essential oils on the cloth. Apply to the area of most acute pain, breathe deeply, and lie still for 20 minutes.

When the pain is not acute, lukewarm (not hot) baths and aromatherapeutic massage are helpful. For a bath, put 2 drops of one of the above oils or 1 drop each of two or three different oils in the water. For the massage, put 1 drop each of two or three of the oils or 1 drop of one oil alone in 2 tablespoons of a carrier oil such as sweet almond or apricot kernel oil. Massage into the area affected by your sciatica. Having a friend give you a massage is preferable. Inhale deeply during the bath and massage.

Flower Essences

As with backache, sciatica often involves emotional tension, so flower essence therapy is most effective when remedies are selected to address the individual's emotional blockages, states flower essence therapist Patricia Kaminski of Nevada City, California. That said, Arnica Alleve flower oil compresses can be used for symptom relief, she notes. Rub 1–2 tablespoons of Arnica Alleve flower oil on the affected area and cover with a hot or cold compress, depending on the condition. Do 2–4 applications daily, or as needed. Self-Heal can aid the sciatica sufferer in looking at the specific healing issues in his or her life, adds Kaminski. Take 4 drops, 2–4 times daily, as needed.

Food Therapy

For their anti-inflammatory and pain-relieving effects, eat ginger, turmeric, pineapple, papaya, foods rich in omega-3 and omega-6 essential fatty acids, and foods high in calcium and magnesium, advises Nick Buratovich, N.M.D., a naturopathic physician from Tempe, Arizona. (For a list of foods containing these nutrients, see part 3, "Food Therapy," pp. 376, 377.) Eat pineapple and papaya by themselves, not with other foods, to get the anti-inflammatory effect of the enzymes these fruits contain. Also get plenty of fiber, as blocked bowels can contribute to back pain. Eat small rather than large meals.

Avoid coffee and other forms of caffeine (aside from green tea) because caffeine blocks endorphin receptors in the brain, says Dr. Buratovich. As endorphins facilitate pain relief, people who consume a lot of caffeine tend to have a low threshold of pain. He also recommends avoiding animal products because they contain arachidonic acid, which promotes inflammation.

Herbal Medicine

Although St. John's wort (*Hypericum perforatum*) has become known primarily as an antidepressant, it has other powerful properties, according to herbalist Teresa Boardwine of Washington, Virginia. As a nerve rejuvenator, it is excellent for nerve inflammation, as in sciatica. You can take it as a tea, in capsules, or as a tincture. To make the tea, use 1 tablespoon of the herb per cup of boiled water. Cover and let steep for 15–20 minutes, then strain. For the pain of sciatica, drink a quart daily. Alternatively, you can take 1 capsule of St. John's wort 3 times daily or up to 1 teaspoon (5 ml) of tincture 3 times daily. Use a whole-plant product rather than standardized hypericin (an active constituent of the herb), so you get the nutrients and anti-inflammatory properties of the whole plant.

Homeopathy

The following are common homeopathic remedies for sciatica:[1]

Belladonna: When the sciatica involves sudden onset of debilitating pain on the right side made worse with motion, jarring, standing, or coughing.

Kali carb: When the sciatica pain gets the patient up at night, is particularly on the right side, extends into buttocks or sole of the foot, is worse at night (2–3 A.M. is typically the bad time), worsened by cold, eating, motion, lying on it, and improved by sitting bent forward, moving, and pressure.

Kali iod: For excruciating and disabling sciatica, particularly on the left side, worsened by nighttime, lying on it, heat, pressure, sitting, and standing, and improved by motion and flexing legs.

Nux vom: For severe sciatica down either leg, accompanied by sensitivity and anger, worse at night and in the morning, worsened by cold, turning in bed, standing, and motion, and improved by heat, pressure, and lying down.

Rhus tox: For sciatica, particularly left-sided, accompanied by restlessness, worse in the morning, worsened by long sitting, cold and dampness, and getting wet, and improved by heat and motion.

Tellurium: For right-sided sciatica with severe pain extending down from the sacrum into the thigh, worsened by jarring, coughing, laughing, sneezing, touch, and straining to defecate, and improved by standing and during urination.

Take the appropriate remedy in a 30c potency 2 times daily for 2–3 days. You will generally experience improvement in that time if it is the correct remedy.

Nutritional Supplements

To relieve the pain and inflammation of sciatica, the following supplements can be helpful, according to Dr. Buratovich.

DLPA (D,L-phenylalanine): 750 mg 3 times daily before meals for 3 weeks; a pain-relieving amino acid.

Tryptophan: 2–4 g 3 times daily for up to 1 month. This amino acid has been shown to reduce pain, perhaps by raising the pain threshold, although the exact mechanism is unknown.[2] To ensure uptake, avoid protein for 90 minutes before and after taking.

Bromelain: 2 capsules on an empty stomach 3 times daily until the pain is resolved; an anti-inflammatory enzyme compound found in pineapple.

Calcium lactate or calcium citrate: These chelated forms of calcium are the most easily absorbed. Take 1,000 mg 3 times daily until you get relief. Calcium relaxes the contracted muscles that produce pain by addressing both the nervous and biochemical components of muscle contraction.

Magnesium glycinate: This form of magnesium is most easily absorbed and less likely to cause the diarrhea some people get when they take magnesium. Take 1,000 mg 3 times daily until you get relief. Magnesium is an antispasmodic and smooth muscle relaxant.

Reflexology

Sciatic nerve, hips, groin, lymphatic system, lumbar spine, tail-bone, knee/leg

Stone/Crystal Therapy

Green (and black) tourmaline, blue kyanite, and smoky quartz can be useful for sciatica, states Katrina Raphaell, crystal healing therapist and author of the crystal reference series *The Crystal Trilogy*. Place the stone directly on the site(s) of pain. Keep it in place for 5 minutes while visualizing your health goal. Do this 3 times daily. You may also want to wear the stone, hold it, or carry it in your pocket for continual healing benefits.

Shingles (*Herpes Zoster*)

Shingles, also known as herpes zoster, is an acute inflammatory condition caused by the varicella-zoster virus (the same virus that causes chickenpox). An attack usually begins with severe pain and itching along the pathway of a nerve, typically on the torso and especially around the waist. The skin in the area can be almost unbearably sensitive. The condition progesses to an outbreak of painful, itchy blister-like bumps along the same pathway. Like other herpes sores, the open blisters are contagious. Though the blisters usually clear up within a few weeks, the pain sometimes lasts for months or even as long as a year (a condition called postherpetic neuralgia).

Herpes zoster occurs most frequently in middle age. The chicken-pox virus, dormant in the body, reemerges as shingles as a result of weakened immunity due to physical or emotional stress.

Seek medical care if your shingles attack is severe or occurs on your face (it can affect the eyes). You may want to get medical attention in any case, but the following remedies can help ease the pain and itching of shingles, and speed the healing of the blisters. To prevent further attacks or the possibility of another disorder developing, you need to take measures to strengthen your immune system. A qualified alternative medicine practitioner can aid you in determining what measures are appropriate for you.

Essential Oils

Bergamot, Eucalyptus, and Tea Tree (*Melaleuca alternifolia*) essential oils are both pain-relieving and antiviral and work well for shingles, says Patricia Davis, founder of the London School of Aromatherapy. They seem to produce better results when they are used in combination, she notes. Bergamot is also a potent antidepressant, which is useful for shingle sufferers as well, given that many report being anxious or depressed before the shingles attack occurred. Davis recommends blending equal parts of Bergamot and Tea Tree, and applying it to the affected area, using a soft paintbrush. If the area is large, you may want to put the oils in an alcohol solution (use the highest grain of vodka you can find) or use them in baths. Topical application 2–3 times daily along with a nightly bath seems to be the most effective, says Davis. She adds that use of these oils can reduce both the healing time and the severity of pain.[1]

Flower Essences

Self-Heal can serve as a foundational healing agent for shingles. Other flower essences to address the specific emotions, mental attitude, and environmental conditions of the individual are recommended, states Patricia Kaminski, a flower essence therapist and codirector of the Flower Essence Society. Self-Heal supports the body's innate healing ability. Take 4 drops 2–4 times daily, or as needed.

Food Therapy

Eat:

Kelp, garlic, cayenne, yogurt, foods high in lysine (this amino acid inhibits the herpes virus), alkalinizing foods.

Avoid:

Processed foods, food additives and preservatives, foods high in arginine (this amino acid aids and abets the herpes virus), acid-forming foods.

(For a list of foods containing the substances cited above, see part 3, "Food Therapy," pp. 376, 377.)

Herbal Medicine

For shingles, a two-pronged approach is most effective, says David Winston, A.H.G., a clinical herbalist and consultant from Washington, New Jersey. Take antiviral herbs internally to help the body suppress the virus, but more important, use antiherpetic herbs topically.

Oral antiviral formula:

St. John's wort (*Hypericum perforatum*): 2 parts
Lemon balm (*Melissa officinalis*): 2 parts
Meadowsweet (*Filipendula ulmaria*): 2 parts
Rosemary (*Rosmarinus officinalis*): 1 part

Combine tinctures of these herbs in the proportions noted and take orally at a dosage of 5 ml (1 teaspoon) 3–4 times daily. You can also just take St. John's wort alone. In that case, the dosage is 40 drops (2 ml, or roughly 2/5 teaspoon) 3 times daily.

Topical application:

Make a very strong herbal tea. Start by putting 2 teaspoons of licorice root in 1 cup of boiling water. Cover, simmer for 15 minutes, and remove from the heat. Add 2 teaspoons each of lemon balm and St. John's wort (preferably the flowers and buds) and let steep for 40 minutes. Soak a cloth with the tea and gently rub into the affected area. It's safe to use this if you have open lesions. Do this twice daily for as long as you are experiencing pain. St. John's wort is a pain reliever as well as an antiherpetic herb. You can also simply apply St. John's wort oil to affected areas.

Kathi Head, N.D., a naturopathic physician from Sandpoint, Idaho, has found the following herbal program effective for shingles:

Licorice root (*Glycrrhiza glabra*): Take internally, 2 capsules twice daily. People who suffer from high blood pressure or water retention should not use pure licorice root, which can aggravate these conditions, but use DGL (deglycrrhizinated licorice; licorice from

which glycrrhizinic acid has been removed) instead; follow manufacturer's recommended dosage. Also use licorice root topically.
You can purchase salves containing a combination of licorice root,
lysine, and zinc; follow the directions on the individual product.
Echinacea root (*E. spp.*): Take 400 mg in capsules, 3 times daily.
Olive leaf extract: Take a standardized 15 percent extract; 500 mg 3
times per day.

Follow this program for 1–2 weeks or until the lesions have dried up.

If you develop postherpetic neuralgia, capsaicin (derived from
cayenne pepper) cream can be quite effective in easing the pain, says
Dr. Head. This is available in health food stores. Rub the cream into the
skin of the affected area, but don't put it directly on any remaining
lesions. You can use this several times a day, as needed.

Homeopathy

In cases of shingles, "Homeopathic medicines can help the body
restore health to the irritated nerves and permanently relieve pain," say
Stephen Cummings, M.D., and Dana Ullman, M.P.H. It still may take
7–10 days for the rash to heal, but without treatment shingles can last
3–4 weeks. Drs. Cummings and Ullman cite the following homeopathic remedies as indicated for shingles:[2]

Rhus tox: Indicated for painful, intensely itchy eruptions; this remedy
and Ranunc bulb are the main remedies for shingles.
Ranunc bulb: If the eruptions are on the chest or back, there is severe
pain between the ribs, and touch, movement, or deep breathing
produces significant pain; this remedy and Rhus tox are the main
remedies for shingles.
Lachesis: If the eruptions are on the left side of the body, very dark red,
bluish, or purplish, quite painful, and highly sensitive to touch.
Mezereum: If the pain is burning or sharp and lightning-like and
persists after lesions heal.
Iris: If the eruptions are on the right side of the chest or abdomen,
characterized by small blisters with dark points, and accompanied
by digestive disturbance.

Arsenicum: If the eruptions burn intensely, are eased by warmth, and worsened by cold air or cold applications.

Take the appropriate remedy at a potency of 6c(x) or 12c(x) every 8 to 12 hours for 2 days. If your symptoms recur after that, take the remedy again, but do not exceed 2 times a day. If there is no improvement after 2 days of taking the remedy, try a different one.

Nutritional Supplements

Dr. Head recommends zinc and the amino acid lysine as antiherpetic nutrients useful in the treatment of shingles. Take 60–90 mg of zinc daily in divided doses, with food. For lysine, take 1,000 mg 2–3 times daily. Continue supplementation for 1–2 weeks. You can begin to taper off when the lesions are drying up and no new lesions are forming.

Reflexology

Diaphragm, spine, thyroid/parathyroid, adrenal glands, pancreas, ovaries/testes, pituitary

Stone/Crystal Therapy

For shingles, use green tourmaline, angelite, black (and blue) kyanite, or green aventurine, recommends crystal healing therapist Katrina Raphaell of Kapaa, Hawaii. Place the stone directly on the lesion or site of pain. Leave the stone there for 5 minutes while visualizing your health goal. Do this 3 times daily. For ongoing benefits, wear the stone, hold it, or carry it in your pocket.

Shock

Medically, shock is a condition in which blood flow in the body is reduced to the point that normal function is impaired. The symptoms—a suddenly pale or ashen complexion, cold and clammy skin, shallow breathing, and shakiness—result from insufficient oxygen (due to the lowered blood supply) reaching the nervous system and other tissues.

The causes of shock are many, including wounds, burns, or other injury, significant blood loss, reaction to a medication or drug, infection, blood poisoning, and emotional trauma.

Severe shock is a medical emergency; seek medical care immediately. In general, anyone suffering from shock should be kept warm (but not overheated). Having the person lie down with the head lower than the feet can help keep circulation going.

Any injury to the body, be it slight or serious, results in some degree of shock. It is a good idea to aid the body in dealing with both physical and emotional shocks by employing some of the remedies below. These remedies in no way replace the medical attention required for serious shock, however.

Essential Oils

For shock, Patricia Davis, founder of the London School of Aromatherapy, recomends inhaling Peppermint or Neroli essential oil right from a bottle. Or sprinkle a few drops on a handkerchief or tissue and inhale it that way. Repeat as needed.[1]

Flower Essences

"Five Flower Formula (Rescue Remedy) provides immediate calm and emotional neutralizing in any emergency," states flower essence therapist Patricia Kaminski of Nevada City, California. The flower essence Arnica is indicated for all symptoms of shock and post-traumatic stress syndrome. Take 4 drops each of Five Flower and Arnica hourly, or more frequently, until your symptoms subside.

Food Therapy

During the acute stage of an emotional or physical shock, it is best to give your body a break from food and not place the added burden of digestion on the already taxed system. Wait until you've recovered a little from the initital shock before you eat. However, drink warm water to keep your system hydrated, advises nutritionist Ann Louise Gittleman, N.D., C.N.S., M.S. If blood sugar is a problem during the acute stage of shock, a little orange juice in water is a good solution, she says.

Herbal Medicine

Licorice (*Glycrrhiza glabra*) tincture or simply fruit juice with a little salt can ease shock, states Amanda McQuade Crawford, M.N.I.M.H., Dip.Phyto., director of the Ojai Center of Phytotherapy in Ojai, California. Put 1 teaspoon of licorice tincture in 8 ounces of water, or 1/8 teaspoon salt in 8 ounces of fruit juice, and sip slowly. Licorice supports the adrenal glands, which are taxed when the system undergoes shock. Salt prevents a dangerous drop in blood pressure. Both remedies rehydrate the body.

Homeopathy

Homeopathic physician Michael G. Carlston, M.D., of Santa Rosa, California, recommends Aconite napellus or Ignatia amara for emotional shock and Carbo vegetabilis for physical shock. If there is an injury involved, take Arnica, too. Take the appropriate remedy at a 30c or 200c potency every 15 minutes until symptoms subside.

Nutritional Supplements

Taking supplements during the acute stage of shock is not advisable. Supplements are best used to support the body in recovery after the initial shock is over. Since shock is stressful for the adrenal glands, taking B complex vitamins and vitamin C, which support adrenal function, is indicated. Take a B complex supplement (containing 50 mg of each of the primary B vitamins) daily for 4 weeks. The antioxidant vitamin C also supports immune function; take 1,000 mg 3 times daily for 4 weeks.[2]

Reflexology

Spine, solar plexus

Stone/Crystal Therapy

Smoky quartz, black tourmaline, rose quartz, or hematite (amethyst) are beneficial for shock, says Katrina Raphaell, crystal healing therapist and founder of the Crystal Academy of Advanced Healing Arts in Kapaa, Hawaii. Place the stone on the center of your body at the level of the heart or over your solar plexus (top of the abdomen, below the ribs). Leave it in place for at least 5 minutes while visualizing your health goal. You can also take a gem essence of the stone. As ongoing healing, wear the stone, hold it, or carry it in your pocket. (For instructions on making a gem essence, see part 3, "Stone/ Crystal Therapy," p. 403.)

Sinus Congestion/Infection

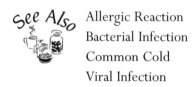 Allergic Reaction
Bacterial Infection
Common Cold
Viral Infection

Sinus congestion refers to when the nasal sinuses (cavities in the bones of the head above the eyes and around the nose, and connected

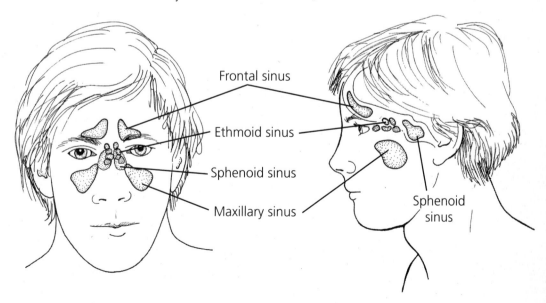

Frontal sinus

Ethmoid sinus

Sphenoid sinus

Maxillary sinus

Sphenoid sinus

to the nasal passages) fill with mucus and their ducts become blocked, impeding drainage. Common symptoms are a stuffed-up nose, a feeling of fullness or stuffiness in the face, and a headache. Such congestion often develops during or after a cold.

Congestion leaves the sinuses vulnerable to infection, creating as it does an ideal bacterial breeding ground. Sinus infection is associated with viral or bacterial infections of the upper respiratory tract. As with congestion, a sinus infection is often preceded by the common cold.

Sinusitis is inflammation of the mucous membrane lining the sinuses. It can be caused by a viral or bacterial infection or by allergies. Over 50 percent of sinusitis cases are due to bacterial infection.[1]

Symptoms of a sinus infection or sinusitis can include those of sinus congestion, along with facial pain, facial swelling, tenderness in the areas where the sinuses are located, nasal discharge, toothache, earache, and sometimes fever. In sinusitis, a nasal discharge may or may not be present.

If you suffer from chronic sinusitis, seek the assistance of a qualified medical practitioner to determine the cause(s) and institute the appropriate treatment.

Essential Oils

Jody E. Noé, M.S., N.D., a naturopathic physician from Brattleboro, Vermont, suggests the following preparation for relief of sinus congestion. Blend 2 ml each of Thyme, Pine, Lavender, and Clove essential oils and add to 100 ml of a fatty acid base oil such as almond or olive oil. Rub this preparation topically on sinus areas and apply to the inside of the nostrils. Use as needed.

Flower Essences

Self-Heal and Yarrow Special Formula can serve as the foundational healing agents for sinus problems. Other flower essences to address the specific emotions, mental attitude, and environmental conditions of the individual are recommended, states Patricia Kaminski, a flower essence therapist and codirector of the Flower Essence Society. Self-Heal supports the body's innate healing ability. Yarrow Special

Formula strengthens and protects against environmental toxicity and stress. Take 4 drops of each 2–4 times daily, or as needed.

Food Therapy

Eat:

Garlic, cayenne, horseradish, foods high in vitamin C (see part 3, "Food Therapy," p. 378). Drink plenty of fluids (diluted vegetable juices, soups, herbal tea, green tea, green drinks, especially barley green).

Avoid:

Sugar (and limit fruit and fruit juices), fried food, mucus-forming foods (dairy, chocolate, eggs, junk food), cold foods, food allergens.

Herbal Medicine

Red root (*Ceanothus americanus*) has a great ability to clear congestion and has a long history of use for that purpose. "Red root is the herb for a lack of movement crisis, which is what sinusitis is," says Michael Cottingham, a clinical herbalist from Silver City, New Mexico.

A fresh root tincture is the most effective form in which to take red root, and relatively large amounts work well, says Cottingham. Red root has no known toxicity, so larger dosages are safe. He suggests combining red root tincture with echinacea (*E. spp.*) tincture to aid the immune system. Use equal parts of the two tinctures, and during the acute stage, take 30–50 drops of the mix up to 5 times daily for a week. Take for another week, reducing the dosage by 10 percent each day. For children 11 to 13 years old, the dosage is half that of adults. For children under 12, cut the dosage in half again. As an astringent, red root tightens and dries tissue. You may feel this sensation in your mouth from taking the tincture.

Homeopathy

For acute sinusitis, two homeopathic remedies are commonly indicated:[2]

Kali bich: When all the sinuses are affected and there is thick, sticky, yellow or yellow-green mucus that is hard to expel and a nasal tone of voice due to complete nasal blockage.

Merc viv: Especially for frontal sinusitis accompanied by a greenish discharge, bad breath, excessive salivation, and no resistance to infection such that you get every cold that comes along and it inevitably turns into sinusitis.

Take the appropriate remedy in a 30c potency 3 times daily for 2–3 days.

Nutritional Supplements

David R. Field, N.D., L.Ac., a naturopathic physician based in Santa Rosa, California, discourages the use of ephedrine products. "People use them chronically, and they are only for very short-term use. If you have any adrenal depletion or have high blood pressure, ephedrine is too stimulating." He recommends instead a protocol of supplements and herbs to ease sinus problems, along with nasal douches (see "Other Remedies" below):

Zinc: 30 mg daily for 1 week.

Vitamin A: 5,000–10,000 IU daily for 1 week.

B vitamins: Take the manufacturer's recommended dosage.

Stinging nettle (*Urtica dioica*): Take 2 freeze-dried capsules 3–4 times daily. You can take nettle indefinitely as a preventive measure if you are prone to sinus congestion and/or infection. Nettle is an astringent and as such cleanses and tightens the tissues of the sinuses. The herb is also a whole body tonic, so can support the immune system.

Reflexology

Sinuses, face, head, neck, adrenal glands, pituitary, ileocecal valve (helps eliminate mucus)

Stone/Crystal Therapy

To support sinus clearing, use azurite, fluorite, amethyst, or kyanite, recommends crystal healing therapist Katrina Raphaell of Kapaa, Hawaii. Place the stone on the skin over the sinuses. Leave the stone in place for 5 minutes while visualizing your health goal. Do this 3 times daily. In between treatments, wear the stone, hold it, or carry it in your pocket for continual healing.

Other Remedies

It is important in conditions of congestion to drink lots of water (at least 8 glasses daily) to aid the body in clearing the blockage. "Water can be one of the ultimate first aid remedies," observes Michael Cottingham.

For sinusitis, in addition to the herbs above, Cottingham suggests nasal washes (douches) with a saline solution, matching the solution to the salinity of the body. "While the red root reduces congestion internally, the saline wash reduces congestion on the surface," he explains. To make the wash, dissolve 1 teaspoon of sea salt to 1 quart of lukewarm distilled water; this is the kitchen approximation of the body's saline level.

There are several ways you can do the wash: use a netty pot, a teapot-like container with a long spout, designed for the purpose of nasal washes and available at health food stores; use a nasal wash bottle, available at drug stores; use a turkey baster; or even pour some of the solution in your hand and snort it up one nostril. Whatever mechanism you use, tilt your head back and to the side, pour 3 tablespoons of the solution in the top nostril, and let it run out the other nostril. Tilt your head the other way and repeat on the other nostril. During the acute stage, do the rinse 2–4 times daily; 4 is preferable. If you tend to develop sinusitis often, do this rinse 1–2 times per week as a preventative measure.

Sore Throat

See Also

Bacterial Infection
Laryngitis
Strep Throat
Tonsillitis
Viral Infection

Pain or soreness in the throat (pharynx) has multiple causes: bacterial or viral infection, irritation from inhalants (such as cigarette smoke), allergies, laryngitis, tonsillitis, or dry air. Most sore throats in adults are due to viral infection, and can be treated with the remedies below. A viral sore throat is usually less painful and comes on more gradually than a strep throat, which is a common bacterial infection. It is also more often accompanied by a cold and cough. If there is a fever, it tends to be lower than that with a strep throat.

If your sore throat persists, seek medical care. If you suspect your sore throat is due to strep, see "Strep Throat." If you have ever had rheumatic fever or there is a history of it in your family, consult your doctor at the first sign of a sore throat.

Essential Oils

Julia Fischer, a medical aromatherapist from Northern California, has a number of suggestions to ease a sore throat. Put 1 drop of Cinnamon Bark essential oil on the back of your hand and lick it off; repeat every 10–15 minutes, as needed. Rub 1 drop of Clove oil on your gums, then gargle with salt water (1/4 teaspoon sea salt to 4 ounces of warm water) 3–4 times daily. Rub Bay Laurel essential oil over the swollen lymph nodes of the neck (below the ears along each side of the neck) 3–4 times daily.

Flower Essences

If you have frequent sore throats and they are connected with issues of low-self esteem and/or performance anxiety when speaking or otherwise performing in public, Larch is the indicated flower essence, according to naturalist Richard Katz of Nevada City, California. Take 4 drops under the tongue, no less than half an hour before eating, at least 4 times daily until your sore throat is gone. During the acute stage, you can take the essence more frequently, as often as hourly if needed.

Food Therapy

Eat:

Garlic, cayenne, horseradish, ginger, bay leaves, miso soup, hot foods, foods high in vitamin C (see part 3, "Food Therapy,", p. 378). Drink plenty of fluids (diluted vegetable juices, soups, herbal tea, green tea).

Eat 2 cloves of crushed garlic 2 times daily as a remedy for a sore throat, says David R. Field, N.D., L.Ac., a naturopathic physician based in Santa Rosa, California. Put the garlic in soup or pasta, or spread it on toast.

Avoid:

Sugar (and limit fruit and fruit juices), mucus-forming foods (dairy, chocolate, eggs, junk food), food allergens, acid-forming foods and cold foods (see below).

Avoid foods and beverages that make the body more acidic, including sugar, caffeine, excessive protein, fried food, and processed food. A sore throat is typically an indication that the system is too acidic, explains nutritionist Ann Louise Gittleman, N.D., C.N.S., M.S.

Avoid cold foods and liquids, advises Julia Fischer. Even though they may feel soothing to the throat, they do not facilitate healing.

Herbal Medicine

For a sore throat, herbalist Teresa Boardwine of Washington, Virginia, recommends a sage gargle. Sage is drying to mucous membranes, which is helpful for a sore throat.

To make the gargle, put 1 cup of dried culinary sage (*Salvia officinalis*) in 1 quart of boiled water. Cover and let steep for 30 minutes. Strain, then while it is still warm, add 2 tablespoons of sea salt. Whisk until the salt is dissolved. Stir in 1 cup of apple cider vinegar and a pinch of cayenne pepper powder (less than 1/8 of a teaspoon). Gargle with this mixture 3 times daily, or as needed, for a sore throat. Make sure you gargle well, so it gets deep into your throat. It is fine to swallow the rinse. As the mixture stores well, you can make a batch and keep it on hand for cold and flu season. You can refrigerate it, but it is not necessary. Note: Pregnant or lactating women should not use this rinse, as it can dry up breast milk.

Boardwine also suggests chewing on osha root. Osha (*Ligusticum porteri*) is in the same family as celery and is similarly porous and fibrous. Its essential oil is abundant and highly antimicrobial, so chewing on a root will bathe your throat with this healing substance. Keep the root in your mouth as long as possible, chewing until it is pulp. You can also make an osha tea or gargle. For the tea (decoction), use 1 teaspoon of the root per cup of water, cover, and simmer for 20 minutes. Strain, and drink 2 cups of the tea daily. For the gargle, use 1/4 cup of the root per quart of water, cover, simmer for 30 minutes, then strain. As with the sage gargle, use this gargle 3 times daily, or as needed, for a sore throat. Again, make sure you gargle well, and you can swallow the rinse if you like.

"The number-one best thing for a sore throat is solid extract of licorice," states Dr. Field. Take 1/4 teaspoon, straight or diluted in 1/4 cup warm water, 3–4 times daily for a week. He also recommends echinacea glycerite (this is a non-alcohol-based tincture) as a natural antibiotic. Take 2 droppersful, directly in the mouth, 4 times daily for a week.

Homeopathy

The following are common homeopathic remedies indicated for a sore throat, according to homeopathic physician Mitchell Fleisher, M.D.:[1]

Belladonna: If the throat is bright red and sensitive to touch, the soreness develops suddenly on the right side of the throat, and there is high fever and thirst.

Lycopodium: If the soreness starts on the right side of the throat and progresses to the left, is eased by drinking warm liquids, and is accompanied by irritability.

Lachesis: If the soreness starts on the left side of the throat and progresses to the right, is aggravated by swallowing saliva, and is eased by eating.

Take the appropriate remedy at a potency of 6c or 12c up to 4 times daily. Discontinue when your symptoms improve; repeat as needed.

Nutritional Supplements

Naturopathic physicians Michael T. Murray, N.D., and Joseph Pizzorno, N.D., recommend the following supplements to support the immune system and help resolve a sore throat:[2]

Vitamin C: 500 mg every 2 hours.

Bioflavonoids: 1 g daily.

Vitamin A: 25,000 IU daily.

Beta-carotene: 200,000 IU daily.

Zinc is another useful supplement for sore throats; zinc lozenges have become a popular cold and sore throat remedy. Dr. Field recommends taking 2 mg of zinc in lozenge form 5 times daily for a week. Do not take zinc for longer than that because it can cause copper deficiency.

Reflexology

Throat, neck, cervical spine, adrenal glands, lymphatic system, spleen

Stone/Crystal Therapy

As a crystal remedy for sore throat, use blue lace agate or blue calcite angelite, suggests Katrina Raphaell, crystal healing therapist and founder of the Crystal Academy of Advanced Healing Arts in Kapaa, Hawaii. Place the stone directly on your neck at the throat. Visualizing your health goal, leave the stone in place for 5 minutes. Do this 3 times daily. You may also want to wear the stone, hold it, or carry it in your pocket for ongoing benefits.

Other Remedies

For sore throat, Dr. Gittleman has found a simple remedy to be quite effective in most cases. Dissolve 1/4 teaspoon of sea salt in 8 ounces of water and drink. Repeat this every 2 hours until the soreness is gone. Use the same mixture to gargle morning and evening. The salt helps neutralize the acidity of the body. You can also make a stronger salt gargle, but don't swallow it.

Sprain/Pulled Ligament

A sprain involves overstretching or tearing joint tissue, typically a ligament (a condition known as a pulled ligament). Ligaments join bone to bone or bone to muscle, and can be injured by overuse or twisting, turning, or falling. Pain, swelling, heat, and limited function of the joint are the symptoms that quickly follow this type of trauma. Bruising may also occur.

The treatment for a sprain is RICE: rest the affected joint, ice it, compress it with an elastic bandage, and elevate it to aid in drainage. Elevate the injured limb and apply cold/ice packs for the first 24 to 48 hours to reduce the swelling and inflammation. When icing an injury, don't place the cold/ice pack directly on the skin. Put a towel between it and the skin. Don't ice continually, but alternate ice on and ice off. Compression also should be alternated with no compression. Wrap the affected area with an elastic bandage, being careful not to wrap it too tight. Leave on for 30 minutes on, then off for 15 minutes. You can wrap the bandage around the ice pack.

Opinion now varies among sports medicine doctors over whether to continue cold applications after the initial 24 to 48 hours or to begin applying heat.[1] Perhaps the best approach is to use whichever eases the pain of your injury at that point.[2] Some doctors recommend alternating heat and cold after the initial cold treatment. In any case, rest of the injured area should continue.

As the intensity of symptoms is not necessarily related to whether the injury involves a fracture rather than only a sprain, seek medical care if you suspect you have broken a bone or if the sprain is severe. If your symptoms persist despite treatment with the methods described here, you should also seek medical care.

Essential Oils

Medical aromatherapist Julia Fischer of Northern California offers a healing essential oil formula for sprains. First, for a wrist or ankle sprain, rub 1 drop each of Peppermint and Clove essential oil into the affected area, then soak in a foot or hand bath. After the soak, apply the following soothing formula. Combine:

Helichrysum: 4 drops
Bay Laurel: 3 drops
Rosemary Camphor: 2 drops
Birch: 1 drop

Arnica fatty oil and/or St. John's wort fatty oil: 6 teaspoons
    (30 ml) total of one or a combination of these fatty oils
    (an herbal fatty oil is a carrier oil that has been infused
    with a given herb, in this case arnica or St. John's wort)

Apply this formula 2–3 times daily. Support the sprained tissue by
wrapping with an elastic bandage, if desired.

Flower Essences

To ease a sprain, alternate topical applications of Arnica Alleve flower
oil with Dandelion flower oil compresses, recommends Patricia Kaminski,
a flower essence therapist and educator from Nevada City, California. Do
2–4 applications daily, or as needed. For the compress treatment, gently
rub 1–2 tablespoons of Dandelion flower oil on the affected area and cover
with a hot or cold compress, depending on the condition.

Food Therapy

Eat:

Whole grains, lean protein, foods high in vitamin C, magnesium,
and silica.

For their anti-inflammatory effects, eat ginger, turmeric, pineapple, papaya, and foods rich in omega-3 and omega-6 essential fatty
acids, suggests Nick Buratovich, N.M.D., a naturopathic physician from
Tempe, Arizona. Eat pineapple and papaya by themselves, not with
other foods, to get the anti-inflammatory effect of the enzymes these
fruits contain.

Avoid:

Coffee and other forms of caffeine (aside from green tea) because
caffeine blocks endorphin receptors in the brain, says Dr. Buratovich.
As endorphins facilitate pain relief, people who consume a lot of caffeine tend to have a low threshold of pain. He also recommends avoiding animal products because they contain arachidonic acid, which
promotes inflammation. Also avoid soft drinks and acid-forming foods.

(For a list of foods containing the substances cited above, see part
3, "Food Therapy," p. 376.)

Herbal Medicine

For a topical application to ease the inflammation and pain of a sprain, combine equal parts of infused oils of arnica (*Arnica montana*), St. John's wort (*Hypericum perforatum*), and lobelia (*Lobelia inflata*) seed, with a few drops of essential oil of Sweet Birch, says David Winston, A.H.G., a clinical herbalist from Washington, New Jersey. (Note that an infused oil is distinct from an essential oil or herbal tincture. It is the herb in a carrier oil such as olive oil, rather than an extract or an essential oil preserved in alcohol or glycerin. Some infused products are labeled olive oil extract.) Lightly massage the blend into the affected area twice daily, for as long as needed. (This oil blend is available as Compound Arnica Oil from Herbalist and Alchemist; see David Winston's listing under "Herbal Medicine" in Appendix B: Resources.)

Winston has also found Chinese medicine remedies excellent for sprains. He highly recommends dit da jows, which are topical preparations that reduce inflammation and promote circulation in the injured area. Tiger Balm and White Flower Oil are common dit da jow formulas.

Bruise plasters are also remarkably effective, says Winston. "A bruise can go overnight from looking fresh to looking three weeks old." Bruise plasters are strips with a tar-like substance on them that you stick onto the area of your sprain and leave on overnight. A bruise plaster is a rubefacient, Winston explains, meaning it increases blood flow, which aids the inflammatory process in clearing toxins and debris from an area of tissue damage.

Both dit da jows and bruise plasters are available in Chinese medicine stores.

Homeopathy

Naturopathic physicians Robert Ullmann, N.D., and Judyth Reichenberg-Ullmann, N.D., cite the following homeopathic remedies for a sprain:[3]

Arnica: "The best medicine to give first for sprains."

Bryonia: Indicated for pain that is worse with motion and joint injuries not helped by Arnica.

Ledum: "The best medicine" if the injured area is cold to the touch and feels better with cold applications.

Rhus tox: If the primary symptom is stiffness that is alleviated by stretching and moving.

Ruta: Indicated for a sprain if there are no clear symptoms suggesting one of the remedies above.

Take the appropriate remedy in a 30c potency every 2–4 hours until your symptoms improve. Stop taking the remedy, repeat if the symptoms return. If there is no improvement with 3 doses, you probably do not have the correct remedy.

Nutritional Supplements

To relieve the pain and speed recovery from a sprain, Dr. Buratovich recommends the following supplements:

DLPA (D,L-phenylalanine): 750 mg 3 times daily before meals for 1–3 weeks; a pain-relieving amino acid.

Tryptophan: 2–4 g 3 times daily for up to 1 month. This amino acid has been shown to reduce pain, perhaps by raising the pain threshold, although the exact mechanism is unknown.[4] To ensure uptake, avoid protein for 90 minutes before and after taking.

Vitamin C: 1,000–2,000 mg three times daily for one month; helps rebuild connective tissue.

Bioflavonoids: These plant substances help stabilize connective tissue and decrease inflammation. Quercetin or citrus bioflavonoids are the best form to take. Take 1000–3000 mg daily for one month.

Bromelain: 2 capsules on an empty stomach 3 times daily for 1 month; an anti-inflammatory enzyme compound found in pineapple.

Curcumin: 100 mg twice daily for one month; an anti-inflammatory substance derived from turmeric. Bromelain and curcumin can be purchased as a combination product.

EPA and GLA: These essential fatty acids (EFAs) are anti-inflammatory. EPA (eicosapentaenoic acid) is an omega-3 EFA found in fish oils; take 300 mg 3 times daily for one month. GLA (gamma-linolenic acid) is an omega-6 EFA found in evening primrose, black currant, and borage oils; take 100 mg 3 times daily for one month.

Reflexology

Treat the area of the foot corresponding to the location of your sprain.

Stone/Crystal Therapy

To help heal a sprain, use green calcite, green aventurine, double-terminated clear quartz, or black tourmaline, notes crystal healing therapist Katrina Raphaell of Kapaa, Hawaii. Place the stone on or as near as possible to the sprained joint. Visualizing your health goal, leave the stone in place for 5 minutes. Do this 3 times daily. In between treatments, wear the stone, hold it, or carry it in your pocket for continual healing.

Other Remedies

"Icing for the first few hours is the most important thing to do for a sprain," states David Winston. He recommends hydrotherapy after that. Soak the affected part for 2 minutes in hot water, then 30 seconds in cold, alternating back and forth about 6 times. This can make a significant difference in reducing swelling and improving range of motion of the joint, says Winston.

Stomachache

 See Also
Colic (Infant)
Food Poisoning
Heartburn/Indigestion
Nausea and Vomiting
Ulcer

As with other gastrointestinal disturbances, an upset stomach or stomachache can be caused by many things, including: overeating or eating too quickly; rich, fatty, or spicy foods; food allergies; food poisoning; stress and anxiety; and flu or other infection. In addition to the pain, a stomachache may be accompanied by bloating, gas, heartburn, nausea, and abdominal cramping.

For the occasional stomachache, the following remedies can be helpful. If you frequently experience stomach pain or your stomachache lasts longer than 48 hours, consult your doctor. Pain in the abdominal region can indicate a range of disorders, among them appendicitis (the pain may be focused in the lower right quadrant of the abdomen), an ulcer, and gallbladder problems.

Essential Oils

Put a drop of Peppermint essential oil on a sugar cube and suck on it to relieve a stomachache. Be sure that you use a high-quality essential oil.[1]

Flower Essences

When your stomachache is accompanied by moodiness or other fluctuating symptoms, take Chamomile flower essence, says Richard Katz, founder of the Flower Essence Society. When it is accompanied by emotional identification with others or absorption of others' emotional toxicity, take Pink Yarrow. The dosage for both is 4 drops under the tongue at least 4 times daily. If needed, you can take the flower essences hourly, or even more often.

Food Therapy

Eat:

Ginger, warm and bland foods, miso and other soups, white basmati rice.

Avoid:

Milk, soft drinks, alcohol, caffeine, spicy foods and raw foods, food allergens.

Herbal Medicine

For stomachache, make a tea using equal parts of chamomile (*Matricaria recutita*) flower, fennel (*Foeniculum vulgare*) seed, and peppermint (*Mentha piperata*) leaf, recommends Mindy Green, A.H.G., M.S., an herbalist from Boulder, Colorado. Use one teaspoon of the mix per cup of boiled water. Steep for 15 minutes, then strain. Drink a cup 1–4 times daily for 1 week or longer. These are all safe herbs for long-term use, states Green. Chamomile alone is also helpful, if you want to keep it simple.

Bitter herbs such as gentian (*Gentiana lutea*) enhance digestion and treat a "sour" stomach, says David R. Field, N.D., L.Ac., a naturopathic physician from Santa Rosa, California. Put 10 drops of gentian tincture in 1/4 glass of water and drink before each meal. You can even use Angostura Bitters, a flavoring used in cocktails and readily available at the supermarket, for the same effect. Take in the same dosage as the gentian tincture. Do this for 2–4 weeks.

Slippery elm *(Ulmus rubra, U. fulva)* capsules are also helpful for easing a stomachache; follow manufacturer's directions.

Homeopathy

See the conditions that indicate a more specific complaint, such as "Heartburn/Indigestion" and "Nausea/Vomiting."

Nutritional Supplements

Digestive enzymes with HCl can help resolve a stomachache, says Dr. Field. Take 2 capsules of plant-based digestive enzymes with HCl (hydrochloric acid, a gastric digestive juice) midway through each meal. Take the supplement for 2–3 days. If you also suffer from heartburn, give yourself a simple test to see if you should take just digestive enzymes or a combination product of enzymes with HCl (see "Heartburn/Indigestion").

Reflexology

Stomach, solar plexus

Stone/Crystal Therapy

For a stomachache, use gold jasper, amber, green calcite, or gold calcite, recommends Katrina Raphaell, crystal healing therapist and author of the crystal reference series *The Crystal Trilogy*. Place the stone on your abdomen directly over the area of greatest distress. Keep it in place for 5 minutes while visualizing your health goal. Do this 3 times daily. At other times, wear the stone, hold it, or carry it in your pocket for ongoing effects.

Other Remedies

Mix 1/2 teaspoon of baking soda in 1 cup of water and drink to ease an acid stomach, suggests Dr. Field.

He also recommends a castor oil pack to ease a stomachache and improve digestion. Put castor oil on a hot towel and place it on the abdomen. Cover with plastic wrap to keep the heat in. Leave it in place until the heat is gone. Do this twice in a day, if needed.

Strep Throat

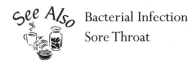 Bacterial Infection
Sore Throat

Strep throat is an infection by the *Streptococcus* bacteria. The symptoms come on suddenly and include a very painful sore throat, high fever, generalized achiness, and tender or hard lymph nodes. A strep throat is usually more painful than a viral sore throat, comes on more quickly, and typically involves a higher fever.

The body is often able to resolve the infection without the aid of antibiotics, but strep throat makes people nervous because of the possibility that it can lead to rheumatic fever, which in turn can permanently damage the heart. Rheumatic fever is no longer common, and can be avoided if the bacteria are killed in the first 10 to 12 days of infection.[1] Some of the remedies below can knock out the infection during that time, but it is up to individuals and their doctors to decide whether antibiotics are indicated. If you have had rheumatic fever, or if your family has a history of rheumatic fever, contact your doctor immediately upon the first indication of a sore throat, even if you're not sure that it's strep throat.

Essential Oils

Melissa essential oil has been shown to exert antibacterial properties against the *Streptococcus* bacteria, according to Jeanne Rose, an aromatherapist and herbalist based in San Francisco, California.[2] Clary sage, Eucalyptus, Geranium, and Lavender are also useful essential oils for strep throat, says aromatherapy authority Robert B. Tisserand.[3]

Use the selected oil or a combination of 2–3 oils as an inhalation, in baths, or in a diffuser. A diffuser placed in the sickroom helps prevent the spread of bacterial infection to other household members. When used topically, Melissa oil can cause a reaction in people with skin problems or who have very sensitive skin (infants are in this category). Even 5 drops in a bath can produce a reaction.[4] To be safe, you may want to use Melissa in inhalation or diffusion only.

Flower Essences

Self-Heal and Yarrow Special Formula can serve as the foundational healing agents for a strep throat. Other flower essences to address the specific emotions, mental attitude, and environmental conditions of the individual are recommended, states Patricia Kaminski, a flower essence therapist and codirector of the Flower Essence Society. Self-Heal supports the body's innate healing ability. Yarrow Special Formula strengthens and protects against environmental toxicity and stress. Take 4 drops of each 2–4 times daily, or as needed.

Food Therapy

Eat:

Garlic, cayenne, horseradish, ginger, bay leaves, foods high in vitamin C (see part 3, "Food Therapy," p. 378). Drink plenty of fluids (diluted vegetable juices, soups, herbal tea, green tea).

Avoid:

Sugar, dairy, alcohol, and caffeine.

Herbal Medicine

According to medical herbalist Chanchal Cabrera, M.N.I.M.H., A.H.G., of Vancouver, British Columbia, if you catch strep throat early and take high doses of the following herbs and supplements, you can usually get rid of it. "But you can't be wishy-washy about it," she says. "You need to be vigilant with the treatment." Here is her protocol:

Herbal mouth rinse: Combine equal parts of tinctures of cooking sage (*Salvia officinalis*), rosemary (*Rosmarinus officinalis*), myrrh (*Commiphora molmol*), goldenseal (*Hydrastis canadensis*), echinacea (*E. spp.*), bloodroot (red root, *Ceanothus americanus*), and peppermint (*Mentha piperata*) for flavoring. Add 1 teaspoon of this blend to 1/2 cup of water. Gargle with and swallow the rinse as often as you can, hourly if possible. Myrrh works on contact, so do not rinse your mouth out afterward. Continue the procedure as long as symptoms are present. A commercial preparation of this mouth rinse, called Orcln, is available through the Gaia Garden Herbal Dispensary and Clinic in Vancouver, British Columbia (see Cabrera's listing under "Herbal Medicine" in Appendix B: Resources).

Echinacea: Take high doses of tincture, 1 teaspoon 3–4 times daily.

Garlic: Take fresh garlic orally. Odorless garlic pills are worthless, according to Cabrera, because the active ingredient in garlic is carried in its essential oil, which is what smells. To lessen the strong odor, chop up a clove of garlic, put it on a teaspoon, and swallow it like a pill, without chewing it. Take as much garlic as you can throughout the day.

Zinc lozenges: Take in 5-mg doses, as much as you can be bothered to suck on, up to 50 mg daily. Don't take on an empty stomach.

If your glands are swollen as well, take cleavers (*Galium aparine*), which is best consumed as a tea. To make an infusion, pour boiled water over the herb (1 teaspoon of dried cleavers per cup of water or 1 ounce of the herb per pint of water), cover the mixture, and let it steep for 10 minutes. Drink 2–3 cups daily; the more the better. Cleavers is a lymphatic flusher, meaning it helps the lymph system drain.

Finally, Cabrera offers a soothing topical treatment for swollen glands, using mullein leaf. Mullein (*Verbascum thapsus*) reduces swelling. Bruise a fresh leaf with a rolling pin, wrap it around your neck like a scarf, then tie a wool scarf over it. The added warmth aids the process. You can speed the process more by placing a hot pack over the leaf and then tying the scarf around both. Leave the leaf in place for an hour. Do 1–2 times daily.

Homeopathy

As homeopathy does not prescribe remedies on the basis of the causal bacteria but on the characteristics of the malady as it is experienced by the individual, see "Sore Throat."

Nutritional Supplements

As a program for strep throat, naturopathic physician Bradley Bongiovanni, N.D., of Independence, Ohio, suggests the following combination of supplements and herbs:

Vitamin C: 1,000 mg 3 times daily for 10–14 days.
Zinc: 30 mg twice daily for 10–14 days.
Thymus gland extract: 500 mg 3 times daily; immune support.
Garlic (fresh extract): 400 mg twice daily for 10–14 days.
Echinacea and astragalus: 1,000 mg (capsules) or 2 ml (extract) 3 times
daily for 10–14 days.

Reflexology

Throat, neck, cervical spine, adrenal glands, lymphatic system, spleen

Stone/Crystal Therapy

Sylvanite placed upon the throat and taken in elixir form (3–5 drops 3 times daily) can bring relief from strep throat in 2 days, states Melody, author of the crystal reference series *Love Is in the Earth*. You can attach the stone with hypoallergenic tape or wear it on a choker-style necklace. Wear it for two days, or less if the symptoms abate. (For instructions on making an elixir, see part 3, "Stone/Crystal Therapy," p. 403.)

Other Remedies

The "apple cider vinegar cure" can be very effective for strep throat, states natural medicine practitioner David Carroll, adding, "[It] has been known to cure strep throat in less than four days." To take the cure, stir 2 teaspoons of apple cider vinegar into a glass of warm water. Take a sip, gargle, and spit it out. Take another sip and swallow it.

Continue this routine, alternating between gargling and swallowing, until you have emptied the glass. Repeat the whole procedure every hour for several days. It may sound like a bit of a commitment, but if that's all it takes to get rid of strep, isn't it worth it?[5]

Stye

A stye, or hordeolum, is a small blister on the eyelid, resulting from an inflammation of a sebaceous (oil-producing) gland in an eyelash follicle. It is caused by an infection, usually of the *Staphylococcus* bacteria. The condition begins with redness, swelling, and tenderness in the area of the infected follicle. A blister then forms, which may subside or burst in the process of healing. Styes can also be internal, forming under the eyelid. Internal styes may require medical attention.

Applying frequent hot compresses is a basic treatment to ease the pain of a stye, promote drainage, and speed healing.

Essential Oils

Medical aromatherapist Julia Fischer of Northern California recommends putting a pinch of goldenseal powder in Lavender, Myrtle, or Rose hydrosol (hydrosol is aromatic water that is a coproduct of the essential oil distillation process) and letting it sit for 10 minutes. Then strain the liquid through an unbleached coffee filter. With an eye cup, hold the solution on the affected eye for a few seconds. Do this 4–5 times daily, or as needed, until the stye is resolved. The hydrosol is soothing; and goldenseal is a strong antimicrobial, so can help fight infection.

Flower Essences

Self-Heal and Yarrow Special Formula can serve as the foundational healing agents for styes. Other flower essences to address the specific emotions, mental attitude, and environmental conditions of the individual are recommended, states Patricia Kaminski, a flower essence therapist and codirector of the Flower Essence Society. Self-Heal supports the body's innate healing ability. Yarrow Special Formula strengthens and protects against environmental toxicity and stress. Take 4 drops of each 2–4 times daily, or as needed.

Food Therapy

Eat:

Garlic, more vegetables and fruits, raw foods. Drink plenty of fluids.

Avoid:

Sugar, processed foods.

Herbal Medicine

Herbalist David L. Hoffman, M.N.I.M.H., recommends treating a stye both internally and externally:[1]

Internal: For an antimicrobial, detoxifying, and tonifying tea, combine equal parts blue flag (*Iris versicolor*), cleavers (*Galium aparine*), echinacea (*E. spp.*), eyebright (*Euphrasia officinalis*), and poke root (*Phytolacca americana*). Use 1 teaspoon of the herbal mixture per cup of water. Simmer for 10–15 minutes. Strain and drink 1 cup 3 times daily.

External: Put 1 tablespoon of eyebright in 1 pint of water and simmer for 10 minutes. Let cool, then use as an eyewash or soak gauze with the decoction and place the gauze on the stye for 15 minutes. You should do the external treatment 2–3 times daily.

Homeopathy

"The best remedy for a stye is homeopathic Staphysagria," states Matthew Wood, an herbalist from Minnetrista, Minnesota. "I have never seen this remedy fail to cure promptly and completely." Take in a 6x or 12x potency 2–3 times a day when the stye is aggravated. Stop taking when your symptoms improve.

Nutritional Supplements

To help resolve a stye, naturopathic physician Linda Rector Page, N.D., Ph.D., recommends the following:[2]

Vitamin A: 25,000 IU daily.
Vitamin D: 400 IU daily.
Flaxseed oil: 1 tablespoon daily.

Continue taking until the stye is resolved. You can use aged garlic extract topically as well, says Dr. Page. Combine 1 drop of the extract with 4 drops of distilled water and use as daily eyedrops in the affected eye.

Reflexology

Treat the eye area on your right foot if the stye is on your right eye, or on the left foot if the stye is on your left eye.

Other Remedies

A potato poultice is a traditional treatment for styes, notes naturopathic physician Susan Roberts, N.D., of Portland, Oregon. Grate potato, put it in gauze, and hold it on the affected area of the eye for 15 minutes. Do this 4 times daily, using fresh potato each time, until the stye is resolved. The potato draws out the infection.

Dr. Page cites another kitchen remedy for styes. Spread the white of an egg on a cloth or bandage and apply it to the affected area.[3]

Sunburn

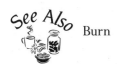 *See Also* Burn

Sunburn arises from overexposure of the skin to the sun's radiation (ultraviolet rays). It is usually a first-degree burn, which is a burn that involves superficial damage, affecting only the epidermis, or outer layer of the skin, and producing redness and mild pain. The development of swelling and blisters signals a second-degree burn, which means the damage has extended deeper into the skin. If you have this degree of burn, talk to your doctor. A very bad sunburn can be a third-degree burn, which requires immediate medical attention.

The redness of sunburn results from capillaries clogged and swollen by the overexposure. Though your sunburn may not seem severe, if it covers a large percentage of your skin area, it is stressful for your body. Using the remedies below can reduce the trauma to your body and aid it in reversing the damage of the burn.

Essential Oils

Essential oils work well for sunburn, notes naturopathic physician Boyer B. Cole, N.M.D., of Cottonwood, Arizona. Put equal parts of Lavender and German Chamomile essential oils in cold water (5 drops of each per ounce of water). Put the solution in a spray bottle, shake well, and spray it on the skin. Do this as often as you like. "It works especially well for kids," says Dr. Cole.

Flower Essences

For sunburn, alternate applications of St. John's Shield flower oil with Calendula Caress flower oil, recommends Patricia Kaminski, an herbalist and flower essence therapist from Nevada City, California. Treat the affected area 2–4 times daily for as long as needed.

Food Therapy

Eat:

Foods high in vitamins A and C (see part 3, "Food Therapy," p. 378). Drink plenty of water.

Avoid:

Sugar, processed foods.

Herbal Medicine

St. John's wort (*Hypericum perforatum*) infused oil is excellent for sunburns, according to herbalist David Hoffmann, M.N.I.M.H. "This is nature's answer for bad sunburn and it will leave the skin in better shape than it started," he says.[1] An infused oil is a carrier oil in which an herb has been steeped. As the oil used is often olive oil, some commercial infused oil products are labeled as olive oil extract.

Herbalist Penelope Ody uses St. John's wort infused oil with Lavender essential oil added for extra sunburn relief. Add 40 drops of Lavender to 2 tablespoons of the infused oil.[2]

Aloe vera gel has become such an accepted treatment for sunburn that drugstores now stock tubes and bottles of it in their suntan lotion section. However, the most effective forms are the gel fresh from the aloe plant (simply cut off a piece and squeeze the gel onto your sunburn) or the type of commercial gel that requires refrigeration. Apply to your sunburn as needed.

Homeopathy

For sunburn, homeopathic physician Mitchell Fleisher, M.D., recommends Calendula officinalis or Urtica urens at a 6c or 12c potency, taken every 2–3 hours as needed. If the skin is swollen, bothered by heat, and alleviated by cold application, take Apis mellifica 12c or 30c every 2–3 hours as needed. You can apply a topical treatment instead of or in addition to the oral remedy, says Dr. Fleisher. Add 20 drops of Calendula tincture to 4 ounces of water and bathe the skin with the mixture until the pain disappears. You can follow the same procedure with Urtica tincture if the sunburn is prickly, stinging, and itchy.[3]

Nutritional Supplements

Taking antioxidants prior to sun exposure can help protect your skin against damage from the sun, which is actually caused by the free radicals the exposure generates in your body. Research has demonstrated that topical application of these nutrients is more effective, but oral supplementation helps as well. Take 50–200 mcg of selenium and 400 IU of vitamin E before going out in the sun. Apply vitamin C (10 percent) lotion with your sunscreen. After sun exposure, apply vitamin E (5 to 100 percent) cream or oil topically and take 5 oral doses of vitamin E (400 IU each) over the next day or two. (Caution: do not take vitamin E supplements if you are on anticoagulant medication.)[4] Take more vitamin C than you usually take to aid in skin healing and support immunity (healing from sunburn requires heightened immune activity).

Stone/Crystal Therapy

Carrollite, quartz, and rose quartz are useful for sunburn, notes Melody, author of the crystal reference series *Love Is in the Earth*. Apply carrollite in elixir form 3 or more times daily as needed to diminish and soothe the burn; improvement generally begins about 3 hours after the onset of treatment. (For instructions on making an elixir, see part 3, "Stone/Crystal Therapy," p. 403.)

To eliminate pain and relieve blistering, place the quartz termination on the burn area for 5–10 minutes. To relieve and lessen blistering, place rose quartz on the sunburned area for 30 minutes.

Other Remedies

Apple cider vinegar is a home remedy for sunburn. Apply as needed to remove the sting.

Surgery (Pre-op and Post-op Support)

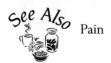 Pain

Surgery, like injury, is a trauma to the body. You can reduce the impact of this trauma and accelerate recovery by taking steps such as those detailed here prior to and following your surgery.

Even minor surgery is a stress on the body, but the trauma is compounded if the surgery requires general anesthesia. Both surgery and anesthesia place a burden on the immune system. If your immunity is already challenged by illness, it is particularly important for you to provide your body with pre-operative and post-operative support to bolster your immunity and aid in the healing process.

Although general anesthetics are better than in the days of ether, they still linger in the body and continue to exert an effect, sometimes producing tiredness and lethargy long after surgery. Using some of the remedies here can help draw the anesthesia out of your body and speed your return to feeling like yourself.

Essential Oils

Medical aromatherapist Julia Fischer of Northern California recommends the following regenerative formula to be used after surgery to prevent infection and speed healing of an incision, as well as reduce scarring:

Helichrysum essential oil: 3 ml

Spike Lavender essential oil: 2 ml

Mugwort essential oil: 2 ml

Sage essential oil: 1 ml

Calophyllum fatty oil: 3 ml (an herbal fatty oil is a carrier oil
that has been infused with a given herb, in this case calophyllum)

Rose hip seed fatty oil: 5 ml

Hemp seed carrier oil: 5 ml

Sunflower vegetable oil: 69 ml

Combine the above ingredients and gently apply the blend to the incision and the surrounding area 2–3 times daily, beginning immediately after surgery. To get the blood moving through the area to facilitate healing, start gentle massages with these applications as soon as you can comfortably touch the skin around the incision, says Fischer.

Fischer notes that you may be instructed by your doctor not to put anything but antibiotic cream on the incision. The above formula is the natural (and more effective) substitute for that cream, and it is completely safe to put on a fresh incision, she adds. Antibiotic cream doesn't speed healing or reduce the scar resulting from the incision, while this formula does.

Flower Essences

Richard Katz, naturalist and founder of the Flower Essence Society, recommends the following flower essence protocol to help you prepare for and recover from surgery:

Pre-op: Take Five Flower Formula (Rescue Remedy) to calm and stabilize you, beginning 2 days before surgery and continuing until the operation. Take 4 drops fairly frequently, as often as hourly.

Post-op: Take a combination of Echinacea, Self-Heal, and Arnica flower essences beginning as soon as you wake up from surgery if you had general anesthesia, and immediately after surgery if the procedure required only local anesthesia. Take 4 drops of each 4 times daily for at least 3 days after surgery, longer if it was a major surgery. The idea is to take the flower essences during the immediate recovery period, however long that lasts.

Food Therapy

Eat:

In the period before and after surgery (the longer the better on both sides), Nick Buratovich, N.M.D., a naturopathic physician from Tempe, Arizona, recommends using ginger and turmeric, which have anti-inflammatory properties, liberally in your diet. Also eat foods high in vitamin A/beta-carotene, vitamin C, vitamin E, bioflavonoids, vitamin K, and zinc. (For a list of foods containing these nutrients, see part 3, "Food Therapy," pp. 376, 378.) Eat turkey, which is high in pain-relieving tryptophan. You should eat it by itself, not with other foods, to promote uptake of the tryptophan.

After surgery, start with clear liquids (broth, especially barley broth, diluted juices, herbal teas), then eat small, light meals and make sure to get plenty of fiber, as constipation is often a problem after surgery.

Avoid:

For at least 1 week before surgery and 2 weeks after, avoid coffee and other forms of caffeine (aside from green tea) because caffeine blocks endorphin receptors in the brain, says Dr. Buratovich. As endorphins facilitate pain relief, people who consume a lot of caffeine tend to have a low threshold of pain. He also recommends avoiding sugar because it suppresses immune function, and animal products (aside from turkey) because they contain arachidonic acid, which promotes inflammation. If you are having major surgery, eliminating caffeine and these foods from your diet for a longer period than cited above is advisable to provide your body with as much pre-op and post-op support as possible.

Herbal Medicine

Medical herbalist Chanchal Cabrera, M.N.I.M.H., A.H.G., of Vancouver, British Columbia, designed the following protocol as preparation for the trauma of surgery and to aid in recovery afterward. It includes herbal medicine and nutritional supplements that support the immune system, lower the risk of infection, protect the brain from the drugs given during and after surgery, help detoxify the liver of drug residues, and reduce scarring. Take all of the below remedies for 2 weeks before and 2 weeks after surgery.[1]

• Combine these herbal tinctures in the amounts designated and take 1 teaspoon of the blend 3 times daily:

Marigold (*Calendula officinalis*): 15 ml; liver stimulant and antioxidant that helps remove drug residues

Milk thistle (*Carduus marianus*): 15 ml; antioxidant that helps protect liver and brain cells from drugs

Gotu kola (*Centella asiatica*): 15 ml; stimulates blood flow, helps heal tissue, and removes drug residues

Horsetail (*Equisetum arvense*): 15 ml; helps heal tissue

Hawthorn (*Crataegus oxyacantha*): 15 ml; helps heal tissue

Goldenrod (*Solidago vigaurea*): 15 ml; antioxidant that protects the brain from the effects of X rays

Dandelion (*Taraxacum officinalis*) root: 10 ml; aids in liver detoxification

• Take antioxidants:

Vitamin C: take throughout the day to bowel tolerance (just below the amount that produces diarrhea).

Zinc: 50 mg daily

Selenium: 400 mcg daily

Beta-carotene: 30,000 IU daily

Vitamin E: 400 IU daily (Note: if you are on anti-coagulant medication, do not take vitamin E, or garlic).

Also take flaxseed oil, evening primrose oil, and lipoic acid in the daily dosages recommended by the manufacturer of the individual product.

• Take chlorophyll to help pull residues of anesthesia and other drugs from your cells; 2 tablespoons twice daily.

• Apply vitamin E oil on the surgical site once the stitches have been taken out; helps the skin heal and reduces scarring.

See "Pain (Natural Pain Relievers)" for natural pain relievers you can use following surgery.

Homeopathy

As preoperative and postoperative support, Maesimund B. Panos, M.D., recommends the following:[2]

Arnica: Take 2 tablets of Arnica 30c before and after surgery to help control shock, bleeding, and soreness, and aid in the healing of tissue; repeat as needed.

Phosphorus: Take 1 dose of Phosphorus 30c the night before surgery to aid in recovery from anesthesia.

Aconite: If you are acutely anxious and apprehensive about the surgery, take 1 dose of Aconite 30c the night before surgery and another dose the next day before the operation.

Gelsemium: For similar reasons as Aconite, but less panicky than trembling with fear; take in the same way as Aconite.

Nutritional Supplements

For 1 week before your operation and 2 weeks after, take the following supplements to minimize the impact of the surgery and facilitate healing, says Dr. Buratovich. As an alternative, you can up the dosage of your regular multivitamin/mineral supplement (the kind that requires divided doses during the day is preferable) and add extra vitamin C, bioflavonoids, and the anti-inflammatories—bromelain and curcumin—in the dosages below:

Vitamin C: 1–2 g three times daily; speeds tissue repair.

Bioflavonoids: Take 1,000 mg of quercetin or citrus bioflavonoids three times daily; these plant substances stabilize capillary membranes, limit bleeding, and decrease inflammation.

Vitamin A or beta-carotene: 25,000 IU 1–4 times daily; speeds skin healing and builds a stronger scar. Although vitamin A can be toxic when taken at high doses for a prolonged period, the dosage here, taken on a short-term basis, will not produce toxicity.

Vitamin E: 200–400 IU 2 times daily; increases circulation, speeds wound healing, and decreases scarring. You can also apply vitamin E oil to the scar once the wound has closed to facilitate less scarring.

Vitamin K: 70–140 mcg daily, in 3 divided doses; increases blood clotting and therefore lessens bleeding.

Zinc: 30–60 mg 2 times daily; speeds tissue repair.

Bromelain: 2 capsules on an empty stomach 3 times daily for 1 month; an anti-inflammatory enzyme compound found in pineapple.

Curcumin: 100 mg twice daily for one month; an anti-inflammatory substance derived from turmeric. Bromelain and curcumin can be purchased as a combination product.

DLPA (optional): 750 mg 3 times daily before meals for 1–3 weeks; D,L-phenylalanine is a pain-relieving amino acid. Taking this natural pain reliever may enable you to cut your dosage of conventional painkillers.

Tryptophan: 2–4 g 3 times daily for up to 1 month. This amino acid has been shown to reduce pain, perhaps by raising the pain threshold, although the exact mechanism is unknown.[3] To ensure uptake, avoid protein for 90 minutes before and after taking.

Reflexology

Treat the area of the foot corresponding to the organ or part of the body that was involved in the surgery.

Stone/Crystal Therapy

As preoperative healing support, use celestite, green aventurine, or angelite, states crystal healing therapist Katrina Raphaell of Kapaa, Hawaii. Place the stone directly on the body at the site of the upcoming surgery. Leave it there for 5 minutes while visualizing successful surgery. Do this 3 times daily beginning at least 3 days prior to surgery. In between treatments, you may also want to wear the stone, hold it, or carry it in your pocket for ongoing benefits.

For postoperative support, use hematite, nebula stone, and black tourmaline, says Raphaell. Place the stone near the incision rather than directly on it. Leave it on for 5 minutes and visualize healing from the surgery. Do this 3 times daily for as long as you like, and keep the stone near you in between treatments.

Swollen Glands

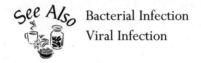 Bacterial Infection
Viral Infection

The condition known as swollen glands refers to a swelling of the lymph nodes in the neck (on the sides, below the ears) and throat. The lymph nodes in the armpits and groin area may also be involved. Attendant symptoms can include redness, hardening, and/or tenderness or pain in the affected nodes, sore throat, and fever.

The swelling of the lymph nodes is most often a sign of infection or allergic reaction. They can also indicate serious disorders such as leukemia, however, so if your swollen glands persist, see your doctor.

With infection or recurrent allergic reaction, the lymph system (the body's filtering system) can become overburdened. Lymph fluid flows between cells in the body, transporting beneficial substances between tissues and the bloodstream and also foreign substances for elimination from the body. The lymph nodes filter the fluid and prevent the foreign substances from entering the bloodstream. Normally, they can keep up with the filtering and elimination demands. During illness or in the case of allergies, however, the load of toxins in the lymph fluid is elevated and the lymph nodes swell with bacteria and bacterial waste or the substances involved in an allergic reaction, and white blood cells are released to destroy the foreign interlopers.

Thus, swollen glands are a condition of toxic overload. The toxins of illness and allergies may have been added on top of a load of toxins (for example, pollutants from food and the environment) the lymph system was already having to filter. To restore health, it's important to reduce the toxic load, take steps to cleanse the body, support the immune system, and get the lymph flowing freely again.

Essential Oils

"Bay laurel oil has astounding effects on swollen glands," states Kurt Schnaubelt, Ph.D., scientific director of the Pacific Institute of Aromatherapy in San Rafael, California. "Its positive effects on the lymphatic system are undeniable." Rubbing a few drops of this essential oil on the swollen glands provides noticeable relief immediately, he says. Apply as needed, but do not use Bay Laurel on the skin for longer than 3 weeks, as it can result in skin irritation with prolonged use.[1]

Flower Essences

Self-Heal and Yarrow Special Formula can serve as the foundational healing agents for swollen glands. Other flower essences to address the specific emotions, mental attitude, and environmental conditions of the individual are recommended, states Patricia Kaminski, a flower essence therapist and codirector of the Flower Essence Society. Self-Heal supports the body's innate healing ability. Yarrow Special Formula strengthens and protects against environmental toxicity and stress. Take 4 drops of each 2–4 times daily, or as needed.

Food Therapy

Eat:

Fresh foods, leafy green vegetables, parsley, garlic, onion, horseradish, miso soup. Drink plenty of fluids (diluted vegetable juices, broths, herbal tea, green tea, green drinks such as chlorella and spirulina).

Horseradish "works great as an antiseptic, decongestant, and cleansing tonic" in cases of swollen glands, says herbalist and nutritionist James Kusick. Mix 1/2 teaspoon of prepared horseradish with a little food 2–3 times daily, or you can take it "straight" and hold it in your mouth, he says. Gradually increase the amount until you are able to take 1 teaspoon at a time.[2]

Avoid:

Sugar, dairy, processed, refined, and fatty foods, excess salt.

Herbal Medicine

Swollen glands reflect the need for lymphatic cleansing. Red root (*Ceanothus americanus*) has a great ability to clear congestion of the lymph glands and has a long history of use for that purpose. "Red root is one of the most important lymphatic plants," says Michael Cottingham, a clinical herbalist from Silver City, New Mexico. The herb can clear dead cell debris and the accumulated waste of bacterial infection, but it may also perform another important function, explains Cottingham. During illness, the normal electrical charge in cell walls is weakened. As a result, the cells can't move fluids as well and congestion ensues. One theory to explain why red root can so drastically reduce congestion is that the herb may help to restore the proper electrical charge to cell walls, thus restoring the body to its natural ability to clear itself.

A fresh root tincture is the most effective form in which to take red root, and relatively large amounts work well, says Cottingham. Red root has no known toxicity, so larger dosages are safe. He suggests combining red root tincture with echinacea (*E. spp.*) tincture to aid the immune system. Use equal parts of the two tinctures, and during the acute stage, take 30–50 drops of the mix up to 5 times daily for a week. Take for another week, reducing the dosage by 10 percent each day. For children 11 to 13 years old, the dosage is half that of adults. For children under 12, cut the dosage in half again. As an astringent, red root tightens and dries tissue. You may feel this sensation in your mouth from taking the tincture.

It is important in lymph conditions to drink lots of water (at least 8 glasses daily) to aid the body in breaking up the congestion. "Water can be one of the ultimate first aid remedies," observes Cottingham.

Homeopathy

Naturopathic physicians Robert Ullmann, N.D., and Judyth Reichenberg-Ullmann, N.D., cite the following remedies for swollen glands:[3]

Bromium: If the glands on the left side of the neck are stony and hard.

Calc carb: Indicated for swollen glands in a chubby baby whose head sweats.

Hepar sulph: If the glands are highly sensitive to touch and accompanied by chilliness.

Mercurius: Indicated for swollen glands accompanied by toxic symptoms such as a bad taste in the mouth, bad breath, body odor, and heavy perspiration.

Phytolacca: Indicated for swollen glands accompanied by a dark red sore throat and pain radiating to the right ear with swallowing.

Take the appropriate remedy in a 30c potency every 4 hours until your symptoms improve. Stop taking the remedy; repeat if the symptoms return. If there is no improvement with 4 doses, you probably are not using the correct remedy and need to try another.

Nutritional Supplements

Naturopathic physician Bradley Bongiovanni, N.D., of Independence, Ohio, recommends the following supplemental program to help alleviate swollen glands; take the designated amounts until your condition is resolved:

Beta-carotene: 50,000 IU twice daily.

Zinc: 25 mg twice daily.

N-acetylcysteine (NAC): 750 mg twice daily; a powerful antioxidant form of the amino acid cysteine.

Selenium: 200 mcg twice daily.

Fish or flaxseed oil: 2,000 mg twice daily; for anti-inflammatory essential fatty acids.

Reflexology

Neck, lymphatic system, adrenal glands, spleen

Stone/Crystal Therapy

To help resolve swollen glands, use moonstone or clear crystal, says Daya Sarai Chocron, a vibrational healer based in Northampton, Massachusetts. Hold the stone or crystal, wear it, carry it in your pocket, or lay it over your swollen glands for 15–20 minutes daily, as needed, until the swelling has subsided.

Other Remedies

Apply witch hazel (available in drugstores and supermarkets) over the swollen gland area.[4] Witch hazel has anti-inflammatory properties, which can help reduce swelling.

Teething

Babies get their first teeth between six and eight months of age, with a new tooth typically coming in monthly. The whole process lasts two or three years. It can be mildly uncomfortable to painful for the baby. Attendant symptoms include gum redness and swelling in the area where the new tooth is coming in, fever, more drooling than usual (which can lead to chapped skin on the lower face), sleep disruption, and emotional and behavioral changes such as fussiness, restlessness, and irritability. Sometimes diarrhea occurs during teething as well.

Your baby does not have to endure the pain or discomfort of teething. Natural medicine remedies are particularly effective for children and tend to work quickly. Some doctors posit that this is because children are a relatively clean slate. Having been here for only a short time, they are carrying less of a toxic load than are adults, who have had ample time to be filled with toxins from our food and environment. Children have also not had the chance to accumulate the emotional and psychological baggage that interferes with healing in adults. Natural remedies can do their work without much impediment in the body of a child.

Essential Oils

Naturopathic physician Boyer B. Cole, N.M.D., of Cottonwood, Arizona, has used the following essential oil remedy with children for fifteen years and found it consistently effective. "They get a look of surprise at the flavor," he says, "which is an added benefit of the remedy—

it distracts them." Combine the following essential oils in 1/4 ounce vegetable glycerin (available at health food stores; do not use the pharmaceutical variety):

Peppermint: 7 drops
Clove: 2 drops
German Chamomile: 1 drop

Rub 1 drop into the gums 2–3 times daily, or as needed.

Flower Essences

Five Flower Formula (Rescue Remedy) can bring emotional calm to a teething child, notes flower essence therapist Patricia Kaminski of Nevada City, California. Add 4–6 drops of Chamomile flower essence to the bottle of Five Flower Formula. Put 2 drops under the child's tongue 2–4 times daily, and rub 4–6 drops on the child's gums 2–4 times daily.

Food Therapy

If the child is on solid food, cold foods (yogurt is good) can be soothing to sore gums. Foods high in vitamin A and bioflavonoids can help by supporting tissue healing. (For a list of foods containing these nutrients, see part 3, "Food Therapy," pp. 376, 378.)

Herbal Medicine

Lobelia (*Lobelia inflata*) extract applied to the gums, 1–2 drops every few hours as needed, can provide relief during teething, according to Sue Reynolds, M.S.W., L.M.T., a certified herbalist and aromatherapist from Goleta, California. Alternatively, rub oil of clove on the gums to numb them.

Homeopathy

"More people have become homeopathic patients because of teething than from any other condition," states Michael G. Carlston, M.D., of Santa Rosa, California. In other words, it works. You can get homeopathic teething tablets or use one of the following remedies:

Chamomilla: If the child is restless, irritable, and wants something, but when you give it to her, she throws it down; the child wants to be carried and moving, but is squirmy and angry; these manifestations of teething are highly frustrating for parents.

Calc phos: For an older child who has digestive upset with teething, and is more whiny than irritable, and more pathetic than frustrating.

For both, give the child 2–3 pellets of 12c or 30c, up to every 4 hours. It is very important to pay attention to the patient. Don't keep giving the remedy if the child is doing well, says Dr. Carlston. He has seen a number of kids in his practice whose parents have brought them in because they got better, then worse, on a homeopathic remedy for teething. That happened because the parents kept giving the child the remedy after the symptoms improved, explains Dr. Carlston. Continuing to give a homeopathic remedy after it is no longer needed can cause a return of the original complaints. The remedy works with the body, so you need to pay attention to symptoms. "Remember, homeopathy is not like a conventional prescription medicine such as antibiotics where you are supposed to take the whole course regardless of how you feel."

Nutritional Supplements

Nutritional supplements are not appropriate for a child of 6 months, which is when the first, most problematic teeth come in.

Reflexology

Teeth and gentle work on the whole foot

Stone/Crystal Therapy

Amber is a useful stone for teething, according to Katrina Raphaell, crystal healing therapist and founder of the Crystal Academy of Advanced Healing Arts in Kapaa, Hawaii. Place the stone in the baby's bathwater. As an extra measure of caution, use a stone large enough that the baby can't swallow it, in the unlikely event that he or she gets hold of the stone.

Other Remedies

Freeze carrot sticks and give them to the baby to gnaw on, suggests Sue Reynolds. This numbs the gums and provides productive activity in the problem area. A frozen teething ring is preferable if the child has any teeth already; he or she might bite off a piece of the carrot and choke on it.

Tendonitis

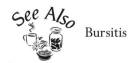 Bursitis

Inflammation of a tendon (fibrous connective tissue that joins muscle and bone), or tendonitis, can produce severe pain and restrict motion and function of the affected joint. Common sites of tendonitis are the back of the ankle (Achilles tendon), knee, shoulder (rotator cuff), and thumb. More people are now suffering from tendonitis of the wrists and forearms due to the repetitive motion of computer keyboard work.

The inflammation of tendonitis is usually the consequence of overuse, as occurs in athletics or repetitive motion. The primary symptoms of the condition are the pain and limited range of motion. Swelling may also occur. Chronic tendonitis can involve the deposit of calcim salts in tendon fibers, which makes the condition more painful and further restricts motion. Consult your doctor if you have chronic tendonitis or your acute tendonitis is severe.

The general practice to follow with tendonitis is the same as for a sprain. It is known as RICE: rest the affected joint, ice it, compress it with an elastic bandage, and elevate it above the heart to aid in drainage. When icing an injury, don't place the ice directly on the skin. Put a towel between the ice pack and the skin. Apply ice for 20- to 30-minute periods, followed by no ice for 15–20 minutes. Continue this for the first few hours after injury. Compression also should be alternated with no compression. Wrap the affected area with an elastic bandage, being careful not to wrap it too tightly. Leave on for 30 minutes on, then off for 15 minutes. You can wrap the bandage around the ice pack.

The remedies here can ease the pain and inflammation, and aid in the healing of the injured tendon.

Essential Oils

For tendonitis, aromatherapist Valerie Ann Worwood recommends the following massage formula: blend 10 drops each of essential oils of Rosemary, Lavender, and Peppermint in 2 tablespoons of vegetable oil. Use the blend as a massage oil on the affected area as needed.[1]

Flower Essences

Dandelion flower oil used in massage and/or with hot compresses can help alleviate tendonitis, according to naturalist Richard Katz of Nevada City, California. Do one or the other 2–4 times daily. For the compress treatment, gently rub 1–2 tablespoons of Dandelion flower oil on the affected area and cover with a hot compress. (For instructions on using flower essences in massage oil, see part 3, "Flower Essences," "Directions for Use," p. 372.)

Food Therapy

Eat:

Dark green vegetables and other alkalinizing foods.

For any "itis" condition (which means "inflammation of"), foods that contain anti-inflammatory substances are recommended, states Nick Buratovich, N.M.D., a naturopathic physician from Tempe, Arizona. To that end, eat pineapple, papaya, ginger, turmeric, and foods rich in omega-3 and omega-6 essential fatty acids. Eat pineapple and papaya by themselves, not with other foods, to get the anti-inflammatory effect of the enzymes these fruits contain.

Avoid:

Sugar, nightshade vegetables (they can be inflammatory for some people), acid-forming foods.

Avoid coffee and other forms of caffeine (aside from green tea) because caffeine blocks endorphin receptors in the brain, says Dr.

Buratovich. As endorphins facilitate pain relief, people who consume a lot of caffeine tend to have a low threshold of pain. He also recommends avoiding animal products because they contain arachidonic acid, which promotes inflammation.

(For a list of foods containing the substances cited above, see part 3, "Food Therapy," pp. 376, 377.)

Herbal Medicine

Take ginger (*Zingiber officinale*) and licorice (*Glycrrhiza glabra*) in combination to help resolve tendonitis, recommends herbalist James A. Duke, Ph.D. Both are anti-inflammatory herbs with a history of use for joint ailments.[2] Slice fresh ginger and boil in water for 15 minutes to make a tea. Prepare licorice root in the same way, using 1 teaspoon of the herb per cup of water. You can drink as much ginger tea as you like. You need to limit your intake of licorice tea to no more than 3 cups daily, however, and drink it on a short-term basis only. Prolonged use can result in headaches and other symptoms. If you suffer from high blood pressure, do not take licorice.

Dr. Duke also suggests willow (*Salix spp.*) as an herbal aspirin. The herb contains salicylates, pain-relieving substances from which aspirin was originally derived. Take as a tea or tincture. For the tea, use 1–2 teaspoons of the dried herb per cup of water, boil for 20 minutes, strain, and drink 1 cup 2–3 times daily, as needed for pain. Or you can take 1 teaspoon of willow tincture 3 times daily. Dr. Duke cautions that if you are allergic to aspirin, it's probably not advisable to take willow.[3]

As a topical treatment for tendonitis, Tei Fu lotion or Tiger Balm (Chinese herbal formulas containing Camphor, Cajeput, and other essential oils) can be quite effective and even remarkable, says Joanne B. Mied, N.D., a naturopath and herbalist based in Novato, California. Tendonitis is a condition of toxic accumulation in the affected area, and these remedies help pull out the toxins, explains Dr. Mied. For optimal results, follow the topical protocol and also take a vitamin B complex supplement to support nerve function and the formation of anti-inflammatory substances. Take 1 capsule 3 times daily of a product that contains 100 mg of each of the main B vitamins (10 mg of B6 and 100 mcg of B12), along with the other members of the B family.

One of Dr. Mied's patients, a longtime computer programmer with serious tendonitis, took B vitamins and used Tei Fu lotion as a nightly treatment, and within two weeks his pain was gone. Apply either the lotion or the balm each night before bed and pin a towel around the area to keep the heat up. Tiger Balm is widely available in health food and other stores. You can purchase Tei Fu lotion via the Internet.

Homeopathy

For tendonitis, the following homeopathic remedies are indicated, according to Maesimund B. Panos, M.D.:[4]

Rhus tox: If there is pain with onset of movement, the pain eases with continued motion, and the condition is worse in damp weather.

Ruta: If there is a lame feeling and the tendonitis does not have the characteristics cited for Rhus tox.

Take the appropriate remedy in a 6x potency 3–4 times daily, or more often if needed. As symptoms improve, decrease the frequency. Stop taking the remedy when the improvement is well established.

Nutritional Supplements

To aid in the healing of tendonitis and to relieve the pain, the following supplements can be effective, says Dr. Buratovich:

Vitamin C: 1–2 g three times daily for one month; helps rebuild connective tissue.

Bioflavonoids: These plant substances help stabilize connective tissue and decrease inflammation. Quercetin or citrus bioflavonoids are the best form to take. Take 1–3 g daily for one month.

Bromelain: 2 capsules on an empty stomach 3 times daily for 1 month; an anti-inflammatory enzyme compound found in pineapple.

Curcumin: 100 mg twice daily for one month; an anti-inflammatory substance derived from turmeric. Bromelain and curcumin can be purchased as a combination product.

EPA and GLA: These essential fatty acids (EFAs) are anti-inflammatory. EPA (eicosapentaenoic acid) is an omega-3 EFA found in fish oils; take 300 mg 3 times daily for one month. GLA (gamma-linolenic acid) is an omega-6 EFA found in evening primrose, black currant, and borage oils; take 100 mg 3 times daily for one month.

DLPA (D,L-phenylalanine): 750 mg 3 times daily before meals for 1–3 weeks; a pain-relieving amino acid.

Tryptophan: 2–4 g 3 times daily for up to 1 month. This amino acid has been shown to reduce pain, perhaps by raising the pain threshold, although the exact mechanism is unknown.[5] To ensure uptake, avoid protein for 90 minutes before and after taking.

Reflexology

Treat the adrenal glands and the area of the foot corresponding to the part of the body where the tendonitis is located.

Stone/Crystal Therapy

For tendonitis, tape holmquistite on the afflicted joint using hypoallergenic tape, and leave it on for 1–2 weeks or until the condition abates, whichever comes first, recommends Melody, author of the crystal reference series *Love Is in the Earth*. You can also use the stone for ongoing maintenance.

Thrush (Oral)

See Fungal Infection.

Tinnitus (Ringing in the Ears)

Although commonly called ringing in the ears, tinnitus actually encompasses a whole range of sounds, from tinkling, buzzing, and chirping to hissing, roaring, and rushing. The sounds are imperceptible to others and come from inside the ears or head. Tinnitus commonly occurs in both ears. In many cases, hearing is not affected. In some instances, however, hearing loss can follow tinnitus.

Science and medicine do not have a clear understanding of why people develop tinnitus. Causal factors may include head injury, wax buildup, food allergies, infections or diseases of the exterior, middle, or inner ear, and prolonged use of certain drugs, notably quinine and salicylates such as aspirin. Salicylate-containing foods, such as apples, grapes, tomatoes, and cucumbers, are also implicated in the disorder.[1] Loud noises such as explosions can trigger tinnitus. Finally, research has found a link between tinnitus and aluminum or lead toxicity.[2]

Essential Oils

For tinnitus, Kurt Schnaubelt, Ph.D., scientific director of the Pacific Institute of Aromatherapy in San Rafael, California, recommends Helichrysum (Everlasting) or Cypress. Gently rub a diluted solution, 3–4 drops of essential oil to 1 teaspoon of carrier oil, around the affected ear—on the outer rim, lobe, and behind the ear. Apply at bedtime and once during the day, as needed for symptoms.

Flower Essences

Self-Heal can serve as a foundational healing agent for tinnitus. Other flower essences to address the specific emotions, mental attitude, and environmental conditions of the individual are recommended, states Patricia Kaminski, a flower essence therapist and codirector of the Flower Essence Society. Self-Heal supports the body's innate healing ability. Take 4 drops 2–4 times daily, or as needed.

Food Therapy

Eat:

Safflower, sunflower, and olive oils, high-arginine foods, foods high in magnesium, manganese, choline, and vitamin B6 (see part 3, "Food Therapy," pp. 376, 377, 378).

Avoid:

Caffeine, alcohol, salicylate-containing foods, mucus-forming foods, food allergens.

Food allergies are often behind tinnitus that is not caused by damage resulting from loud noises, says Karen Vaughan, E.M.T, A.H.G, a clinical herbalist from Brooklyn, New York. Further, certain foods tend to be related to the right and left ears in one-sided tinnitus, she notes. Allergies to rice, cinnamon, blueberries, grapes, strawberries, watermelon, wine, and pumpkin are more often associated with tinnitus in the left ear, while allergies to wheat tend to be associated with right-ear tinnitus. As a result, Vaughan's first recommendation for treatment is to go off the foods related to the ear in which you have tinnitus. She cites the case of a woman who suffered from tinnitus in her right ear for seven years. Within ten days of giving up wheat, upon Vaughan's suggestion, the tinnitus was gone.

If you have tinnitus in both ears, go off all the foods listed above. Vaughan cautions to watch out for hidden wheat in foods; soy sauce, for example, contains wheat. If you experience an improvement after giving up these foods, it is likely that allergies are a factor in your tinnitus. After the tinnitus abates, gradually reintroduce the foods one at a time to see which ones you are allergic to.

If you have left-ear tinnitus, look at your diet to see if you are getting enough foods that contain manganese, vitamin B6, and the amino acid arginine, advises Vaughan. A deficiency in these nutrients can cause left-ear tinnitus.

For right-ear tinnitus, look at your dietary intake of niacin (vitamin B3), zinc, lecithin, and magnesium.

(For a list of foods containing the substances cited above, see part 3, "Food Therapy," pp. 376, 378)

As a general practice for wheat-allergy tinnitus, use safflower, sunflower, and olive oils in your diet, says Vaughan, and consider sources of other essential fatty acids, such as evening primrose, hemp, or borage oil.

Along with these dietary steps, take the nutritional supplements below. You can add the herbal remedy to your program, too, if you like.

Herbal Medicine

As ginkgo (*Ginkgo biloba*) improves blood flow, it can open the blood vessels to the ears and resolve tinnitus, according to herbalist

Teresa Boardwine of Washington, Virginia. Ginkgo has become popular and there are a lot of products to choose from. Not all are good quality. Look for tinctures derived from the whole plant. Take 1 dropperful 3 times daily for 4–6 months to determine whether it is beneficial for your particular tinnitus. When you see improvement, you can reduce to a maintenance dose of 1/2 dropperful twice daily. Note: If you are on blood-thinning medication, you shouldn't use ginkgo. Active consituents in the herb called ginkgosides can act as blood thinners.

When your tinnitus is due to loud equipment operation, black cohosh tincture is useful, states Boardwine. Follow the manufacturer's recommended dosage.

Homeopathy

The following are some of the numerous homeopathic remedies for tinnitus, according to Dr. Barry Rose of the Royal London Homeopathic Hospital:[3]

Carb sulph 12c: For buzzing and singing noises with defective hearing.
Chin sulph 12c: For violent ringing, roaring, and buzzing with defective hearing.
Lachesis 12c: For singing, roaring, and excessive ear wax.
Salicyl acid 12c: For ringing, roaring, deafness, and dizziness.
Sanguinaria 30c: For roaring and humming with a headache; the ears feel hot internally.

Take the appropriate remedy (except for Sanguinaria) 2 times daily until your symptoms improve. Sanguinaria should be taken 3 times daily for 4 days. If you get no improvement, you may want to consider consulting a homeopath for constitutional treatment.

Nutritional Supplements

In addition to implementing the dietary suggestions above, Karen Vaughan recommends the following nutritional protocol for tinnitus. You can take ginkgo concurrently if you like (see "Herbal Medicine" above). Alleviation of tinnitus can occur within a week of beginning this program, says Vaughan, adding that the standard natural medicine rule of thumb in reversing a health ailment is one month of nutritional correction (diet and supplements) for each year that you have had the condition.

For right-ear tinnitus:

Magnesium: 250–500 mg daily.
Essential fatty acids: Take 2 capsules of evening primrose or borage oil in the morning.
Histadine: Take this amino acid at the manufacturer's recommended dosage.

For left-ear tinnitus:

Vitamin B-6: 50 mg daily.
Manganese: 250 mg daily.
Arginine: Take this amino acid at the manufacturer's recommended dosage.

Applying DMSO (dimethyl sulfoxide) topically around the affected ear 3 times daily can also be helpful, notes Vaughan. DMSO is used to improve circulation and relax muscles. Make sure to use pharmaceutical-grade DMSO, wash your ear and hands before applying it, and take 500 mg of vitamin C when you do the application.

Reflexology

Ear, neck, cervical spine, sinuses, adrenal glands

Stone/Crystal Therapy

An elixir of garnet in sillimanite can help control tinnitus, according to Melody, author of the crystal reference series *Love Is in the Earth*. Take 3–5 drops of the elixir twice daily for 4–6 months. (For instructions on making and using an elixir, see part 3, "Stone/Crystal Therapy," p. 403.)

Other Remedies

Put cotton balls soaked in onion juice in your ears to alleviate buzzing noises.[4]

Acupuncture can offer significant relief from tinnitus, says Karen Vaughan. "This is especially true of tinnitus caused by stresses and strains in the back or mechanical functions, which may not respond well to the nutritional protocol alone."

Tonsillitis

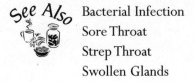

See Also Bacterial Infection
Sore Throat
Strep Throat
Swollen Glands

Tonsillitis is inflamation of the tonsils (masses of lymphatic tissue on each side of the throat). It tends to come on suddenly with symptoms of chills and fever (often high); headache; aches and pains in the limbs and back; and swollen, red, and painful tonsils. Swallowing can be particularly painful. The adenoids, or pharyngeal tonsil, located at the top back of the throat, may be swollen as well, as may be the lymph nodes in the neck.

Tonsils, like lymph nodes, are lymphatic filters. They filter the lymph fluid that flows between cells in the body and prevent bacteria and other foreign substances from entering the bloodstream. They assist the immune system, both in their filtering function and by contributing to white blood (disease-fighting) cell production. Normally, the tonsils can keep up with the filtering demands. As with swollen glands, however, tonsils can become inflamed or infected when the lymph system is overloaded. The bacteria they filter accumulate in their tissue and produce infection.

A common source of tonsillitis is the *Streptococcus* bacteria. If strep is responsible for your tonsillitis, the concern about rheumatic fever is the same as it is for strep throat; that is, although rheumatic fever is unlikely to develop, infection with this bacteria is not something to treat casually. If you have had rheumatic fever or there is a history of it in your family, seek medical attention immediately upon the first indications of a sore throat.

Other causes or contributing factors in tonsillitis include overuse of antibiotics, food allergies, and buildup of toxins due to constipation.

As with swollen glands, it's important to reduce the load on the lymphatic and immune systems by taking steps to cleanse the body, bolster immunity, and get the lymph flowing freely again.

Essential Oils

For tonsillitis, Julie Oxendale, C.M.T., an aromatherapist based in San Francisco, California, recommends the following essential oil blend, which is safe for children as well as adults:

Lavender: 10 drops
Tea Tree (*Melaleuca alternifolia*): 15 drops
Ginger: 5 drops
Lemon: 2 drops

If you don't like the smell of Tea Tree oil, you can substitute 5 drops of Roman Chamomile instead.

Put 4 drops of the blend on a warm compress, lay it over the throat area, and leave it on for 10 minutes. Do this twice a day. You can also use this blend in an aromatherapy diffuser placed in the patient's room. Oxendale recommends using a nonelectric diffuser to avoid the effect of electromagnetic fields on the oils. She also recommends using a diffuser that has a large container (one that holds about a cup of liquid) for the oil and water. Put half of the above blended amount in the water and keep the diffuser burning all the time.

For a massage blend, combine 5 drops each of the same oils in 2 teaspoons of vegetable oil. Massage into the abdomen and entire back. The tension in the shoulder, chest, and neck area, which constricts the throat, often stems from the lower back muscles being "switched off" and the abdomen being held tightly, explains Oxendale. The upper body is forced to carry the load of posture, and tension results. Massage with essential oils can activate the back muscles and help release the abdomen. The result is a lessening of tension and improved circulation in the throat, which is beneficial in healing tonsillitis.

Flower Essences

Self-Heal and Yarrow Special Formula can serve as the foundational healing agents for tonsillitis. Other flower essences to address the specific emotions, mental attitude, and environmental conditions of the individual are recommended, states Patricia Kaminski, a flower essence therapist and codirector of the Flower Essence Society. Self-Heal supports the body's innate healing ability. Yarrow Special Formula strengthens and protects against environmental toxicity and stress. Take 4 drops of each 2–4 times daily, or as needed.

Food Therapy

Eat:

Fresh foods, vegetables, fruit, fiber. Drink plenty of fluids (diluted vegetable juices, broths, herbal tea, green tea, green drinks such as chlorella and spirulina).

Avoid:

Sugar, dairy, processed, refined, and fatty foods.

Herbal Medicine

Like swollen glands, tonsillitis reflects the need for lymphatic cleansing. Red root (*Ceanothus americanus*) has a great ability to clear congestion of the lymph glands and has a long history of use for that purpose. "Red root is one of the most important lymphatic plants," says Michael Cottingham, a clinical herbalist from Silver City, New Mexico. The herb can clear dead cell debris and the accumulated waste of bacterial infection, but it may also perform another important function, explains Cottingham. During illness, the normal electrical charge in cell walls is weakened. As a result, the cells can't move fluids as well and congestion ensues. One theory to explain why red root can so drastically reduce congestion is that the herb may help to restore the proper electrical charge to cell walls, thus restoring the body to its natural ability to clear itself.

A fresh root tincture is the most effective form in which to take red root, and relatively large amounts work well, says Cottingham. Red root has no known toxicity, so larger dosages are safe. He suggests combining red root tincture with echinacea (*E. spp.*) tincture to aid the immune system. Use equal parts of the two tinctures, and during the acute stage take 30–50 drops of the mix up to 5 times daily for a week. Take for another week, reducing the dosage by 10 percent each day. For children 11 to 13 years old, the dosage is half that of adults. For children under 12, cut the dosage in half again. As an astringent, red root tightens and dries tissue. You may feel this sensation in your mouth from taking the tincture.

It is important in lymph conditions to drink lots of water (at least 8 glasses daily) to aid the body in breaking up the congestion. "Water can be one of the ultimate first aid remedies," observes Cottingham.

Homeopathy

For tonsillitis, Drs. Andrew Lockie and Nicola Geddes recommend the following homeopathic remedies:[1]

Belladonna: If the tonsillitis involves burning pain that shoots into the head, high fever, red face, and pain spasms upon moving; take 30c every 2 hours for up to 10 doses.

Hepar sulph: If the tonsillitis is characterized by stabbing pain in the throat as if there is a fishbone stuck in it, chills and shivering, and possibly voice loss; take 6c every 2 hours for up to 10 doses.

Mercurius: Indicated for tonsillitis with bad breath, a dark red color to the throat, and painful swallowing with a burning sensation as saliva is swallowed; take 6c every 2 hours for up to 10 doses.

Nutritional Supplements

To help resolve tonsillitis, James F. Balch, M.D., and Phyllis A. Balch, C.N.C., recommend what they call an ascorbic acid flush. Flushing the body with this form of vitamin C is an effective treatment for bacterial, viral, and other infections. To do the flush, drink 1,000 mg (1 teaspoon) of ascorbic acid (use calcium ascorbate or other buffered form) in a glass of water or juice every half hour, adding up how much you take, until you have diarrhea. Subtract 1 teaspoon from the total number you took and that is your bowel tolerance dosage. For example, if diarrhea occurred after your fifth dose, your bowel tolerance dosage is 4 teaspoons. Take this amount in one drink every 4 hours for 1–2 days thereafter. If your stool becomes more watery than tapioca, lower the dosage by another teaspoon.

Zinc gluconate lozenges are also an important supplemental treatment, say the Balches. Zinc stimulates the immune system and aids in tissue healing. Suck on a lozenge every 2–3 hours.[2]

Reflexology

Throat, neck, cervical spine, adrenal glands, lymphatic system, spleen

Stone/Crystal Therapy

Petrified palm, placed on the throat and taken as an elixir, can relieve the symptoms of tonsillitis in about 36 hours, states Melody, author of the crystal reference series *Love Is in the Earth*. You can attach the stone with hypoallergenic tape or wear it as a choker-style necklace. For the elixir, take 3–5 drops 3 times daily. Continue the remedy as long as needed. (For instructions on making an elixir, see part 3, "Stone/Crystal Therapy," p. 403.)

Tooth Extraction
(Pre-op and Post-op Support)

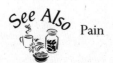 Pain

Like surgery, tooth extraction is a trauma to the body. The effects can be mitigated and the recovery time shortened by preparing your body beforehand (preoperative support) and providing healing assistance afterward (postoperative support). Pre-op and post-op support can also reduce the likelihood of infection of the gums following the tooth extraction.

Note: Dental work can antidote homeopathic remedies. If you use homeopathy, talk to your homeopath before having any dental work done, aside from manual cleaning (ultrasonic cleaning may be a problem as well).

Essential Oils

"Clove essential oil is not only useful for relieving pain and swelling, but is also a very powerful broad-spectrum antimicrobial, so it can help prevent infection after a tooth extraction," says medical aromatherapist Julia Fischer of Northern California. On the day before you get your tooth pulled, put 1 drop of undiluted Clove on the gums of that tooth; do this 3 times that day. Try to avoid your lips and tongue; Clove produces an intense sensation in tissue. Some people are sensitive to Clove, so if it is too strong for you, mix equal parts of Clove and vegetable oil and put 2 drops of that on the site. For children, mix equal parts of Clove and vegetable glycerin (which is sweet-tasting). After the tooth extraction, start the applications right away and continue as needed. You don't need to be concerned about overdoing it, says Fischer.

Flower Essences

The following flower essence protocol can help you prepare for and recover from a tooth extraction, states Patricia Kaminski, a flower essence therapist and educator from Nevada City, California.

Pre-op: Take Five Flower Formula (Rescue Remedy) to calm and stabilize you, beginning 2 days before the tooth extraction and continuing until the procedure. Take 4 drops fairly frequently, as often as hourly.

Post-op: Take a combination of Self-Heal and Arnica beginning immediately after your tooth extraction. Take 4 drops of each 4 times daily for at least 3 days after the procedure. The idea is to take the flower essences during the immediate recovery period, however long that lasts. If there is excessive bleeding, take 4 drops of Yarrow at least 4 times daily. You can take it as frequently as hourly, or more often if needed.

Food Therapy

Eat:

Foods high in vitamin A/beta-carotene, vitamin C, vitamin E, bioflavonoids, vitamin K, and zinc (see part 3, "Food Therapy," pp. 376, 378).

Avoid:

Sugar.

Herbal Medicine and Nutritional Supplements

Medical herbalist Chanchal Cabrera, M.N.I.M.H., A.H.G., of Vancouver, British Columbia, recommends the following protocol as preparation for tooth extraction and to aid in recovery afterward. The protocol supports the immune system, lowers the risk of infection, protects the brain from the drugs given during and after surgery, helps detoxify the liver of drug residues, and reduces scarring. Take all of the below remedies for 2 weeks before and 2 weeks after having a tooth pulled.[1]

• Combine these herbal tinctures in the designated amounts and take 1 teaspoon of the blend 3 times daily:

> Marigold (*Calendula officinalis*): 15 ml; liver stimulant and antioxidant that helps remove drug residues
>
> Milk thistle (*Carduus marianus*): 15 ml; antioxidant that helps protect liver and brain cells from drugs
>
> Gotu kola (*Centella asiatica*): 15 ml; stimulates blood flow, helps heal tissue, and removes drug residues
>
> Horsetail (*Equisetum arvense*): 15 ml; helps heal tissue
>
> Hawthorn (*Crataegus oxyacantha*): 15 ml; helps heal tissue
>
> Goldenrod (*Solidago vigaurea*): 15 ml; antioxidant that protects the brain from the effects of X rays
>
> Dandelion (*Taraxacum officinalis*): 10 ml; aids in liver detoxification

• Take antioxidants:

> Vitamin C: take throughout the day to bowel tolerance (just below the amount that produces diarrhea).
>
> Zinc: 50 mg daily.
>
> Selenium: 400 mcg daily.
>
> Beta-carotene: 30,000 IU daily.
>
> Vitamin E: 400 IU daily (Note: if you are on anticoagulant medication, do not take vitamin E, or garlic).
>
> Also take flaxseed oil, evening primrose oil, and lipoic acid in the daily dosages recommended by the manufacturer of the individual product.

• Take chlorophyll to help pull residues of anesthesia and other drugs from your cells; 2 tablespoons twice daily.

• Herbal mouth rinse:

For an antimicrobial rinse to help prevent infection after a tooth extraction and promote healing, combine equal parts of tinctures of cooking sage (*Salvia officinalis*), rosemary (*Rosmarinus officinalis*), myrrh (*Commiphora molmol*), goldenseal (*Hydrastis canadensis*), echinacea (*E. spp.*), bloodroot (red root, *Ceanothus americanus*), and peppermint (*Mentha piperata*) for flavoring. Add 1 teaspoon of this blend to 1/2 cup of water. Swish it around in your mouth for 1 minute, then gargle. It's fine to swallow the mixture. Do this 2–3 times a day. Myrrh works on contact, so do not rinse your mouth out afterward. Continue the procedure until the extraction site is healed. A commercial preparation of this mouth rinse, called Orcln, is available through the Gaia Garden Herbal Dispensary and Clinic in Vancouver, British Columbia (see Cabrera's listing under "Herbal Medicine" in Appendix B: Resources). Note: The herbal mouth rinse is not intended to be used in lieu of dental treatment.

See "Pain (Natural Pain Relievers)" for natural pain relievers you can use following a tooth extraction.

Homeopathy

If you are nervous about the impending tooth extraction, Aconite napellus or Gelsemium sempervirens can help, say Drs. Andrew Lockie and Nicola Geddes. Take Aconite 30c every hour, as needed, if you feel acute panic at the prospect of the dental visit. Take Gelsemium 30c in the same way if your apprehension is causing you to tremble and feel weak in the knees.[2]

To reduce the shock to the system and help heal the tissue, Judith Lewis, N.D., R.N., recommends taking Arnica montana 30c before and after you have your tooth pulled. Take a dose 30–60 minutes before the dentist anesthetizes you. Take another dose right after the tooth has been pulled, and several more over the next 12 hours.[3]

The following remedies are also helpful after a tooth extraction, according to Stephen Cummings, M.D., and Dana Ullman, M.P.H.:[4]

Ruta: "The first medicine for pain after most dental procedures."
Hypericum: Indicated for shooting or persisting pain following a dental procedure.
Phosphorus: If bleeding, particularly of bright-red blood, continues after a tooth is pulled; you can also take Phosphorus to help pull the anesthesia out of your body.[5]

Take the appropriate remedy at a potency of 6c(x) or 12c(x) every 2–3 hours for a few days. As your symptoms improve, take the remedy less often.

Reflexology

Teeth, pituitary (for pain relief)

Stone/Crystal Therapy

Clear crystal is useful in cases of tooth extraction, states Daya Sarai Chocron, a vibrational healer and author of *Healing with Crystals and Gemstones*. Lay it on the outside of your cheek over the site of the problem tooth for 15–20 minutes daily for a few days before the procedure. After the tooth has been pulled, do the same daily until the gums have healed. To further prepare the body and facilitate healing after the extraction, you can also hold the crystal, wear it, or carry it in your pocket.

Toothache

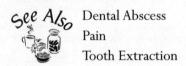 See Also
Dental Abscess
Pain
Tooth Extraction

Pain in a tooth or the area around a tooth can be excruciating. Chewing can make it worse, as can hot or cold. The causes of a toothache (odontalgia) are many, including a cavity (decay), fracture, dental abscess, gum infection, dental work, sinusitis or ear infection (the pain is referred to a tooth), injury to the mouth or face, and neuralgia (pain along a nerve, such as the facial nerve). Given the multiple causes of toothache, it is advisable to seek dental care to determine the source of the pain and apply appropriate treatment. Meanwhile, the remedies here can help ease the pain of toothache.

Essential Oils

Clove essential oil rubbed into the gums is an old remedy for a toothache. While it is quite effective for many people in easing the pain until they can get to the dentist, it can be irritating to some because the oil is so concentrated, notes naturopathic physician Boyer B. Cole, N.M.D., of Cottonwood, Arizona. Stop using it if you find it too irritating, he advises.

The following essential oil blend reduces the likelihood of irritation from Clove and is more effective due to the additional cleansing and healing properties of Cajuput and Helichrysum, according to Dr. Cole. Combine:

Clove: 1 drop
Cajuput: 30 drops
Helichrysum: 10 drops

Apply 1 drop of this blend on the gums of the affected tooth 2 times daily. You can use it neat or mix it with 1/4 ounce vegetable glycerin (available at health food stores; do not use the pharmaceutical variety). Use the blend until the pain resolves or you get to the dentist.

Flower Essences

Self-Heal can serve as a foundational healing agent for toothache. Other flower essences to address the specific emotions, mental attitude, and environmental conditions of the individual are recommended, states Patricia Kaminski, a flower essence therapist and codirector of the Flower Essence Society. Self-Heal supports the body's innate healing ability. Take 4 drops 2–4 times daily, or as needed.

Food Therapy

Eat:

Green vegetable drinks.

Avoid:

Sugar, caffeine, alcohol, soft drinks, dairy, red meat.

Herbal Medicine

"I have treated many cases of dental caries; infected, abscessed roots; gum disease; and infection of the jaw without recourse to dentistry," states Matthew Wood, an herbalist from Minnetrista, Minnesota. "In many cases where the patient went to the dentist after herbal treatment, work was canceled because the X rays showed cavities, abscesses, and decalcified bones repaired." Here are Wood's herbal protocols for common causes of toothache:

For jaw infection and decalcification: Gargle with tinctures of dandelion (*Taraxacum officinalis*) root and white oak (*Quercus alba*) bark. Put a half-dropperful in 1 cup of water. Swish the mixture around in the mouth for about a minute and gargle. Do this once or twice daily. For the first week, spit the gargle out. After that, swallow it.

For gum deterioration: Gargle with tinctures of white oak bark and myrrh (*Commiphora molmol*). Follow the same procedure as above.

For severe toothache, before the white oak bark has produced effect, add a half-dropperful of tincture of prickly ash (*Zanthoxylum americanum*) or echinacea (*E. spp.*) to the gargle. Use only for 3 days.

For abscesses with threatened root canal: Chew up a wad of fresh plantain (*Plantago major* or *P. lanceolata*) leaf and stick it by the tooth. Leave it in place for 10–15 minutes. Do this twice daily. Or you can gargle with plantain tincture following the above procedure.

For nutritional treatment of toothache or any other dental problem, it can help to take horsetail (*Equisetum arvense*) powder, which is high in silica, an important bone and teeth nutrient, says clinical herbalist Karen Vaughan, E.M.T, A.H.G, of Brooklyn, New York. Take 3 capsules daily. You can take horsetail on a long-term basis if you have an ongoing bone or tooth problem, says Vaughan.

Oatstraw (*Avena sativa*) is also very good for your teeth and bones, and can be taken indefinitely. As it is rich in minerals, Vaughan recommends an infusion as "food" for your teeth and bones. Pour 1 quart of boiled water over 1 ounce of dried oatstraw in a bottle. Cap the bottle and leave overnight. Strain it in the morning and drink 2–4 cups daily. The infusion doesn't keep longer than 2 days. Alternate the oatstraw infusion with an infusion of 1/2 ounce of dried oatstraw combined with 1/2 ounce of nettle (*Urtica dioica*), red clover (*Trifolium pratense*), or red raspberry (*Rubus idaeus*), and 1/4 ounce of horsetail.

Homeopathy

The following are some of the many homeopathic remedies for toothache, as cited by London homeopath Miranda Castro:[1]

Coffea: Indicated for shooting and/or spasmodic pain worsened by heat and hot food and beverages, and improved by cold water; indicated for children and nervous people with toothache.
Lachesis: If the pain is throbbing, the cheeks are swollen, and the tooth is sensitive to touch, warmth, and cold water.
Chamomilla: Indicated for unbearable pain made worse by warmth, chewing, and hot foods or drinks, and for children with toothache.
Aconite: If the pain is tearing and excruciating, and occurring in a good tooth.

Take the appropriate remedy in a 6c or 12c potency every 1–2 hours, as needed. Discontinue the remedy when there is improvement. Repeat if necessary.

Nutritional Supplements

For any dental problem, Karen Vaughan recommends supplementing with magnesium and calcium, mineral building blocks of teeth and bone. Take twice as much magnesium as calcium. A typical daily dosage is 500 mg of calcium and 1,000 mg of magnesium.

Naturopathic physician Bradley Bongiovanni, N.D., of Independence, Ohio, recommends the following combination treatment for toothache:

Bromelain: 400 mg 3 times daily on an empty stomach; anti-inflammatory enzyme compound derived from pineapple.

Quercetin: 500 mg 3 times daily on an empty stomach; anti-inflammatory bioflavonoid.

Clove oil: Apply topically as needed for pain relief.

White willow, feverfew, kava-kava, or oatstraw: 1,000 mg (capsules) or 2 ml (extract) 3 times daily for pain relief.

Take or use all until your symptoms abate.

Reflexology

Teeth, pituitary (for pain relief)

Stone/Crystal Therapy

Use amethyst, herkimer diamond, green tourmaline, green aventurine, or green fluorite for a toothache, recommends crystal healing therapist Katrina Raphaell of Kapaa, Hawaii. Place the stone on your cheek directly over the site of the toothache. Keep it in place for 5 minutes while visualizing your health goal. Do this 3 times daily. In between treatments, wear the stone, hold it, or carry it in your pocket for added healing benefit.

Other Remedies

Green clay poultices may be all you need to resolve your toothache, depending on what the underlying problem is, says Karen Vaughan. Pack green clay powder around the gums of the problem tooth; saliva makes it into a poultice. Leave it in place for as long as you can stand it. Repeat a few times daily. "I know people who have removed a dental abscess simply with green clay," notes Vaughan.

Ulcer (Stomach)

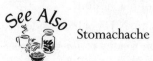 See Also Stomachache

A stomach, or gastric, ulcer is an open sore or lesion in the mucosal lining of the stomach. A peptic ulcer can be a gastric ulcer or a duodenal ulcer (an ulcer in the upper part of the small intestine, the duodenum). An ulcer develops when gastric acid (hydrochloric acid, or HCl) and the digestive enzyme pepsin eat away at the mucosal lining, as they do at food. This occurs when the lining, which normally has built-in protection against these acidic substances, has been compromised by infection, irritation, or other cause. The lining may not be producing enough mucus to provide protection.

The symptoms of a stomach ulcer are pain or burning in the stomach after eating, belching, abdominal bloating, nausea, vomiting, and loss of appetite.

A common cause of stomach ulcers is the bacterium *Helicobacter pylori,* which weakens the mucosal lining. Irritating substances can also weaken the lining. Among the culprits are coffee, alcohol, tobacco, and NSAIDs (nonsteroidal anti-inflammatory drugs) such as aspirin and ibuprofen.[1] Allergies are also implicated in ulcers; one study found that 98 percent of patients suffering from a peptic ulcer also had respiratory allergies.[2]

Stress is not the clear-cut factor it was once thought to be in the development of an ulcer. Certainly, it is beneficial in general to attempt to reduce the stress in your life, but it is important to attend to the other possible causes of your ulcer.

The conventional treatment of antacids, aimed at reducing the level of stomach acids eating away at the stomach lining, does not address the source of the problem. You may have perfectly normal levels of stomach acid and pepsin. Taking antacids disturbs that balance and does not treat the cause of the lining's loss of its protective coating. Although you may get relief from the pain of your ulcer, as soon as you stop taking the antacids, it will likely return. Research has shown that taking antacids actually increases the rate of ulcer recurrence.[3]

The natural medicine remedies here can help ease the pain, heal the ulcer, and strengthen the mucosal lining of your stomach to reduce the risk of developing another ulcer. Ulcers can develop complications, however, so it is advisable to work with your doctor to determine the cause and design treatment for your ulcer.

Essential Oils

Aromatherapy authority Robert B. Tisserand cites Chamomile and Geranium essential oils for ulcers. Chamomile is "especially good for peptic ulcers because of its antiphlogistic [anti-inflammatory] and vulnerary [tissue-healing] properties, and because of its general sedative action," he states, while Geranium "is renowned for its efficacy on wounds and all types of ulcers."[4] Use singly or in combination. For a massage oil, use 5 drops of essential oil per 2 teaspoons of vegetable oil. Massage the abdomen in a clockwise direction 1–2 times daily. You can also inhale the oil directly or use it in baths or a diffuser.

Flower Essences

If your ulcer is due to external stress and tension, take a combination of Dandelion, Indian Pink, and Lavender flower essences, recommends Richard Katz, founder of the Flower Essence Society. If your ulcer is accompanied by emotional repression or other emotional holding patterns, take a combination of Bleeding Heart, Pink Yarrow, and Chamomile. In both cases, take 4 drops of each at least 4 times daily until your symptoms subside. During a flare-up of your ulcer, you can take the essences as frequently as hourly, or even more often.

Food Therapy

Eat:

Fiber, green vegetables, ginger, plantains, bananas, foods high in vitamin K (see part 3, "Food Therapy," p. 378). Drink cabbage juice.

Cabbage juice is high in the amino acid glutamine, which has been shown to aid in the healing of ulcers.[5] To make it more palatable, you can mix it with carrot and potato juices, which are also beneficial for ulcers, suggests Kathi Head, N.D., a naturopathic physician from Sandpoint, Idaho. If you want to drink the juice instead of taking a glutamine supplement, drink 1 quart daily.

If *H. pylori* bacteria are the source of your ulcer, garlic, which is antimicrobial, may be helpful, says Dr. Head.

Avoid:

Coffee, alcohol, sugar, citrus, spicy foods, milk, saturated fats, food allergens.

Although spicy foods are generally to be avoided, there is some evidence that cayenne pepper can actually help heal an ulcer, notes Dr. Head. As individuals differ in what foods make their ulcer worse, the best approach is to pay attention to how you feel after eating and adjust your diet accordingly.

Herbal Medicine/Supplements

The following program of herbs and supplements can be effective for a stomach ulcer, according to Dr. Head:

Slippery elm (*Ulmus rubra, U. fulva*): Take 200 mg in capsules 3 times daily.

Marshmallow (*Althea officinalis*) root: Take 200 mg in capsules 3 times daily.

DGL (deglycrrhizinated licorice): Licorice root from which the potentially irritating glycyrrhizinic acid has been removed has been shown to be quite effective in healing stomach ulcers.[6] Take 300 mg in capsules or chewable tablets 3 times daily. While some practitioners believe that the licorice needs to be mixed with saliva in order to achieve the healing effects, Dr. Head has not seen a difference in the results between capsules and chewable tablets.

Glutamine (amino acid): Take 1,000 mg powder 3 times per day. Mix with water and drink.

This program should produce improvement in a few weeks to 2 months. Continue treatment, as needed. If you are not getting results, you need to pursue other treatment.

If testing has revealed that *H. pylori* bacteria are the source of your ulcer, Dr. Head has found berberine (an extract of Oregon grape, goldenseal, or barberry) to be helpful. You should, however, be under medical care. Take 100 mg of standardized 80 percent berberine on an empty stomach 4 times daily. This should be used only on a short-term basis; take for 8 weeks.

Jody E. Noé, M.S., N.D., a naturopathic physician from Brattleboro, Vermont, suggests another herbal protocol for an ulcer caused by *H. pylori*. Take 50–100 mg 3 times daily of each of the following herbs: wild indigo (*Baptisia tinctoria*); cranesbill (American, *Geranium maculatum*); goldenseal (*Hydrastis canadensis*); ginger (*Zingiber officinale*); and cayenne (*Capsicum spp.*), enteric coated capsules to prevent stomach irritation.

Homeopathy

While constitutional treatment may be in order if you suffer from an ulcer, the following simple remedies are commonly indicated for the condition, according to Dr. Barry Rose of the Royal London Homeopathic Hospital:[7]

Anacardium: If there is dull pain that radiates to the back 2 hours after eating, and tasteless or sour burps, and eating provides relief.

Arg nit: If the stomach pain is gnawing, radiates in all directions, and worsens after eating and with pressure.

Arsenicum: If the stomach pain is burning and worsens after eating, accompanied by loss of appetite, inability to digest food, nausea, and vomiting.

Bryonia: If there is sharp, cutting pain after eating, the pain radiates to the shoulders and back, food sits like a stone in the stomach, the mouth is dry with a bitter taste, and there is constipation and frontal headaches.

Nux vom: If the pain occurs about an hour after eating and after mental overwork, is worse in the morning, and is accompanied by nausea, nonproductive retching, sour burping, and bad temper.

Phosphorus: If there is sour burping, a white-coated tongue, and a craving for cold food and liquids, which temporarily relieve the stomach pain before they are vomited up.

Take the appropriate remedy in a 12c potency 4 times daily until your symptoms improve. Repeat as needed.

Nutritional Supplements

Take aloe vera gel as a healing agent for your ulcer, suggests Joanne B. Mied, N.D., a naturopath, herbalist, and iridologist from

Novato, California. She does not recommend taking the juice, because it is more astringent than the gel. Get a high-quality aloe vera gel, the kind that needs to be refrigerated and is not whole-leaf aloe vera. Do not use the drugstore variety shelved with suntan lotions as a remedy for sunburn. Take 1 tablespoon on an empty stomach, in the morning and before going to bed, until your ulcer is resolved.

If stress is a contributing factor to your ulcer, Dr. Mied recommends taking a vitamin B complex supplement and additional vitamin B5 (pantothenic acid). B complex supports nerve function, and B5 is known as the antistress vitamin because it supports adrenal gland function. Take 250 mg daily of vitamin B5 in addition to 1 capsule 3 times daily of the B complex supplement, which should contain 100 mg of pantothenic acid and each of the main B vitamins (10 mg of B6 and 100 mcg of B12), along with the other members of the B family. Supplementation is not a substitute for addressing the stress in your life and taking steps to reduce it, however.

Reflexology

Stomach, solar plexus, diaphragm, adrenal glands

Stone/Crystal Therapy

For a stomach ulcer, green and blue smithsonite, lepidolite, green aventurine, or chrysocolla can be helpful, according to Katrina Raphaell, crystal healing therapist and author of the crystal reference series *The Crystal Trilogy*. Place the stone on your abdomen directly over the area where the pain is focused. Leave the stone there for 5 minutes while visualizing your health goal. Do this 3 times daily. At other times, wear the stone, hold it, or carry it in your pocket for ongoing healing.

Urinary Tract Infection

See Bladder Infection (Cystitis).

Vaginal Yeast Infection

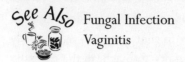

See Also Fungal Infection
Vaginitis

A vaginal yeast infection is actually an overgrowth of a yeast-like fungus—*Candida albicans*—normally found in the body. It is the most common form of vaginitis, inflammation of the lining of the vagina.

Overgrowth can occur when the balance of the vaginal environment is disturbed. The main culprit in throwing off the balance is antibiotics, which kill all the beneficial bacteria that keep potentially harmful flora such as *Candida* in check. Weakened immunity can also result in a yeast overgrowth. Other factors or conditions that can change the vaginal environment and lead to a yeast infection are birth control pills, steroids, pregnancy, diabetes, and wearing tight clothing, nylon underwear, and/or pantyhose. Women who wear nylon undergarments are three times as likely to get a yeast infection as women who wear cotton.[1] If you have recurrent infections, your sexual partner, particularly if he is uncircumcised, may be reinfecting you.

The symptoms of a vaginal yeast infection are a cottage cheeselike discharge, itching, and burning. Redness and swelling of the tissue in the vagina and vaginal area can also accompany the infection.

Effective treatment of a vaginal yeast infection needs to address the infection and strengthen the immune system as well. If you suffer from chronic yeast infections, you may have a systemic yeast overgrowth (candidiasis). This is a serious condition that requires medical treatment. Seek medical help.

Essential Oils

"Yeast infections are very short-lived" using the following treatment, says herbalist Colleen K. Dodt. Put 10–15 drops of Tea Tree (*Melaleuca alternifolia*) essential oil on a tampon, insert in the vagina, and leave in overnight. Do this nightly for a week. Tea Tree is a potent antifungal. "Tea tree is safe to use neat on the most delicate parts of the body," notes Dodt, adding, "There is *no* other essential oil that I would recommend applying in this manner."[2]

Flower Essences

Take a combination of Tiger Lily, Easter Lily, and Alpine Lily flower essences if you suffer from chronic yeast infections and they are related to emotional issues of sexuality and femininity, recommends Patricia Kaminski, an herbalist and flower essence therapist from Nevada City, California. Take 4 drops of each at least 4 times per day. During an acute episode, you can take the essences as frequently as hourly.

Food Therapy

Eat:

Yogurt, garlic, onion, shitake mushrooms, green vegetables, nuts, seafood, egg yolks, organ meats, legumes.

Advising women with a vaginal yeast infection to avoid all fermented foods, as is common practice, is giving bad advice, says Karen Vaughan, E.M.T, A.H.G, a clinical herbalist from Brooklyn, New York. It is only foods that can be further fermented by the yeast, such as vinegar, bread, and wine, that are the problem. Other fermented foods such as miso, yogurt (full-fat, live culture), cheese, sauerkraut, kim chee, and unpasteurized pickles provide competition to the *Candida* and prevent its overgrowth. One of the best foods to eat to help reestablish the vaginal (as well as intestinal) flora is unpasteurized blue cheese, notes Vaughan.

Avoid:

Sugar, fruit or fruit juice, white flour, pasta, mashed potatoes, baked goods and other yeast foods, soy sauce, vinegar, alcohol, caffeine.

Herbal Medicine

White oak (*Quercus alba*) tea used as a douche or external wash exerts astringent effects and can help pull out the discharge of a vaginal yeast infection, says herbalist Teresa Boardwine of Washington, Virginia. To prepare the tea, put 1 tablespoon of the herb per quart of water, cover, and simmer for 20 minutes. You will need several quarts for the external wash. Let the tea cool sufficiently to use it as a douche or in a bath. Douche every other day when the infection is acute. For the external wash, put the tea in a sitz bath (tub in which water covers your hips when you sit in it) or washbasin big enough for you to sit in with your legs draped over the side. The idea is to immerse your genital area in the tea. Cleanse and splash your genital area with the tea. Do this daily until the symptoms disappear.

Fireweed (*Epilobium angustifolium*), which grows in North America, is as potent an antifungal as the Amazon rain forest herb pau d'arco, according to Karen Vaughan. Take as a tea. Put 1/2 cup of dried fireweed in a quart of boiled water, cover, and let steep for 15–25 minutes. Drink 1 cup 4–5 times daily until your yeast infection symptoms have been gone for a few weeks. You can also douche with a cup of the fireweed tea daily for a week.

Homeopathy

Although there are a wide range of remedies for vaginal infections, Pulsatilla nigricans and Sepia are often indicated in cases of yeast infection. Take Pulsatilla if the vaginal discharge is white and creamy, there is soreness, burning, and/or stinging, and symptoms worsen around menstruation. Take Sepia if the discharge is yellow, stinging, and foul-smelling, there is a bearing-down sensation in the pelvis, and symptoms worsen just before menstruation or midway between periods. Take the appropriate remedy at a 6c or 12c potency 1–3 times daily for up to 3 days. As your symptoms improve, take the remedy less often. If there is no improvement after 2–3 days of taking the remedy, it is probably not the correct one for your infection.[3]

Nutritional Supplements

Taking probiotics (friendly bacteria) can help restore the balance of flora in the vaginal environment. *Lactobacillus acidophilus* and *Bifidobacterium bifidum* are the most important, says Ann Louise Gittleman, N.D., C.N.S., M.S., nutritionist and author of *Super Nutrition for Women*. Make sure when you buy probiotic capsules that these two strains are included in the product, and also that each capsule contains 1–5 billion organisms. Dr. Gittleman's recommended dosage is 1 capsule before meals, 3 times daily. After your vaginal infection has cleared up, take 1 capsule daily as maintenance, to help prevent the infection from recurring.

Stone/Crystal Therapy

Blue sodalite may be helpful for a vaginal yeast infection. Place the stone in the area of your pubic hair and rest quietly several times a day for 10–15 minutes. You can also benefit from the stone's properties in the form of an elixir; drink a few sips 3 times daily.[4] (For instructions on making an elixir, see part 3, "Stone/Crystal Therapy," p. 403.)

Other Remedies

Wear cotton underwear. Avoid wearing nylons and tight clothing.

Douching with cider vinegar or inserting yogurt in the vagina is a good corollary to dietary and supplement protocols, states Dr. Gittleman. Use 2 tablespoons of cider vinegar in 8 ounces of water for the douche. Cider vinegar balances the pH of the vaginal tract, which inhibits yeast overgrowth. For the yogurt treatment, use a large syringe or funnel to insert 1/2 cup of plain yogurt (make sure it contains live yogurt cultures) in the vagina. Do this while lying down. It's best to do it at bedtime and leave the yogurt in overnight; use a sanitary pad to avoid mess. For extra probiotic (beneficial bacteria) punch, you can open acidophilus capsules and mix the powder with the yogurt you insert. Dr. Gittleman recommends doing either the douche or the yogurt treatment every third day until your yeast infection disappears.

Vaginitis

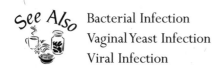 Bacterial Infection
Vaginal Yeast Infection
Viral Infection

Vaginitis is inflammation of the mucosal lining of the vagina. The symptoms of vaginitis are a discharge (often smelly), reddened vaginal tissue, vulval and vaginal itching and irritation, pain with sexual intercourse, increased urination, and pain with urination. The pain with urination differs from that associated with urinary tract infections, in that it results from the acidity of urine passing over the inflamed genital tissue, rather than resulting from inflamed tissue in the urethra (urinary passageway).

Vaginitis has many causes, including bacterial, viral, protozoal, or fungal infection; irritation, as from chemical douches; prolonged presence of a tampon or contraceptive diaphragm; and sexually transmitted disease (STD). Infection can result from a foreign microbe or an overgrowth of microorganisms normally found in the vagina (such as *Candida albicans;* see "Vaginal Yeast Infection"). A disturbance of the vaginal environment allows both foreign and normally-present microbes to create infection. Taking antibiotics, birth control pills, or steroids can change the vaginal environment and lead to vaginitis, as can wearing tight clothing and/or synthetic undergarments. Diabetes and pregnancy also increase your risk of vaginitis.

The most common kinds of vaginitis are caused by *Candida albicans* (yeast-like fungus), *Gardnerella vaginalis* (bacteria), and *Trichomonas vaginalis* (protozoa). The last kind of infection is categorized as an STD because it is typically spread by sexual contact.

Since the causes of vaginitis are multiple, it is advisable to see your doctor to culture the vaginal discharge so you know the proper treatment to implement. An untreated vaginal infection can spread upward through the reproductive system and become pelvic infammatory disease, an infection that can damage the fallopian tubes. If you suffer from recurrent vaginitis, it may be a sign of a weakened immune system or other disorder. Seek medical care.

Essential Oils

Taking daily baths with a blend of essential oils of Eucalyptus (4 drops), Bergamot (4 drops), and Lavender (2 drops) can help alleviate vaginitis, according to natural healer Diane Stein. Remain in the bath for 20 minutes, allowing the water into the vagina. Daily douching with Tea Tree (*Melaleuca alternifolia*) oil is also effective, particularly for vaginitis caused by *Trichomonas*. Use 1 tablespoon of Tea Tree to a quart of warm water.[1]

Flower Essences

Take Easter Lily, Tiger Lily, and Crab Apple flower essences for prolonged or frequent bouts of vaginal infection, especially if there are emotional issues regarding sexual activity, states flower essence thera-pist Patricia Kaminski of Nevada City, California. Put 4 drops of each in a glass of water. Take 4 drops of each at least 4 times per day. During an acute episode, you can take the essences as frequently as hourly.

Food Therapy

Eat:

Yogurt, garlic, onion. Drink plenty of fluids (coffee, black tea, and soft drinks do not count).

Avoid:

Sugar, caffeine, dairy, wheat, yeast, refined foods, alcohol; limit fats.

Herbal Medicine

Sweet leaf (*Monarda fistulosa*), yellow dock (*Rumex crispus*) root, lady's mantle (*Alchemilla vulgaris*), and archangelia (*Lamium album*) are all excellent herbs for the treatment of vaginitis, according to herbalist Matthew Wood of Minnetrista, Minnesota. "My dosage is small," he says, recommending 3 drops of tincture of one or a combination of the herbs, 3 times daily, and less as improvement sets in.

If your vaginitis is bacterial, clinical herbalist Karen Vaughan, E.M.T, A.H.G, of Brooklyn, New York, recommends treating it both orally and with douches. Take an antimicrobial herb—myrrh (*Commiphora molmol*), St. John's wort (*Hypericum perforatum*), cleavers (*Galium aparine*), or echinacea (*E. spp.*). Choose one and take 3–5 cap-sules 3 times daily. For a douche, use 1/4 teaspoon of Tea Tree (*Melaleuca alternifolia*) essential oil or 1/2 teaspoon of a triple (full-spectrum) echinacea tincture to a douche bag of water. Douche daily for a week.

Homeopathy

The following are common remedies for vaginitis, according to naturopathic physicians Robert Ullmann, N.D., and Judyth Reichenberg-Ullmann, N.D.:[2]

Caladium: Indicated for horribly itchy vaginitis during pregnancy.
Kreosotum: If the vaginal discharge is yellow, burning, very itchy, and

produces rawness in the mucous membranes, and is worse just before menstruation.

Sanicula: If the discharge smells fishy, the body odor resembles old cheese, and there is a bearing-down feeling in the pelvis.

Take the appropriate remedy in a 30c potency every 4 hours until your symptoms improve. Stop taking the remedy, repeat if the symptoms return. If there is no improvement after 3 doses, take a different remedy.

Nutritional Supplements

As a treatment program for vaginitis, the following can be effective, states Bradley Bongiovanni, N.D., a naturopathic physician from Independence, Ohio:

Vitamin C: 1,000 mg 3 times daily for 10–14 days.

Garlic (fresh extract): 400 mg twice daily for 10–14 days.

Acidophilus: 5–10 billion organisms 3 times daily for 10–14 days.

Boric acid suppositories: Insert 1 into the vagina in the morning and again in the evening for 10–14 days.

Stone/Crystal Therapy

Blue sodalite may help ease vaginitis. Place the stone in the area of your pubic hair and rest quietly several times a day for 10–15 minutes. You can also benefit from the stone's properties in the form of an elixir; drink a few sips 3 times daily.[3] (For instructions on making an elixir, see part 3, "Stone/Crystal Therapy," p. 403.)

Other Remedies

Change underwear frequently (wear cotton only) or go without underwear while treating vaginitis. Urinate after sexual intercourse. Wipe yourself from front to back following urination; wiping from back to front risks the transferral of bacteria from the anus or vagina to the urethra. Shower rather than take baths, and especially avoid bubble baths. Dry well after bathing, and use a hair dryer on warm to dry the external tissues of the genital area. Karen Vaughan also suggests applying a thick barrier cream, such as zinc oxide, unpetroleum jelly, or shea butter, to the external tissues to protect them from urine burns while you are treating the infection.

Viral Infection

Viruses, a class of microorganisms, are normally present throughout our bodies and the environment. Normally, the immune system prevents a virus from multiplying to a level that produces infection. When immunity is weakened, however, a virus can flourish and create infection. Stress, poor nutrition, toxic exposure, lack of exercise, lack of sleep, and overuse of antibiotics and other drugs can all contribute to suppressed immunity. Since we live in a toxic world, lead stressful lives, and eat food grown in depleted soil or a diet of processed food, most of our immune systems are compromised to some degree.

Common symptoms of a viral infection are fever, chills, headache, and general achiness. Other symptoms depend on the type of virus. For example, viruses that affect the upper respiratory tract produce respiratory symptoms such as cough, congestion, and a runny nose. Flu and the common cold are caused by viruses, as are many childhood illnesses.

Antibiotics are ineffective against viruses. There are numerous natural antivirals that can help fight a viral infection, however. Another important component of treatment is to strengthen your immune system to help restore your body's ability to heal itself.

Essential Oils

Research has established the antiviral activities of essential oils. Bergamot, Eucalyptus, Geranium, and Lemon are among the more well-known antiviral oils.[1] However, Tea Tree (*Melaleuca alternifolia*), Manuka, and Ravensara are even more powerful, according to aromatherapist Patricia Davis. "They also stimulate the body's immune response to the infection," notes Davis. She recommends baths and diffusing as the preferred methods of delivery because viral infections often involve fever; massage is contraindicated when fever is present. If the infection is a respiratory one, steam inhalation is useful. Diffusion has the added benefit of decreasing the likelihood of infectious transmission to other household members.[2] (For instructions on using essential oils, see part 3, "Essential Oils," pp. 366–68.)

Flower Essences

For a viral infection, take Yarrow Special Formula to rebuild the immune system and provide greater protection from intrusive elements, says Richard Katz, founder of the Flower Essence Society. Take 4 drops under the tongue, no less than half an hour before eating, at least 4 times daily. During the acute stage of infection, you can take it as often as hourly, if needed.

Food Therapy

Eat:

Garlic, sage, seaweed, apples, black currants, blueberries, cranberries, barley, collard greens.

Avoid:

Sugar, soft drinks, caffeine, alcohol, refined foods.

Herbal Medicine

Among the many natural antivirals, the following are especially useful, notes Chanchal Cabrera, M.N.I.M.H., A.H.G., a medical herbalist from Vancouver, British Columbia:

Garlic: Take fresh garlic orally. Odorless garlic pills are worthless, according to Cabrera, because the active ingredient in garlic is carried in its essential oil, which is what smells. To lessen the strong odor, chop up a clove of garlic, put it on a teaspoon, and swallow it like a pill, without chewing it. Take at night, and again in the day if you can tolerate it.

Osha (*Ligusticum porteri*): Traditionally used by Native Americans to treat flu, colds, and respiratory infections, this herb is good for both viral and bacterial infections, especially those deep in the lungs and involving sticky mucus. Take 1/2 teaspoon of tincture 2–3 times/day.

Lomatium (*Lomatium dissectum*): Another traditional Native American herb, lomatium is also good for viral infection that strikes the lungs. Take 1 teaspoon of tincture 2–3 times/day.

You shouldn't need osha and lomatium for more than a week to 10 days. If you're not getting results, it can be for three reasons: the quality of the product is poor, you aren't taking enough, or the infection you have is not viral.

Astragalus (*Astragalus membranaceus*): This herb is a deep immune tonic, which can help strengthen a weak immune system. It should not be used for the occasional sudden infection, but reserved for more deep-seated immune problems. If you have a history of suffering recurring colds or other viral infections in the winter, take astragalus from early fall to late spring as a preventive. Take 1 teaspoon of tincture 1–2 times daily during that period.

Homeopathy

See the particular type of viral infection.

Nutritional Supplements

"Virtually all known vitamins and minerals are essential for normal functioning of white blood cells," state naturopathic physicians Michael T. Murray, N.D., and Joseph Pizzorno, N.D. (White blood cells carry out the work of the immune system in fighting infection.) However, they cite zinc and vitamins A, B6, and C as possibly the most important nutrients for the immune system. Selenium is also vital for proper immune function.[3] When you have a viral infection, you may want to consider taking at least this group of vitamins and minerals.

Grapefruit seed extract (GSE) is another supplement that is beneficial to take for a viral infection. A powerful antimicrobial agent, GSE has proven effective against viruses, bacteria, fungi, and protozoa, says clinical nutritionist Allan Sachs, D.C., C.C.N.[4] Tablets are a palatable way to take the extract; some people object to the taste and drying sensation of the liquid form. Take as directed for your particular infection.

Reflexology

Treat the spleen area and the area of the foot corresponding to the part of the body where the symptoms are most pronounced.

Stone/Crystal Therapy

Chevron amethyst, marble, and wad are all useful for a viral infection, says Melody, author of the crystal reference series *Love Is in the Earth*. Place the amethyst on your third eye (forehead between the eyes) for 4 hours. You can attach it with hypoallergenic tape. Take the marble or wad as an elixir, 3–5 drops 3 times daily or up to 5 times daily for 24–30 hours. (For instructions on making an elixir, see part 3, "Stone/Crystal Therapy," p. 403.)

Wart

Note

Venereal warts are a different problem and not covered in this discussion. Do not apply these treatments to venereal (genital) warts.

A common wart, or verruca, is a raised, rough skin growth caused by the papillomavirus. Warts range from barely visible to a quarter of an inch in diameter, and may grow in clusters. They typically appear on the face, hands, arms, and feet.

Although the common wart virus is contagious, it is also omnipresent, so exposure to it is nearly inevitable. The good news about that is that someone with common warts need not be concerned about giving them to others, and those without such warts need not be concerned about getting them from someone who has them. If your immune system is strong, you are unlikely to develop warts.

Many warts disappear on their own. Avoid picking at a wart; that can cause it to spread. Some people have their doctor remove their warts by cutting them off or freezing them with liquid nitrogen. Unfortunately, warts may return after removal.

There are some effective natural remedies that can help dissolve a wart without the pain of medical procedures. As with any viral infection, treatment should also include strengthening the immune system.

If a wart changes shape or color or is painful, see your doctor.

Essential Oils

Many practitioners cite Thuja essential oil as an effective treatment to get rid of a wart. Put 1 drop of Thuja essential oil on the wart every day until the wart dries up or falls off, says naturopathic physician Boyer B. Cole, N.M.D., of Cottonwood, Arizona. Be patient, he warns; it usually takes several weeks.

Flower Essences

Self-Heal can serve as a foundational healing agent for warts. Other flower essences to address the specific emotions, mental attitude, and environmental conditions of the individual are recommended, states Patricia Kaminski, a flower essence therapist and codirector of the Flower Essence Society. Self-Heal supports the body's innate healing ability. Take 4 drops 2–4 times daily, or as needed.

Food Therapy

Eat:

Foods high in vitamin A/beta-carotene, vitamin E, sulphur, and zinc (see part 3, "Food Therapy," p. 378).

Avoid:

Refined sugar and flour.

Herbal Medicine

Fresh celandine (*Chelidonium majus*) can effectively dissolve warts, according to Jody E. Noé, M.S., N.D., a naturopathic physician from Brattleboro, Vermont. Break off a leaf or stem of the fresh plant and apply the latex (fluid in the plant; in this case, orange-yellow) directly in the center of the wart; be sure to get it in the center. Do this twice daily for about two weeks.

Homeopathy

As warts reflect a systemic condition, they are best treated by a constitutional remedy. You may want to consult a homeopath for individualized treatment. However, homeopathic Thuja occidentalis is commonly used to get rid of warts; indicated for the fleshy, cauliflower-like variety found on any part of the body. Drs. Andrew Lockie and Nicola Geddes recommend taking Thuja 6c every 12 hours for up to 3 weeks.[1]

Nutritional Supplements

Grapefruit seed extract (GSE), which is both acidic and antiviral, can dissolve a wart, says Allan Sachs, D.C., C.C.N., an authority on GSE. He notes that warts are one of the few conditions for which you can use the highly concentrated extract undiluted. Dr. Sachs cautions, however, to be sure before using this treatment that the growth in question is actually a wart and not something else. Use a cotton swab to apply GSE to the wart, being sure to "paint" the whole wart, including the base and stem if possible. Put an adhesive bandage over the wart to prevent getting the GSE in your eyes via the fingers after inadvertently touching the treated wart. Do this 2–3 times daily. It may take several weeks to achieve the desired result, notes Dr. Sachs.[2]

Stone/Crystal Therapy

For warts, use pyrite included quartz or labradorite, recommends Melody, author of the crystal reference series *Love Is in the Earth*. Use hypoallergenic tape to secure the stone on the wart; keep it in place until the wart disappears, which is usually in 4–14 days.

Other Remedies

For warts, naturopathic physician Susan Roberts, N.D., of Portland, Oregon, has found green clay poultices effective. The poultice draws the virus out of the wart, so it disappears. Before going to bed, mix a little green clay powder (available at health food stores) with enough water to produce a mud consistency. Apply the "mud" to the wart and cover or wrap with gauze, depending on where the wart is. If it's on your foot, put a sock on over the gauze wrapping. Leave on overnight. Repeat nightly until the wart is gone. Typically, you'll notice improvement in a week.

Part III
About the Therapies

Essential Oils

Throughout the book, I purposely cite protocols for these potent plant extracts under the heading "essential oils" rather than "aromatherapy" because the latter label has contributed to the devaluing of this field of medicine. Essential oils are far more than nice smells, and their therapeutic effects extend far beyond the power of aroma. While aroma in itself is therapeutic (by stimulating the olfactory sense, it can relax, soothe, energize, or serve to lift one's mood, among many other actions), aroma is also a means of delivering essential oil molecules, with their healing properties, into the body via the lungs. From the lungs, the molecules enter the bloodstream and are dispersed throughout the body, to all the organs and tissues, where they exert the particular healing actions of the plants from which they are derived.

Another reason that "aromatherapy" is not the most accurate name for this form of medicine is that absorption of the oils through the skin is as important a transmittal method as aroma. Again, the molecules travel throughout the body. The fact that they penetrate the skin and tissue and stay there for a time before being eliminated makes essential oils a potent means of delivering herbal medicine to the body. As evidence of the body-wide dispersal and lasting power of essential oils, naturopathic physician Boyer B. Cole, N.M.D., notes that days after someone has given you an essential oil massage, if you bite one of your fingernails, you will taste the essential oil.

Names for this therapy that are perhaps more reflective of its powerful healing abilities are "medical aromatherapy," "aromatic medicine," and "essential oil therapy."

An essential oil comprises the aromatic, volatile oils of a plant—its essence—extracted through distillation with water or steam. (Hydrosol, or aromatic water, is a coproduct of the essential oil distillation process, and also is used in aromatherapy.) All essential oils are antiseptic to some degree, but each has other particular healing qualities. Research has demonstrated, among numerous other properties, the potent antiviral, antibacterial, antifungal, and antispasmodic effects of specific oils.[1] As essential oils possess the properties of the plants from which they are extracted, they cover the whole range of medicinal function, from analgesic to vasodilator.

Aromatic medicine is an ancient form of healing, used around the world for thousands of years. The actual name "aromatherapy" was conceived in 1937 when French perfume chemist René Maurice Gattefossé discovered the skin-healing effects of Lavender essential oil

Essential Oils: Directions for Use

Measurements: 1 dropperful equals about 20 drops equals about 1 ml.

Bath: Use essential oils as directed or 3–8 drops of essential oil to a tub of warm water. When the tub is half full, add the oils, then fill the tub the rest of the way. Add the oils to the stream from the faucet or mix them with water in a plastic container and then add to the faucet stream. Stir with your hand to ensure dispersion. Keep the bathroom door closed while you are running the bath and during soaking so you get the full benefit of inhaling the aroma in addition to immersion in the oils. Soak in the tub for at least 20 minutes. Rest afterward, as the essential oils continue to work.

Compress: Use as directed or put 4–5 drops of essential oil (do not use oils that irritate the skin) on a hot or cold compress, lay it over the affected area, and leave it on for 10 minutes. For a compress, you can simply immerse a washcloth in hot or icy-cold water, then squeeze it out. Alternatively, you can add the essential oils to the water into which you dip the cloth.

Diffusion: Use an aromatherapy burner, an electric diffuser, or simply put 1–2 drops on a light bulb and turn on the light. The heat of the bulb sends the aroma wafting through the room (do not apply the oil to a heated light bulb, as essential oils are flammable). The aromatherapy burner consists of a tealight candle under a container in on a bad laboratory burn, began to study the medicinal use of oils, and dubbed the practice "aromatherapy."

Today, in the boom of alternative medicines, aromatherapy is becoming increasingly popular. While this means that essential oils are now readily available in health food stores everywhere, it also means that there are many inferior oils on the market along with the good ones. In this case, you get what you pay for. High-quality oils can be expensive, but you will need far less than you will of a lower-quality oil to get the therapeutic benefits; one drop of a good oil is often sufficient. With the cheaper oils, you may use many drops and still not get comparable effects. To ensure optimal results, use high-quality essential oils, organic if possible. The essential oil should be in a brown/amber bottle to preserve the oil's qualities. Store out of the sun at room temperature. Some practioners recommend using an essential oil within six to nine months.

which you put water and essential oil drops. As the water heats, the aroma is released. It works best if you get a burner that has a large container for the water. The water in the smaller containers evaporates more quickly. As for electric diffusers, some practitioners recommend using other diffusing methods because they believe the electromagnetic field of an electric diffuser interferes with the energetic properties of the essential oils.

Inhalation: Sniff directly from the bottle; put a few drops of the essential oil on a handkerchief or tissue and inhale from that; or put a drop on your hands (if the essential oil is safe to use on the skin), rub them together, and inhale.

Massage: Use the amount indicated or 5 drops per teaspoon of carrier oil. The carrier oil can be sweet almond, apricot kernel, avocado, or olive or other vegetable oil. Carrier oils are also called base or fatty oils. A vegetable oil is more neutral when using blends of numerous oils, although almond oil is fine, too. Carrier oils can be infused oils, meaning oils in which an herb has been steeped. Calendula fatty oil, for example, is not an essential oil. It is a carrier oil that has been infused with the herb calendula, whereas essential oil is an extract of an herb or plant.

Misting bottle: Mix 4 or more drops of essential oil per 1 cup of water in a spray bottle. Shake the bottle before spraying around your body and in your environment.

Steam inhalation: Add 2–3 drops of the selected essential oil to a bowl of boiled water. Drape your head and the bowl with a towel and inhale the steam.

Caution

Test an essential oil before using it on your skin by putting a drop on the inside of your elbow to make sure you aren't allergic to it.

Do not use Bergamot essential oil on your skin if you are going to be in the sun or otherwise exposed to UV rays because it increases the sensitivity of the skin to ultraviolet rays.

If you are pregnant, do not use essential oils of Anise, Camphor, Cedar, German Chamomile, Eucalyptus, Hyssop, Myrrh, Marjoram, Niaouli (MQV), Rosemary (Corsica or camphor type), Sage, Spike Lavender, Thuja, Thyme, or Yarrow.

Do not use Cinnamon or Clove on your skin in any way—direct application, massage, or baths. These essential oils can seriously irritate the skin.

Use Thuja only in small external applications, such as dabbing on a wart. It contains a high level of ketones, neurotoxic substances that can also induce abortion.

Julie Oxendale, C.M.T., among other aromatherapists, doesn't believe in blending more than three essential oils in one mix because, with more than that, the properties of the individual oil get lost, she says. Some oils, such as lemon, don't count as one, however, but are added to a blend to magnify the potency of the other oils. In that case, three essential oils plus lemon are fine, says Oxendale.

In choosing from a selection of oils in any of the protocols in this book, experiment to find the oils that best suit you. Essential oil treatment is a very individualized therapy, as smell is highly personal. Aromas exert a strong effect on the central nervous system. That is why an aroma can vividly recall to your mind past experiences—pleasant and unpleasant. The odor is stored in your body memory and unalterably linked to those experiences. Consider aromatherapy an ongoing interactive experience and modify it to suit your individual needs.

Flower Essences

Like essential oils, flower essences are often dismissed in the United States, even by some alternative medicine practitioners, as a "lightweight" therapy that may be pleasing, but that has little therapeutic value. As with essential oils, this view is completely mistaken. Perhaps, as with aromatherapy, the problem arises in part from the name and the common attitude that anything pleasant-sounding can't be potent medicine. A perhaps stronger reason for the misconception, however, is the general lack of understanding in this country about energetic medicine. You may not be aware of it, but magnetic resonance imaging (MRI), the scanning technique used in conventional medicine, is a form of energy medicine. Flower essence therapy is another form.

To clarify another common misunderstanding, essential oils and flower essences are two very different kinds of medicine. While essential oils contain the biochemical components of the plants from which they are extracted, flower essences are closer to homeopathic remedies in nature, in that they are energetic imprints of their source. Another way of saying this is that a flower essence contains the life force of the flower.

A flower essence is made by sun-infusing the blossoms of a particular plant, bush, or tree in water. (This is a simplistic summary of the process, which involves timing the picking of the flowers according to life cycle, environmental, and other factors.) The liquid is then diluted and potentized in a method similar to the preparation of homeopathic remedies, and preserved with brandy. The result is a highly diluted, potentized substance that embodies the energetic patterns of the flower from which it is made. This means that the therapeutic effects of flower essences are vibrational, or energetic.[2]

Despite Einstein and solid science demonstrating that matter is energy, the fact that you can contain energy in a liquid and influence human energy fields to help resolve physical ailments is not widely known. Yet, that is precisely what flower essence liquids do: influence your energy fields. When you take flower essences, the energy they contain affects your energy fields, which in turn has an impact on your physical, mental, emotional, and spiritual condition, as these aspects are all energy based.

Although flower essences are included in this book as first aid remedies, this in no way implies that they simply address your physical symptoms. As with some of the other therapies covered here, they are a holistic medicine, meaning they work to bring the whole back into balance and thus health. The specialty of flower essences is the realm of emotions and attitudes, which have come to be accepted as exerting a powerful influence on health and ill health. As Edward Bach, the father of flower essence therapy, stated, "Behind all disease lies our fears, our anxieties, our greed, our likes and dislikes."[3] By promoting energetic shifts in the mind and emotions, flower essences promote a return to health. Put simply, flower essences are "catalysts to mind-body wellness." Or you could say they act as a bridge between the realms of the physical and the spiritual, the body and the soul.[4]

In the 1930s, Dr. Bach, an English physician and homeopath, developed thirty-eight different flower essences to address thirty-eight different emotional-soul, or psychological, types. As an example of the "profile" associated with a remedy, the flower essence Willow is indicated for someone who, when out of balance, feels resentful, bitter, and envious of others, and adopts a "poor me" victim stance. Dr. Bach's remedies are still available today—the Bach Flower Remedies seen in health food stores everywhere.

The Flower Essence Society in Nevada City, California, has expanded on the work of Dr. Bach and significantly furthered the field of flower essences. The Society's codirectors, Patricia Kaminski and Richard Katz, provided the flower essence protocols for this book. The protocols are not derived from their clinical experience alone, but are the result of extensive research compiled by the Society. Founded in 1979 by Katz, the Society has become renowned for its pioneering flower essence research, including an extensive collection of case studies and practitioner reports. Thus, the remedies cited throughout this book reflect the work of thousands of flower essence practitioners from all over the world and have been clinically correlated with positive effects on the condition involved.

In addition to research, Kaminski and Katz expanded on Bach's remedies, developing a line of more than one hundred flower essences derived from North American plants. They developed the line for several reasons: to expand the emotional repertoire of flower essences; to provide North Americans with essences derived from indigenous plants, which might better resonate with their healing issues; and to address the more complicated emotional and psychological makeup of people today. Many of the flower essences cited in this book are from the Flower Essence Society's line.

For some conditions in this book, the flower essence protocol calls for Self-Heal, Five Flower Formula, and/or Yarrow Special Formula. These are foundational healing agents:

• Self-Heal supports the body's innate healing ability; the essence of the herb self-heal (*Prunella vulgaris*), also known traditionally as heal-all and heart of the earth.

• Five Flower Formula (also known as Rescue Remedy), which brings immediate calm and emotional neutralizing, is indicated for physical and/or emotional trauma; the five flower essences in this formula are Rock Rose, Clematis, Impatiens, Cherry Plum, and Star of Bethlehem.

• Yarrow Special Formula strengthens and protects against environmental toxicity and stress, and is excellent for travel and working near computers; combines essences of Yarrow, Echinacea, and Arnica.

For conditions in which these remedies are indicated, further flower essence therapy, based on a more tailored approach, can address the specific emotions, mental attitude, and environmental conditions of each person. Consult a flower essence repertory or a qualified practitioner to determine the additional remedies uniquely suited to you.

Flower Essences: Directions for Use

In flower essence therapy, it is not the amount of the essence taken but the frequency of application that increases the effect. So for acute conditions, take or apply flower essences frequently. For ongoing or chronic situations, the rate of dosage is less frequent. As for how long you should keep taking the remedy, for acute conditions, take it until the acute symptoms are alleviated.

In some cases, a longer application may be needed. Anxiety, insomnia, and depression, for example, are almost always associated with deeper issues in the emotional self that require taking essences for a longer period for the full effect. "A month is a typical cycle to clear out emotional residue," says Patricia Kaminski. In those cases, you can take the flower essences for a month and then reevaluate.[5]

Use high-quality flower essences to ensure optimal results.

Internal: Take directly from the bottle, putting 4 drops under the tongue, no less than half an hour before eating, 2–4 times daily. During the acute stage of a condition, 4 times daily is the minimum. For an acute emergency situation, such as a sudden shock or an anxiety attack, you can take 4 drops every 15 minutes to 1 hour, as needed.

If you don't want to take the flower essences straight, mix them with a little water, stir for 1 minute, and sip slowly. The exception is Yarrow Special Formula, which should always be taken undiluted, directly from the bottle.

Topical: Apply 2–4 times daily. Once in the morning and again at night is still effective, if that's all you can manage. The ratio for adding flower essences to a carrier substance for topical application is 6–10 drops of each flower essence per 1 ounce of cream, oil, or lotion.

Bath: Add 20 drops of each flower essence to a tub of warm water. Stir the water, using a figure-eight motion, for at least 1 minute. Soak in the tub for 20 minutes. After the bath, wrap yourself in large towels or a blanket and rest. This helps to anchor the patterns you received from the flower essences.

Compress: Gently rub 1–2 tablespoons of the selected flower oil (note oil, not essence) on the affected area and cover with a hot compress. Leave in place until the compress has cooled.

Massage: Apply a flower essence directly on the skin, use a selected flower oil for massage, or prepare your own massage oil according to the instructions under "Topical."

Misting bottle: Mix 4 drops of each flower essence per 1 ounce of water in a spray bottle. Shake the bottle before spraying around your body and in your environment.

This approach is similarly applicable to all the conditions in this book. While the specific flower essences (aside from the general foundational ones) cited under a given condition have a demonstrated clinical correlation with that condition, flower essence therapy, like all alternative therapies, treats the person, not the symptoms. Each case is unique and must be given individual consideration. The essences indicated for each condition are a key or pivotal essence for turning the healing in another direction, and are intended as a starting point for an individualized path of therapy. The physical symptoms for which you are seeking treatment are only one component in the complete picture of you and the state of your health.

While flower essences work subtly, their effects can be quite powerful. As a tool for healing, they can aid you in learning the lessons of your health problem and stimulate health-enhancing inner transformation. For example, you can use flower remedies to help you deal with your anger issues, clear creative stagnation, clarify career direction, and find your way out of depression. As flower essences are working on the mind-body, you can facilitate their effectiveness by tuning in to your inner world. When you take them, don't do so on the run. Use your dosings as a time for reflection, even if it is just for a few minutes. These moments of mindfulness may begin to expand to more moments during the day, and assist the essences in their transformative work.

Flower essences engender stages of healing. You may experience immediate results, and then these shifts will in turn precipitate other ones. Kaminski likens it to tossing a stone in a lake and seeing the ever-expanding circles. "The first circles are small and immediate," she says, "then they get larger and larger until they are assimilated in the whole of the lake (or our entire body-soul being)."

Food Therapy

Food is powerful medicine, both preventive and curative, but it is often overlooked as a therapy. Too few doctors inquire about your diet when you come to them with a health problem. In the view of naturopathic physicians, among other alternative medical practitioners, that should be one of the first questions. Food provides the basic foundation of health—or disease, if you are eating a nutrient-deficient diet of refined, processed foods.

Aside from the recommendations given for the individual conditions in this book, a general recommendation for everyone, in sickness and in health, is to eat a wholesome diet with an emphasis on fresh vegetables, whole grains, and unprocessed food. Your body runs on nutrients, and if you are not supplying them, your body can't function at an optimal level. While there is some debate over whether or not we need to take nutritional supplements if we are eating a good diet, there is no debate over the fact that supplements can't make up for a lousy diet.

Most of us could improve our diets: cut out sugar, stop drinking so much coffee, eat breakfast, get more fiber, eat more salads. More than one doctor has commented that it's more difficult for people to change their diet than their religion. Given that, here are four basic dietary practices that can make a difference to your health. If you do nothing else, at least adopt these four:

1. Eat organic whenever possible.

2. Eat plenty of fresh vegetables (emphasize vegetables over fruit because fruit contains a lot of sugar).

3. Avoid trans-fatty acids (found in margarine and other hydrogenated and partially hydrogenated oils).

4. Drink eight glasses of water daily, more when you are sick.

There are a few food therapy recommendations that appear under many of the conditions in this book. Drink plenty of water is one of them. Water is a medicine in itself because our bodies are, like the planet on which we live, nearly three-quarters water. Keeping our body well-supplied with pure water supports the optimal functioning of all cells, tissues, organs, and systems.

Eating garlic and avoiding sugar are two other recommendations that appear repeatedly. Garlic is a natural antibiotic that also boosts immunity. Sugar suppresses immunity and depletes the body of nutrients.[6] While it may be a good practice to avoid sugar all the time, it is particularly advisable when you are sick, injured, or otherwise weakened.

Avoiding caffeine is another common prescription. Like sugar, caffeine depletes the body of vitamins and minerals.[7] It is a diuretic (increases urine flow) and tends to dehydrate the body. If you drink caffeinated beverages, you need to drink more than eight glasses of water daily to compensate for the dehydration effect. Note that green tea is not included in this caffeine taboo. Research has shown that green tea has a number of healing properties. It is high in catechins, chemical compounds with antioxidant action that is far more potent than that of vitamin E. Green tea has also been shown to support the immune system, lower cholesterol, and inhibit cancer.[8]

Perhaps less often, but still frequently, the suggestion to eat yogurt appears. Note that this means plain yogurt with live acidophilus cultures, not the highly sweetened product full of artificial flavoring, gelatin, and other additives that passes as yogurt. Yogurt made from organic milk is preferable because of the many undesirable substances in milk today, including bovine growth hormone and antibiotics passed on from the cow. Goat's milk yogurt is a good option for avoiding the problems associated with cow's milk.

The following is a guide to the many categories of food and dietary sources of nutrients referred to throughout the book.

A Dietary A-to-Z

Acid-forming: Alcohol, soft drinks, coffee, cocoa, black tea, chocolate, cranberries, prunes, tomatoes, Brussels sprouts, peanuts, beans, legumes, oatmeal, eggs, milk, cheese, poultry, fish, seafood, meat, vinegar, sugar, pasta, processed foods, most condiments (catsup, mustard, olives, pepper).

Alkalinizing: Corn, dates, most fresh fruits and vegetables (especially citrus), sprouts, brown rice, millet, honey, maple syrup, molasses, raisins, soy, goat's milk, green drinks (spirulina, barley greens, chlorella, blue-green algae).

Arginine: Nuts, chocolate, peanuts, beer, raisins, cereals, gelatin, sesame seeds, lentils, flaxseed, bacon.

Bioflavonoids: Citrus fruit (rind), dark blue-black fruit, blueberries, hawthorn berries, buckwheat, onion, green tea.

Biotin: Brewer's yeast, rye, whole grains, egg yolks, soy, oatmeal, split peas, sunflower seeds, walnuts, lentils, cauliflower, liver, poultry.

***Brassica* family of vegetables:** Broccoli, cauliflower, Brussels sprouts, kohlrabi, kale, collards, cabbage.

Calcium: Kale, turnip greens, collards, mustard greens, parsley, tofu, kelp, brewer's yeast, blackstrap molasses, cheese, egg yolk, almonds, filberts, sesame seeds, sardines.

Carbohydrates: Complex carbohydrates are whole grains, legumes, fresh fruit and vegetables; refined or simple carbohydrates are white flour, white rice, sugar.

Choline: Soy lecithin, egg yolks, legumes, whole grains, milk, liver.

Cold-water fish: Salmon, cod, mackerel, sardines, herring.

Common allergenic foods: milk, wheat, eggs, citrus, corn, peanut butter, chocolate, tomatoes, soy, shellfish.

Essential fatty acids (EFAs): The primary omega-3 EFAs are ALA (alpha-linolenic acid) found in flaxseed, canola oil, soybeans, and walnuts; and DHA (docosahexaenoic acid) and EPA (eicosapentaenoic acid) found in the oils of cold-water fish, such as salmon, mackerel, herring, and sardines. The primary omega-6 EFAs are linoleic acid or cis-linoleic acid found in many vegetables and safflower, sunflower, corn, peanut, and sesame oils; and GLA (gamma-linolenic acid) found in evening primrose, black currant, and borage oils.

Folic acid: Brewer's yeast, green leafy vegetables, wheat germ, soybeans, legumes, asparagus, broccoli, oranges, sunflower seeds.

Immune-suppressing: Sugar, refined carbohydrates, food allergens.

Inositol: Citrus, nuts, seeds, legumes.

Iron: Spinach, asparagus, soybeans, prunes, raisins, sea vegetables, blackstrap molasses, pumpkin seeds, sesame seeds, eggs, fish, liver.

Lecithin: Soy, wheat germ, nuts, sunflower and pumpkin seeds, whole grains, cold-pressed vegetable oils, eggs, dandelion greens.

Lysine: Soybeans, milk, potatoes, brewer's yeast, fish, chicken, beans.

Magnesium: Parsnips, tofu, buckwheat, beans, leafy green vegetables, wheat germ, blackstrap molasses, kelp, brewer's yeast, nuts, seeds, bananas, avocado, dairy, seafood.

Manganese: Whole grains (especially buckwheat and bulgur), nuts, sunflower seeds, leafy green vegetables.

Mucus-forming: Dairy, chocolate, eggs, refined sugar, junk food.

Nightshade family: Eggplant, tomato, green pepper, potato, paprika, cayenne, tobacco.

Nitrite-cured meats: Hot dogs, salami, bacon, sausage, bologna.

Oxalates: Spinach, Swiss chard, beet greens, parsley, rhubarb, peanuts, baked beans, cocoa, black tea, instant coffee.

Pantothenic acid (vitamin B5): Brewer's yeast, dairy, fish, poultry, liver and other organ meats, whole grains, soybeans, sweet potatoes, peanuts, broccoli.

Phosphorus-containing foods: found in most foods, especially whole grains and seeds, bran, brewer's yeast, eggs, fish, poultry, dried fruit, corn, garlic.

Potassium: Bananas, apricots, avocado, blackstrap molasses, dried fruits, brewer's yeast, potatoes, dairy.

Purine: Meats, organ meats, shellfish, brewer's and baker's yeast, herring, sardines, mackerel, anchovies.

Salicylate: Strawberries and other berries, raisins, prunes, tomatoes, nuts; salicylates are also added as flavoring to many commercially prepared sweet goods, such as cake mixes, puddings, licorice candy, chewing gum, and soft drinks. Salicylates are natural compounds from which salicylic acid, the active compound in aspirin, is derived.

Saturated fats: Butter, animal fat, coconut oil, palm oil.

Sea vegetables: Arame, bladderwrack, dulse, hijiki, kelp, kombu, nori, sea palm, wakame.

Selenium: Brazil nuts, whole grains, wheat germ, soybeans, oats, red Swiss chard, seafood.

Silica (silicon): Alfalfa, beets, soy, oatmeal, brown rice, root vegetables, leafy greens, bell peppers.

Sulphur: Brussels sprouts, cabbage, garlic, onions, green pepper, cucumber, turnips, dried beans, kale, wheat germ, oats, eggs, fish, meats.

Trans-fatty acids: Found in hydrogenated oils in margarine and many processed/packaged foods such as crackers and cookies (often listed on the label as "partially hydrogenated" oil), trans-fatty acids interfere with the absorption of the beneficial fats such as essential fatty acids and promote inflammation.

Tyramine: Red wine, cheese, pickled herring, yeast baked goods, chicken livers, peanuts, sunflower seeds, pumpkin seeds, sesame seeds, lima beans, pinto beans, navy beans, lentils, snow peas.

Vitamin A/beta-carotene: Yellow and green fruits and vegetables (particularly carrots, parsley, spinach, turnip greens, dandelion greens, broccoli, pumpkin, apricots, canteloupe, and mangoes), liver, fish liver oil.

Vitamin B complex: Includes all the B vitamins, biotin, choline, folic acid, and inositol.

Vitamin B1 (thiamin): Brewer's yeast, wheat germ, sunflower seeds, soybeans, peanuts, liver and other organ meats.

Vitamin B2 (riboflavin): Brewer's yeast, wheat germ, whole grains, almonds, soybeans, green leafy vegetables, liver and other organ meats, milk, cottage cheese.

Vitamin B3 (niacin): Brewer's yeast, rice bran, peanuts, eggs, milk, fish, legumes, avocado, liver and other organ meats.

Vitamin B5: See "Pantothenic acid."

Vitamin B6 (pyridoxine): Brewer's yeast, wheat germ, bananas, seeds, nuts, legumes, avocado, leafy green vegetables, potatoes, cauliflower, chicken, whole grains.

Vitamin B12 (cobalamin): Liver, kidneys, eggs, clams, oysters, fish, dairy.

Vitamin C: Green vegetables (particularly broccoli, Brussels sprouts, green peppers, kale, turnip greens, and collards), fruits (particularly guava, persimmons, black currants, strawberries, papaya, and citrus; citrus contains less vitamin C than the other fruits).

Vitamin D: fatty fish or fish oils (anchovies, bass, cod, herring, mackerel, salmon, sardines, tuna), fortified milk and other dairy products.

Vitamin E: Wheat germ and wheat germ oil, sunflower and other seeds, nuts, whole grains, green leafy vegetables.

Vitamin K: Green tea, dark green leafy vegetables (particularly kale, turnip greens, and spinach), cabbage, cauliflower, broccoli, alfalfa, soybeans, liver.

Zinc: Oysters, herring, sunflower seeds, pumpkin seeds, lima beans, legumes, soybeans, wheat germ, brewer's yeast, dairy.

Herbal Medicine

In the 1800s, herbal medicine, along with homeopathy, was mainstream medicine in the United States. The advent in the twentieth century of the pharmaceutical industry with its ability to reap enormous profits caused a transformation of medicine in this country. Herbs cannot be patented, so their money-making potential paled next to chemical drugs. Herbal medicine and homeopathy were systematically discredited, as the medical machine we know today was mobilized.

In the twenty-first century, however, we are in the midst of a resurgence of natural medicine. People are becoming increasingly disheartened with the conventional medical model of treating only the body, and that in parts, and using chemicals to suppress symptoms. As herbal medicine answers the need for a more holistic approach, the public is returning to its roots, so to speak. In this, we are simply rejoining the rest of the world. Herbal medicine has always been and still is the primary medicine for most of the Earth's population,[9] and it is a recognized, respected, and widely used form of medicine in Europe. As herbalist Karen Vaughan states, "Using herbs as medicine brings us back to a much richer, deeper way of approaching medicine. They work on a psychological and spiritual level as well as on a physical level."

There are different traditions in herbalism, and these are increasingly reflected in the range of products available in stores that stock herbal medicines. Ayurvedic herbs, Chinese medicine herbs, and so-called Western herbs are three prominent herbologies. Ayurveda (the traditional medicine of India) and traditional Chinese medicine are complex medical systems, of which herbalism is one component. While this book recommends the occasional Ayurvedic or Chinese medicine herb, most of the protocols focus on Western herbs.

Note In the Latin names for the herbs that appear throughout the text, *spp.* means species, indicating that multiple species of the plant genus are appropriate to use as the common herb.

The word "herb" as it is employed in herbal medicine refers to any part of any plant, from delicate flowers to the bark of trees. The plant world is filled with healing agents, and the medicinal properties of herbs are well documented. From adaptogens to vasodilators, different plants exert specific actions in the body (see "Herbal Properties" below). Rather than suppressing symptoms, herbs heal by addressing underlying imbalances and stimulating the body's innate capacity to heal itself.

As with essential oils, however, the quality of the herbs you use bears a significant relationship to the results. The resurgence of interest in herbs has led to a flood of commercial herbal products. (While herbs can't command the huge profits engendered by chemical pharmaceuticals, they constitute a sizable market.) The good news is the increased availability of herbs in convenient forms for usage, such as tinctures, capsules, and powders. The bad news is, there are a lot of products out there that contain little to none of the active constituents of the herb. This means that many people never experience the true power of herbal medicine and may end up concluding that herbs don't work. While using a fresh plant may be optimal, a quality herbal extract or tincture can produce similarly strong results.

Knowing the reputation of an herbalist or company that sells herbal preparations is one way to ensure quality. By asking around about who produces quality products, usually you can get this information readily. If you informally poll health food stores, alternative medicine practitioners, friends, and community members, the same names will keep popping up. Another method for ensuring quality in commercial products is to buy only standardized (or guaranteed potency) extracts. This means that the product contains a standardized level of the active constituents of the plant. A nonstandardized product may contain little to none of what makes the herb work as a medicine.

A moral note on herbal consumption: With the increasing popularity of herbs, rampant wild-crafting (harvesting of plants growing in

Herbal Properties

The following is a selection of the many healing categories of herbs, according to the specific action the herb exerts in the body.

Adaptogen: An herb that increases the body's adaptability; these herbs are often those that support the adrenal glands, as this system regulates the stress response.

Alterative: An herb that helps restore the body to balance; these herbs (previously called blood-cleansers) are often detoxifying herbs and promote elimination.

Analgesic: An herb that relieves pain.

Anti-inflammatory: An herb that reduces inflammation, most commonly through increasing circulation and aiding the body in metabolism and elimination of inflammatory products.

Antimicrobial: An herb that inhibits the growth of or helps the body destroy bacteria, viruses, fungi, and protozoa.

Astringent: An herb that tightens tissue, reduces secretions, and checks inflammation; commonly used to contain irritation or inflammation, as in wounds, ulcers, and hemorrhoids.

Bitter: An herb with a bitter taste resulting from chemical constituents that also give bitters the medicinal properties of stimulating appetite, aiding in digestion, supporting the liver and gallbladder, and promoting repair of the lining of the gut.

Demulcent: An herb that can soothe and protect inflamed or irritated tissues; usually rich in mucilage (sliminess).

Diuretic: An herb that promotes the flow of urine.

Nervine: An herb that tones and strengthens the nervous system.

Tonic: An herb that restores the health (tone) of an organ, a system, or the whole body; its actions are nourishing, supportive, and restorative.

Vasodilator: An herb that opens (dilates) the blood vessels, facilitating circulation.

the wild) has placed some plants in danger of extinction. Goldenseal is one of these. To support the survival of this precious plant, buy only products that use cultivated goldenseal rather than the wild-crafted herb. And if you gather herbs yourself, be respectful of the natural world. A friend in Montana told me what happens to the wooded hills near her house when the coneflower is in season. Mad echinacea hunters make a sweep through the area, heedlessly trampling and damaging all vegetation in their path as they denude the hills of coneflowers. Help preserve the plant kingdom by harvesting only where it's appropriate to do so, picking sparingly, and leaving no footprint.

Herbs: Directions for Use

INTERNAL REMEDIES

Infusion (tea): Steep an herb in boiled water for 10–15 minutes, or as indicated. Steep means let it sit, in a covered container, not on a heat source. Strain before drinking. Generally, the ratio is 1 teaspoon of dried herb or 3 teaspoons of fresh herb per cup of water. Infusion is used with leaves and flowers, from which the healing substances are readily extracted.

Decoction (tea): Simmer the herb for 15–20 minutes, or as indicated. Simmer means keep it at a low boil in a covered pot. Strain before drinking. A typical ratio is 1 teaspoon of dried herb or 3 teaspoons of fresh herb per cup of water. Decoction is used with the tougher parts of a plant such as the root, bark, or hard seeds, from which extraction of the active components is not as easy as it is from the leaves or flowers.

Tincture: This is a concentrated liquid herbal extract, usually preserved in alcohol, but you can also get vegetable-glycerin-based tinctures. Tinctures are much stronger than dried or fresh herbs taken in tea form. They are widely available in health food stores.

TOPICAL TREATMENTS

Compress: Soak a washcloth or a piece of cotton or flannel in a hot or cold herbal infusion, decoction, or diluted tincture. Squeeze some of the liquid out and lay the compress on the affected area. Leave in place for 10–15 minutes and repeat as needed. In the case of a hot compress, reapply when the compress cools.

Infused oil: This is a carrier oil in which an herb has been steeped. As the oil used is often olive oil, some commercial infused oil products are labeled as olive oil extract. This is not to be confused with a tincture, in which the liquid is alcohol as opposed to oil. Infused oils are generally used as a base for massage.

Poultice: Mash fresh herbs by hand or put them in a blender or food processor to make a pulp. Apply the mixture directly on the skin or spread it on gauze or a cloth and apply that way. You can also use powdered herbs. In that case, mix them with enough water to make a paste and apply it in the same manner as the fresh herb. Poultices are generally used to reduce inflammation, draw out infection, or pull debris from a wound.

Homeopathy

To understand homeopathy, it is helpful to consider the derivation of the word as well as that of allopathy, both of which were coined by the father of homeopathy, Dr. Samuel Hahnemann, in the late 1700s. A German physician who became increasingly frustrated with conventional medical practice, Dr. Hahnemann devoted himself to developing a safer, more effective approach to medicine. The result was homeopathy, which arose out of his discovery that illness can be treated by giving the patient a dilution of a plant that produces symptoms resembling those of the illness when given to a healthy person. He called this principle "let likes be cured with likes," and it became known as the law of similars. He named this system of healing "homeopathy," a combination of the Greek *homoios* (similar) and *pathos* (suffering). At the same time, he dubbed conventional medicine "allopathy," or "opposite suffering," to reflect that model's approach of treating illness by giving an antidote to the symptoms, a medicine that produces the opposite effect from what the patient is suffering. (A laxative for constipation is an example of the allopathic approach; it produces diarrhea.)[10]

Homeopathy became a widely accepted and practiced medicine throughout Europe and the United States. In fact, in the 1800s, homeopathy was mainstream medicine in this country, as was herbalism. The American Medical Association (AMA) bears much of the responsibility for the marginalization of this safe and effective form of medicine. The AMA "was created largely to slow the growth of homeopathy, the success of which was threatening the livelihood of orthodox physicians. . . . [T]he AMA's efforts at discrediting and suppressing homeopathy eventually began to take effect."[11] Homeopathy continued strong in Europe, however, and is still strong today; as one example of its cachet, it has long been publicly sanctioned and used personally by Britain's royal family. Fortunately, as with herbal medicine in the United States, frustration with conventional medicine has led to the resurgence of interest in and use of homeopathy.

The homeopathic remedies presented in this book can be employed with excellent results as single episodic remedies to address a certain ailment. First aid is kindergarten for homeopathy, however, as it is for the other therapies in this book. Full homeopathic treatment involves a homeopath identifying the constitutional remedy that will address the whole cluster of physical, psychological, and emotional characteristics of an individual patient. These remedies work on all levels to restore balance and heal pervasively. For ongoing health issues, this deeper treatment is what is required. Some of the conditions in this book fall in this category, and you may want to consult a homeopath for comprehensive healing. Those conditions are noted as such.

You will notice that under general conditions, such as bacterial infection, you are directed to look up your specific kind of infection. This is because homeopathy does not treat an illness or combat a germ. There are no generic natural antibiotics in homeopathy because remedies are tailored to the particular cluster of symptoms manifested by the patient. And, as each person manifests illness differently even within the same conventional medical diagnosis, there are multiple remedies listed for a malady such as a cough, based on the particular kind of cough involved. It's important to select the correct remedy for your individual condition, so observe your symptoms and choose accordingly. But don't worry, you just won't get results with the wrong remedy, and it's fine to switch to one of the other remedies.

Homeopathic remedies are prepared through a process of dilution of plant and other substances, which results in a "potentized" remedy, one that contains the energetic imprint of the plant rather than its biochemical components. Paradoxically, the higher the number of dilutions, the greater the potency and the effects of the remedy. Here's how it works: a remedy with a 6c or 6x (the c and x refer to the two different scales used in dilution; the results are similar) potency has been diluted 6 times. A remedy with a 12c or 12x potency has been diluted 12 times and is more potent. The 30c remedy involves 30 dilutions and is more potent yet. Thus, the higher the potency number, the more powerful the remedy. These are low-potency remedies, however. Dilutions go into the hundreds and even thousands. Homeopaths, when giving a single remedy to a patient, for example, often use a 1M potency, which is a remedy that has been diluted a thousand times. In home care, as in the protocols in this book, the low-potency remedies are the ones cited—mostly 6 and 12; and in some cases, 30.

Generally, a single dose as described in this book is 2–3 pellets of the remedy (but read your product label). Do not touch or pick up the pellets. Shake them into the cap of the bottle and drop them into your mouth from the cap. Do not drink or eat anything for 20 minutes before and after taking a remedy. These steps maintain the energetic purity of the remedy. In taking a remedy, let your symptoms be your guide. As symptoms lessen, reduce the frequency with which you are taking the remedy. When your symptoms disappear, stop taking it. It is not like a course of prescription pills that you are supposed to finish out. In the case of homeopathy, if you keep taking a remedy after your symptoms have subsided, you may bring them back. Remember that the remedy for a given condition is based on the fact that it produces similar symptoms to that condition in a healthy person.

Homeopathic Remedies Cited in this Book

Common Name	Full Name	Derived From
Acetic acid	Acetic acid	acetic acid
Aconite	Aconite napellus	monkshood
Aesculus	Aesculus hippocastanum	horse chestnut
Allium cepa	Allium cepa	red onion
Alumina	Alumina	Aluminum oxide
Ammon phos	Ammonium phosphoricum	ammonia phosphate
Anacardium	Anacardium orientale	marking nut
Ant crud	Antimonium crudum	antimony
Ant tart	Antimonium tartaricum	tartar emetic
Apis	Apis mellifica	bee venom/ honeybee
Apocynum can	Apocynum cannabinum	Indian hemp
Arg nit	Argentum nitricum	silver nitrate

Common Name	Full Name	Derived From
Arnica	Arnica montana	arnica
Arsenicum	Arsenicum album	arsenic
Aurum met	Aurum metallicum	gold
Badiagia	Badiagia	freshwater sponge
Belladonna	Belladonna	deadly nightshade
Bellis	Bellis perennis	daisy
Benzoic acid	Benzoic acidum	benzoic acid
Berberis	Berberis vulgaris	barberry
Borax	Borax	sodium borate
Bromium	Bromium	bromium
Bryonia	Bryonia alba	wild hops
Caladium	Caladium seguinum	American arum
Calc carb	Calcarea carbonica	calcium carbonate
Calc phos	Calcarea phosphorica	calcium phosphate
Calendula	Calendula officinalis	marigold
Cantharis	Cantharis	Spanish fly
Carb sulph	Carboneum sulphuratum	carbon bisulfide
Carbo veg	Carbo vegetabilis	charcoal
Causticum	Causticum	potassium hydrate
Chamomilla	Chamomilla	chamomile
Chin sulph	Chininum sulphuricum	quinine sulfate
China (Cinchona)	China officinalis	cinchona bark
Cocculus	Cocculus indicus	Indian cockle
Coffea	Coffea cruda	coffee
Colchicum	Colchicum autumnale	autumn crocus
Collinsonia	Collinsonia canadensis	horse balm, stone root
Colocynth	Colocynthis	bitter apple
Cyclamen	Cyclamen europaeum	cyclamen
Eupatorium	Eupatorium perfoliatum	boneset
Euphrasia	Euphrasia officinalis	eyebright
Ferrum phos	Ferrum phosphoricum	iron phosphate
Fragaria	Fragaria	wood strawberry
Gelsemium	Gelsemium sempervirens	yellow jasmine
Glonoine	Glonoinum	nitroglycerin
Graphites	Graphites	graphite

Common Name	Full Name	Derived From
Hamamelis	Hamamelis virginica	witch hazel
Hekla lava	Hekla lava	volcano
Hepar sulph	Hepar sulphuris calcareum	calcium sulfide
Hypericum	Hypericum perforatum	St. John's wort
Ignatia	Ignatia amara	St. Ignatius' bean
Ipecac	Ipecacuanha	ipecac
Iris	Iris versicolor	blue flag iris
Kali bich	Kali bichromicum	potassium bichromate
Kali brom	Kali bromatum	potassium bromide
Kali carb	Kali carbonicum	potassium carbonate
Kali iod	Kali iodatum	potassium iodide
Kali mur	Kali muriaticum	potassium chloride
Kali sulph	Kali sulphuricum	potassium sulfate
Kreosotum	Kreosotum	creosote
Lachesis	Lachesis	bushmaster snake venom
Ledum	Ledum palustre	wild rosemary
Lycopodium	Lycopodium clavatum	club moss
Mag phos	Magnesia phosphorica	magnesium phosphate
Medorrhinum	Medorrhinum	gonorrhea
Merc sol (Mercurius)	Mercurius solubilis	mercury
Merc viv	Mercurius vivus	mercury
Mezereum	Mezereum	Daphne mezereum
Nat mur	Natrum muriaticum	sodium chloride (table salt)
Nitric acid	Nitricum acidum	nitric acid
Nux mosch	Nux moschata	nutmeg
Nux vom	Nux vomica	poison nut
Ocimum can	Ocimum canum	alfavaca
Opium	Papaver somniferum	opium poppy
Oscillococcinum	Oscillococcinum	combination formula
Oleander	Oleander	rose laurel
Passiflora	Passiflora incarnata	passionflower
Petroleum	Petroleum oleum petrae	coal oil
Phos acid	Phosphoric acidum	phosphoric acid
Phosphorus	Phosphorus	phosphorus
Phytolacca	Phytolacca decandra	poke root

Common Name	Full Name	Derived From
Pulsatilla	Pulsatilla nigricans	pasqueflower
Ranunc bulb	Ranunculus bulbosus	buttercup
Rhus tox	Rhus toxicodendron	poison ivy
Rumex	Rumex crispus	yellow dock
Ruta	Ruta graveolens	rue
Sabina	Sabina	savin
Salicyl acid	Salicylic acid	salicylic acid
Sanguinaria	Sanguinaria canadensis	sanguinaria
Sanicula	Sanicula aqua	spring water
Sepia	Sepia	cuttlefish ink
Silica	Silicea	flint
Spigelia	Spigelia anthelmia	spigelia, pink root
Staphysagria	Delphinium staphysagria	stavesacre
Sulphur	Sulphur	sulfur
Sulphuric acid	Sulphuric acid	sulphuric acid
Symphytum	Symphytum officinale	comfrey, knitbone
Tabacum	Tabacum	tobacco
Tellurium	Tellurium	the element tellurium
Terebinth	Terebinthina	turpentine
Thuja	Thuja occidentalis	arbor vitae, tree of life
Urtica	Urtica urens	stinging nettle
Veratrum	Veratrum album	white hellebore
Wyethia	Wyethia helenioides	poison weed

Nutritional Supplements

To supplement or not to supplement? Some natural medicine practitioners believe that we should look to whole foods and herbs to meet our nutritional requirements, that if we eat a proper diet, we don't need to take supplements. Other practitioners believe that modern life requires supplements. They point to the dwindling mineral content of the soil in which crops are grown, which translates into food with a lower mineral content than our forebears enjoyed. They also point to the many factors that deplete us of vitamins and minerals, regardless of how well we eat: stress, smoking, alcohol, caffeine, pollution, heavy metals such as the mercury in our dental fillings.

In addition, these practitioners consider the recommended daily allowance (RDA; purportedly, the amount of individual vitamins and minerals our body requires daily, whether from food or supplements) far below our nutritive needs, in most cases. The RDA standard is based on a group norm for preventing nutritional deficiencies. There are two problems with that. One, individual needs diverge widely; and two, the level of deficiency the RDAs are designed to avoid is severe. The systems of the body can begin to be compromised long before that degree of deficiency registers. In other words, if you use the RDAs as your guideline, you could be walking around with moderate nutritional deficiencies. A subclinical deficiency can affect the quality of your health and life, manifesting in fatigue, lethargy, concentration problems, a general lack of well-being, or other vague complaints.[12]

Given these facts, along with the reality that most of us, despite the best of intentions, don't always take the time in our busy lives to eat well, a daily multivitamin/mineral supplement may be a good idea as a preventative, health-promoting practice. While supplements are not a replacement for a healthy diet, they can help ensure that our bodies are getting the nutrients they need to function optimally. You may also want to take antioxidants as a prophylactic against the stresses and toxins of life. Antioxidants have been shown to protect the body from premature aging and degenerative diseases such as cancer and heart disease.[13] They exert a more potent effect when taken together, rather than singly, so take your antioxidants in combination.

In addition to daily supplements as a foundation for health, specific supplements can be used to address health problems when they arise, providing the body with the extra nutrients required during illness or injury. The various properties of supplements discussed in this book as nutritional treatment for common ailments are delineated below.

It is important to use natural rather than synthetic supplements. Synthetic supplements, made from chemicals rather than extracted from natural sources, may not be easily absorbed by the body. They also often contain sugar and additives, which make the supplement a dubious health proposition. Even those of us who make a concerted effort to avoid chemical exposure or ingestion have enough chemicals in our bodies from inescapable environmental sources. Why add to the toxic load by taking synthetic vitamins?

As with other natural medicines, choose high-quality products for best results. In most cases, it's worth the extra money for the increased therapeutic effects. Poor-quality supplements have little to offer your body, will probably not produce the health benefits you're seeking, and may actually do more harm than good.

Don't take the word "natural" at face value, however. It's a popular word to use on a label because companies know that it attracts the growing number of "green" consumers. Read the labels carefully to make sure you aren't getting unhealthy ingredients along with the healthy ones. The vitamin industry is a booming money-maker, and there is a lot of junk out there masquerading as health-inducing supplements.

As a general procedure, take your supplements with meals, unless otherwise directed. Some nutrients require others in order to be absorbed by the body; by taking your supplements with food, your body will likely get the conutrients it needs to absorb the supplement.

Units of Measurement

IU = international unit

mg = milligram

mcg = microgram

g = gram

1,000 mg = 1 g

A Guide to Nutritional Supplements

Acidophilus: See "Probiotics."

Activated charcoal: Binds with toxins and speeds their removal from the body.

Antioxidants: Natural biochemical substances that protect cells and tissue from free-radical damage, or oxidation, which if left unchecked produces premature aging and degenerative illnesses such as arthritis, heart disease, and cancer. Antioxidant nutrients include vitamins A, C, and E, beta-carotene, selenium, coenzyme Q10, pycnogenol, bioflavonoids, the amino acid glutathione, and SOD (superoxide dismutase). Antioxidants exert more potent effects when they are taken in combination, rather than singly.

Arginine: Amino acid that supports the immune system, promotes wound healing, aids in collagen production, increases muscle tone (athletes take it to help prevent injury and build muscles), and is needed for protein synthesis and optimal growth.

Bee pollen/propolis: Bee pollen is antimicrobial and highly nutritious; bee propolis (bark resins collected by bees) stimulates the immune system and is also antimicrobial.

Bioflavonoids: Antioxidant plant pigments found in plants and fruits that also enhance the actions of vitamin C. Formerly called vitamin P, bioflavonoids include citrin, hesperidin, rutin, quercetin, epicatechin, flavones, and flavonols. Citrus bioflavonoids are those derived from citrus fruit.

Biotin: Member of the vitamin B family; aids in cell growth, needed for healthy skin and hair, aids in the metabolism of protein, fatty acids, and carbohydrates.

Bromelain: An anti-inflammatory enzyme compound found in pineapple; take it on an empty stomach so the enzymes will break down inflammatory products rather than digest your food.

Calcium: Mineral that decreases muscular contraction and is a nervous system relaxant.

Capsaicin: The pain-relieving active component in cayenne pepper. Research suggests that it reduces pain by depleting skin cells of substance P, a primary chemical messenger for pain impulses and an activator of inflammation.[14]

Chlorophyll: The pigment in plants used in photosynthesis; aids red blood cell production, is rich in vitamin K, which is needed for blood clotting; a potent detoxifier, it can help remove heavy metals and other toxins from the body.

Choline: Member of the vitamin B family; necessary for proper liver function and boosts brain levels of the neurotransmitter acetylcholine, important for memory and other brain activities.

Chromium: Mineral that aids in circulation and helps to control blood sugar levels.

Coenzyme Q10: Potent antioxidant enzyme, aids in energy production at the cellular level and strengthens the immune system.

Curcumin: An anti-inflammatory substance derived from turmeric.

Digestive enzymes: Plant-based or pancreatic (derived from animals) digestive enzymes with or without HCl (hydrochloric acid, a gastric digestive juice) that improve digestion when taken as supplements. Take the enzymes midway through a meal, which prevents the body from relying on the supplement for its digestive enzyme supply instead of producing its own.

DLPA (D,L-phenylalanine): A pain-relieving amino acid.

DMSO (dimethyl sulfoxide): A sulfur-rich by-product of wood that can help repair damaged tissue, speed healing, reduce pain, swelling, and inflammation, relax muscles, increase circulation, and inhibit bacteria.

Essential fatty acids (EFAs): The primary omega-3 EFAs are ALA (alpha-linolenic acid; found in flaxseed, canola oil, soybeans, and walnuts) and DHA (docosahexaenoic acid) and EPA (eicosapentaenoic acid), found in the oils of cold-water fish such as salmon, cod, mackerel, herring, and sardines. The primary omega-6 EFAs are linoleic acid or cis-linoleic acid found in many vegetables and safflower, sunflower, corn, peanut, and sesame oils, and GLA (gamma-linolenic acid) found in evening primrose, black currant, and borage oils. EFAs are used by the body to manufacture prostaglandins, hormone-like substances involved in numerous metabolic functions, including inflammatory processes. Taking EFAs can therefore produce anti-inflammatory effects.

5-HTP (5-hydroxy tryptophan): A plant extract that behaves like the amino acid tryptophan in the body. While it works similarly to tryptophan in relieving depression, it does not exert the pain-relieving effects of tryptophan.

Folic acid: Member of the vitamin B family that is vital for normal cell development and proliferation; aids in the manufacture of brain neurotransmitters and can be useful in treating depression.

Glutamine: Amino acid that aids in mental performance, reduces sugar cravings, contributes to muscle formation, and facilitates mineral absorption.

Glycosaminoglycans (GAGs): Biochemical substances manufactured in the body that promote the production of mucin (a glycoprotein in mucus), which lubricates and soothes tissues, assisting healing.

Grapefruit seed extract (GSE): Powerful broad-spectrum antimicrobial; useful against bacteria, viruses, fungi, and parasites.

Green foods/drinks: Supplements or drink powders that are high in chlorophyll, minerals, and enzymes; chlorella, spirulina, blue-green algae, barley grass, and/or wheat grass are common green foods.

Histadine: Amino acid that aids in tissue repair and red and white blood cell production. Histamine, the substance that produces the symptoms of an allergic reaction (runny nose and eyes, inflammation) as an immune response to a perceived allergen, is made from histadine; histadine is used to treat allergies.

Inositol: Member of the vitamin B family necessary for proper liver, muscle, nerve, and brain function; required by serotonin and other neurotransmitters.

Lysine: Essential amino acid needed for bone health, collagen production, muscle and other tissue repair, and proper immune function; possesses antiherpetic properties (antiviral effects against the herpes family of viruses).

Magnesium: Antispasmodic and smooth muscle relaxant mineral that is also necessary for bone health, nerve function, and energy and calcium metabolism.

Manganese: Mineral needed for bone health, proper thyroid function, energy metabolism, blood sugar regulation, and other enzymatic actions. As it is required by SOD (see below), taking manganese can increase the activity of that important enzyme.

Melatonin: Hormone produced by the pineal gland that regulates the sleep-wake cycle.

Monolaurin: Fatty acid ester (compound) found in breast milk; it breaks down the protective coating of viruses.

NAC (N-acetyl cysteine): Antioxidant and mucolytic (able to break down mucus) amino acid.

Potassium: An electrolyte mineral that is one half of the sodium-potassium pump that serves to maintain the electrical charge inside cells; needed for nervous system health, proper heart rhythm, acid-base (pH) balance, water balance in the body, and muscle, kidney, and adrenal function.

Proanthocyanidins (PCOs): Potent antioxidants found in grape seed, maritime pine bark, and bilberry; help decrease the fragility of capillaries.

Probiotics: Beneficial bacteria normally found in the intestines; *Lactobacillus acidophilus* and *Bifidobacterium bifidum* are common forms; help restore the proper balance of intestinal bacteria. To ensure that you are getting a quality product, buy powder or capsules that require refrigeration.

Psyllium: A fiber supplement useful for constipation and detoxification (it binds with metabolic waste and bacteria and carries them out of the body).

Pycnogenol: Powerful antioxidant derived from grape seed or maritime pine bark.

Quercetin: Anti-inflammatory flavonoid useful in allergic and inflammatory conditions; its effects are enhanced when used in combination with bromelain; see "Bioflavonoids."

SAMe or SAM (S-adenosylmethionine): A form of the amino acid methionine; involved in numerous metabolic processes, including the production of brain chemicals. People with depression may have low levels of SAMe.

Selenium: Potent antioxidant mineral needed for heart health, skin and other tissue elasticity, proper pancreatic function, and production of thyroid hormone; works synergistically with vitamin E, so take the two supplements together.

Silica (silicon): Mineral required for healthy bones, skin, hair, nails, connective tissue, the thymus gland, and flexible arteries.

SOD (superoxide dismutase): Antioxidant enzyme found in all body cells; contains copper and zinc and works in concert with the enzyme catalase to prevent free-radical damage; may help slow the aging process.[15]

Thymus gland extract: Extract from the thymus gland (typically bovine); in the person taking it, a glandular extract stimulates the gland from which it was derived. In the case of thymus gland extract, it supports immunity since the thymus gland is central to the immune system, activating its worker cells.

Tryptophan: An amino acid precursor to the neurotransmitter serotonin, which regulates mood; tryptophan is a natural pain reliever and can help lift depression.

Vitamin A/beta-carotene: Antioxidant essential for immune function, vision, and healthy skin, hair, and teeth; speeds skin healing. Beta-carotene is converted into vitamin A in the body.

Vitamin B complex: Includes all the B vitamins, biotin, choline, folic acid, and inositol. The members of the vitamin B family work in relationship to each other, so you should take them together. You can take an additional amount of one or more of them, however, to address a specific health issue. In general, the B vitamins are essential for energy production and the metabolism of fats, carbohydrates, and proteins, and help maintain the health of the nervous system, hair, and skin. The following are their individual effects, in addition to those functions.

Vitamin B1 (thiamin): Particularly needed for nerve cell function and carbohydrate metabolism; called the "morale vitamin" due to the effects it exerts on mental state and the nervous system.[16]

Vitamin B2 (riboflavin): Essential for red blood cell formation, aids in protection against free-radical damage, promotes healthy hair, skin, and nails, benefits vision.

Vitamin B3 (niacin and niacinamide): Helps lower cholesterol and maintain blood sugar levels. Niacinamide and niacin are biochemically different, so have different applications. Niacin is the form used to lower cholesterol, while niacinamide is often used in the treatment of arthritis because it decreases joint soreness and increases range of motion.

Vitamin B5 (pantothenic acid): Called the "antistress" vitamin because of its essential role in adrenal gland function, notably the manufacture of adrenal hormones; helps prevent arthritis and high cholesterol.

Vitamin B6 (pyridoxine): Aids in more body functions than any other nutrient;[17] vital for cell formation, normal brain function, RNA and DNA synthesis, immune function, and tissues with rapid cell replication (mucous membranes, skin); useful in treating kidney stones, depression, water retention, and carpal tunnel syndrome, among many other conditions.

Vitamin B12 (cobalamin): Critical to energy production, nerve and immune function, and red blood cell formation; fatigue and anemia are common signs of deficiency.

Vitamin C (ascorbic acid): Antioxidant vital to immune function, the manufacture of collagen (protein comprising connective tissue), wound repair, the health of the gums, and adrenal gland function.

Vitamin D: Essential for calcium absorption and the health of the bones and teeth, supports the thyroid gland. Sunlight on the skin enables the body to manufacture vitamin D, so this "sunshine" vitamin is also considered a hormone.

Vitamin E: Antioxidant vital to immune function, increases circulation, promotes blood clotting, speeds wound and tissue healing, reduces scarring; see "Selenium."

Vitamin K: Essential for blood clotting and bone health, supports liver function.

Zinc: Mineral essential for immune function, cell growth, reproductive health, and vision, taste, and smell; speeds tissue repair.

Reflexology

The foot is a map of the body, according to reflexology. Stimulating an area on the foot that corresponds to a specific part, gland, or organ of the body can exert a healing influence on that part, gland, or organ. The correspondence is based on nerve, or energy, pathways between the point on the foot and the body part. Reflexology works by producing relaxation, reducing tension, promoting circulation, and clearing blockages in energy flow. The result is a restoration of balance in any body part treated via the foot. (Reflexology can also be done on the hands, but the treatments in this book focus on the feet.)

Reflexology is an ancient healing art, with the earliest known reference to the therapy dating as far back as 2500 B.C. and the tomb of an Egyptian physician.[18] While therapeutic foot massage has been practiced for thousands of years, reflexology has its modern roots in the work of Dr. William Fitzgerald, who in the early 1900s developed what he called zone therapy, mapping out zones of the body, each one of which ran from the top of the head to the tip of the fingers and toes. Physiotherapist Eunice Ingham is the founder of reflexology as we know it, however. In the 1930s, she expanded on Dr. Fitzgerald's work by focusing on the zones of the feet, developing the map of the body now used in reflexology and techniques for producing healing effects in areas on the "map."

Many reflexologists still regard the energy lines of the zone system as the source of the effectiveness of reflexology. Others, however, believe that the map of the foot is a map of the termination points of acupuncture meridians (energy channels) and the finger pressure used in reflexology is a substitute for the needles used in acupuncture, as it

Reflexology: Directions for Use

It is more relaxing to have someone else do reflexology on you, but you can do it yourself by sitting cross-legged on the floor or on a chair with one ankle resting on the opposite knee. Hold the foot with one hand while you work on it with the other hand.

It is best not to use massage oil or lotion while doing reflexology because it makes it difficult to maintain a grip on one spot. Apply oil or lotion at the end of your session to give your feet an extra treat.

Consult the maps of the feet to locate the area you want to treat. For body parts that are on both sides of the body, such as an eye or a shoulder, the left foot corresponds with the part on the left side of the body and the right foot for that on the right.

Do the treatment daily or at least 2–3 times weekly during an acute ailment, 1–2 times weekly for chronic conditions. Be sure to treat both feet where appropriate.

Try to keep the pressure at a constant, firm level. For children, the elderly, and people who are sensitive to touch, gentle pressure is recommended.

Use thumb-walking or finger-walking to exert the pressure. For thumb-walking, bend the first joint of the thumb and press the thumb on the spot. The fingers support the foot on the other side. Keeping the thumb flexed, walk it forward, maintaining steady pressure and moving in minute increments, to work the area. Always move forward, not backward or sideways. Cover the area, then switch to the other foot, if appropriate. Make 2–3 passes on each area. For finger-walking, use the thumb for support and the fingers, bent at the first joint, to apply the pressure. This method is good for the tops of the toes and other places where thumb pressure is awkward to apply.

When treatment calls for working the endocrine system, work the points for the thyroid/parathyroid, adrenal glands, pancreas, ovaries/testes, pituitary gland, hypothalamus, and pineal gland.

When treatment calls for working the intestines, work the points for the small intestines and the ascending, descending, transverse, and sigmoid colon.

The solar plexus is a special point. It is the body's "midbrain," a network of nerves that radiate to all parts of the torso and limbs. "If one had to choose only one area on the foot to work, it would have to be this one," say reflexology authorities Kevin and Barbara Kunz.[22]

Working the spleen area helps strengthen immunity and increase resistance to infection.[23]

Note: With reflexology treatments, you may experience more frequent urination and bowel movements, increased perspiration, and an initial worsening of skin conditions. These are signs that the body is detoxifying.

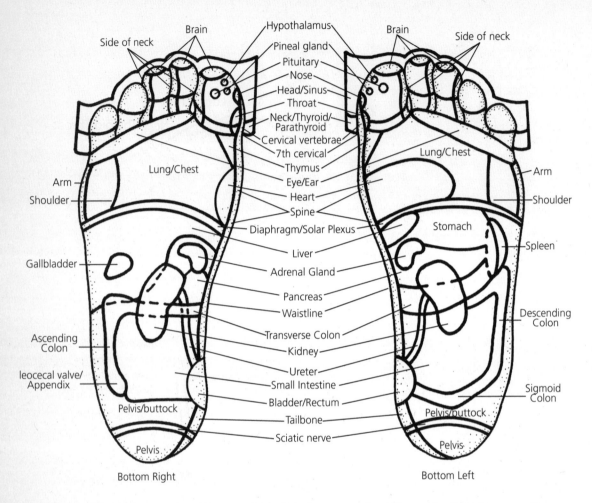

Brain — Hypothalamus — Brain
Side of neck — Pineal gland — Side of neck
Pituitary
Nose
Head/Sinus
Throat
Neck/Thyroid/Parathyroid
Cervical vertebrae
7th cervical
Lung/Chest — Thymus — Lung/Chest
Arm — Eye/Ear — Arm
Shoulder — Heart — Shoulder
Spine
Diaphragm/Solar Plexus
Liver — Stomach
Gallbladder — Adrenal Gland — Spleen
Pancreas
Waistline
Ascending Colon — Transverse Colon — Descending Colon
Kidney
Ileocecal valve/Appendix — Ureter
Small Intestine
Pelvis/buttock — Bladder/Rectum — Sigmoid Colon
Tailbone — Pelvis/buttock
Pelvis — Sciatic nerve — Pelvis

Bottom Right

Bottom Left

is in acupressure.[19] In either case, the effects of reflexology are due to the clearing of energy blockages and improvement of nerve function.

Reflexology receives its name from the fact that the points stimulated produce reflexive, or automatic, responses in the targeted body part.[20] Just as the therapeutic massage of the foot can summon these responses, problems in the foot can have negative effects on the corresponding body parts. For example, accumulations of lactic acid and calcium crystals can interfere with nerve transmission from or to any of the 7,200 nerve endings in each foot. Reflexology can be used as massage to break up these accumulations and clear nerve pathways. Similarly, a bunion is often associated with neck problems, while a

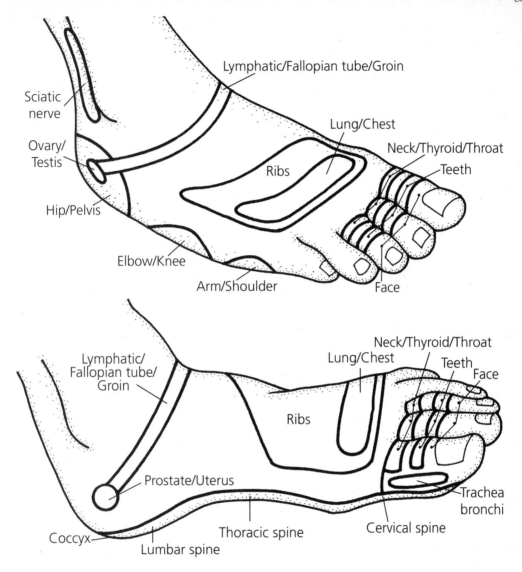

Sciatic nerve

Ovary/Testis

Hip/Pelvis

Elbow/Knee

Arm/Shoulder

Lymphatic/Fallopian tube/Groin

Lung/Chest

Neck/Thyroid/Throat

Teeth

Ribs

Face

Lymphatic/Fallopian tube/Groin

Prostate/Uterus

Coccyx

Lumbar spine

Thoracic spine

Ribs

Lung/Chest

Neck/Thyroid/Throat

Teeth

Face

Trachea bronchi

Cervical spine

toenail ailment, such as an ingrown toenail, may be related to headaches.[21] The ailments exist in a chicken-and-egg relationship, however. Did the bunion or ingrown toenail develop because the person had neck problems or headaches, or vice versa? Regardless of which came first, reflexology can help to resolve the related problems.

While doing reflexology, you will likely encounter sore or tender points in your foot. This indicates a crystal accumulation in the foot, as discussed above, or a problem in the corresponding body part. Often, although not always, you can use the presence of soreness to locate the correct spot to work on. If you want to treat the kidney, for example, go to that area of your foot, as illustrated on the diagram, and press gently in the area until you find the sore point.

In addition to treating the areas specifically indicated for the health conditions in this book, you can give your whole body a treatment by systematically working through both of your feet and thus balancing all the organs, glands, and other parts of the body. Start with your toes and work through the foot to the heel. Be sure to treat both feet. Whole-foot treatment is more in keeping with the holistic nature of reflexology and the holistic principle that all body systems are interrelated.

Caution

Women, especially those with a history of miscarriage, should avoid reflexology in the first 14 weeks of pregnancy.

Do not do reflexology on an injured or painful foot. Consult a qualified reflexologist for treatment.

Stone/Crystal Therapy

Like flower essence therapy and homeopathy, stone/crystal healing is an energy-based medicine. Unlike the other two therapies, stones and crystals are energy in a solid form, although they can be used in essences. Stones and crystals vary in their chemical composition, so each has its own energetic characteristics. The vibrations (which simply means energy) emitted by each stone are the source of the stone's healing properties. Healing occurs through the effect of these vibrations on the electromagnetic field (known as the aura) of a human individual.[24] This is why stone/crystal therapy is also called vibrational healing.

Stones have been employed for their energetic properties since ancient times. For thousands of years, Indians in South America have buried crystals throughout their fields to aid in growing crops; amaranth (a grain) grown in the Andes by this method is known for its amazingly abundant harvests.[25] Early Greeks and Romans wore certain stones for health and protection, as well as to attract virtues.[26] In ancient medical practice, stones were ground into powder and taken orally or applied topically to treat health problems. For example, powdered amber was ingested in a honey, flower, and water mixture as treatment for constipation and kidney or liver ailments. Powdered malachite was made into paste and applied to the eyes to treat cataracts.[27]

Healing stones are variously referred to as crystals, minerals, and gemstones (I use the terms interchangeably). Cutting, polishing, or faceting a stone does not change the nature or impact of its energy, but it does influence the focus or intensity. For example, the energy of a smooth, egg-shaped stone is diffused in all directions, while the pointedness of a faceted stone such as a wand focuses and directs the energy and the facets intensify it, which makes these stones useful for healing.

Cleansing Your Stone/Crystal

Stones and crystals are highly sensitive and pick up vibrations from people and other sources. For this reason, you need to cleanse your stones. Here are some ways to do that:[29]

Saltwater: Take your crystal to the ocean and let the seawater wash over it. As an alternative, completely immerse your crystal in dry sea salt in a glass bowl 7–24 hours, then rinse it off in pure water. After either method, set the crystal in the sun; sunlight is highly purifying and energizing. Or you can submerge the crystal in a saltwater solution (3 tablespoons of salt per cup of water) in a clear glass jar or other glass container, set it in the sun, and let it sit for 1–7 days.

Freshwater: Cleanse your stone in a natural spring, river, or lake. Set the crystal in the sun afterward.

Smudging: Light a smudgestick of sage or sweetgrass or a stick of incense and cleanse the crystal with its smoke.

Flower cleansing: Put the crystal in a bowl of flowers (rose petals or orange blossoms, for example) for 24 hours. Make sure the crystal is covered by the flowers.

Earth cleansing: Bury the stone in some earth overnight. Rinse it off afterward and place it in the sun.

Cluster cleansing: Set the stone on a large quartz crystal cluster for several days; the energy of the large cluster will purify the smaller stone.

The size of the crystal is not important in terms of its healing energy; in other words, bigger is not better. What matters is what's known as the "completeness principle." This is the size needed for the stone to manifest its metaphysical nature, to be complete. Stones differ in this; for example, a very small diamond is complete, while a stone such as a banded agate needs to be much larger in order to represent itself fully.[28]

As each stone's vibrations are as individual as each human's energy field, the main criterion in selecting a stone is that it appeals to you (some say the stone chooses you rather than the other way around). This indicates that its energy is not jarring or unpleasant to your energy field.

Katrina Raphaell, crystal healing therapist, founder of the Crystal Academy of Advanced Healing Arts in Kapaa on the Hawaiian island of Kauai, and author of *The Crystal Trilogy*, provided many of the

Stones/Crystals: Directions for Use

Place the stone on the area of distress or designated location: Keep it in place for 5 minutes 3 times a day, preferably first thing in the morning and the last thing at night while visualizing your health goal and wholeness, says Katrina Raphaell. This is in addition to wearing, carrying, or holding the stone in between treatments.

Place the stone near the body: Rest quietly several times daily for 10–15 minutes, with the stone near the part of the body in need of healing.

Wear/carry/hold the stone: Wearing stones that hang down to the center of the chest (heart and solar plexus area) is a good way to benefit from the healing effects of the stones. You can also hold the stone or carry it in your pocket.

Sleep with the stone: Place the stone under your pillow or hold it in your hand while sleeping. "I have had my best uses of gemstones and crystals over the years by holding them in my hand while I sleep," says natural healer Diane Stein.[30]

Attach with an adhesive bandage: Use an adhesive bandage to keep a small stone in place on or near the area you are treating.

Bath: Place the stone in your bathwater.

Massage: Charge massage oil with the stone's properties. Put the stone in a clear glass bottle of massage oil (such as sweet almond) and place the bottle on a sunny windowsill. Leave it there for a week, shaking it once a day. You can take the stone out of the bottle after a week or leave it in.[31]

Elixir/gem essence: A crystal elixir, also called a gem essence or magnetized or charged water, is made in a similar fashion to flower essences. Like flower essences, it is based on the concept of a transfer of energies, in this case transferring energy from the crystal into water. To make an elixir, place the stone in distilled water in a glass jar or bowl. No metal should contact the liquid. Put the jar or bowl in the sun/moon for 24 hours. Although the healing power of the stone will be transferred to the water without particular intention on your part, conscious programming of the stone enhances the healing focus. Conscious programming is focused intention. Before placing the stone in the water, hold it with both hands and mentally state your healing intention. Katrina Raphaell recommends taking 5 drops of the elixir under the tongue or in a glass of water 2–3 times daily, as needed; as you take the remedy, visualize the stone and your healing intention.[32]

Treating children: Place the stone in the child's bathwater. Or put the stone in the infant's crib, as long as the baby is too young to move around. As an extra measure of caution, use a stone large enough that the baby can't swallow it, in the unlikely event that he or she gets hold of the stone. You can also give a child a gem essence; adjust the dosage according to the child's weight (the dosage above is for an average-size adult).

stone/crystal protocols for this book. "The use of crystals for first aid can be in conjunction with other natural or medical methods," says Raphaell. "Generally, in a full crystal healing, the mental, emotional, and spiritual associations would be attuned to and worked with as well."

In addition to the methods of use described on the previous page, Raphaell recommends meditations with the stones and their placement on an altar or other special site as other means of bringing the crystal's energy into the auric field for healing. She also emphasizes conscious focus, the breath, and visualization as important healing tools in crystal work. This means that you don't do or think of something else while you are engaged in a crystal session, but instead turn your attention to your breathing and to visualizing the health benefit you desire, such as clear skin, easy breathing, or freedom from pain. If you are carrying the stone in your pocket or wearing it, you can do mini-sessions throughout the day. Touch the stone and focus your intention for a few minutes.

Caution:

Never eat a crystal or place it on a mucous membrane.

Appendix A:
Professional Degrees and Titles

A.H.G.	Member of the American Herbalists Guild
C.C.N.	Certified Clinical Nutritionist
C.M.T.	Certified Massage Therapist
C.N.C.	Certified Nutritional Consultant
C.N.S.	Clinical Nutrition Specialist
D.C.	Doctor of Chiropractic
Dip.Phyto.	Diploma in Phytotherapy (medicinal plants)
D.O.	Doctor of Osteopathy
E.M.T.	Emergency Medical Technician
L.Ac.	Licensed Acupuncturist
L.M.T.	Licensed Massage Therapist
M.H.	Master Herbalist
M.N.I.M.H.	Member of the National Institute of Medical Herbalists
M.P.H.	Master of Public Health
M.S.W.	Master of Social Work
N.M.D.	Doctor of Naturopathic Medicine
N.D.	Doctor of Naturopathy
O.M.D.	Oriental Medical Doctor
R.N.	Registered Nurse
R.Ph.	Registered Pharmacist
R.S.Hom.	Registered member of the Society of Homœopaths

Appendix B: Resources

Essential Oils

See also Naturopathic Medicine.

Julia Fischer, Certified Aromatherapist
Kinarome
Northern California
Tel: (415) 457-3673
E-mail: kinarome@aol.com

    Kinarome offers aromatherapy education and consultation to publishers, manufacturers, retailers, spas, and schools; aromatherapy staff trainings and intensives.

Julie Oxendale, C.M.T.
80 Seventh Avenue, Suite 8
San Francisco, CA 94118-1242
Tel: (415) 386-4939
E-mail: olfactor@sirius.com or olfactor@europe.com
Web site: www.aromatherapynow.com

    Aromatherapeutic massage therapist and founder of Direct from Europe, a purveyor of fine-quality essential oils from worldwide plants.

Jeanne Rose
219 Carl Street
San Francisco, CA 94117
Tel: (415) 564-6785
E-mail: diredu@aromaticplantproject.com
Web site: www.aromaticplantproject.com

Aromatherapist, herbalist, and author of *The Aromatherapy Book: Applications and Inhalations, Jeanne Rose's Herbal Body Book*, and *Herbs and Things*.

Kurt Schnaubelt, Ph.D.
Scientific Director
Pacific Institute of Aromatherapy (PIA)
P.O. Box 6723
San Rafael, CA 94903
Tel: (415) 479-9121
Web site: www.pacificinstituteofaromatherapy.com

PIA offers courses, conferences, books, and supplies; including international certification in aromatherapy, quality essential oils (Original Swiss Aromatics/organic oils), and books by Dr. Schnaubelt (*Advanced Aromatherapy* and *Medical Aromatherapy*).

American Aromatherapy Association
P.O. Box 3679
South Pasadena, CA 91031
Tel: (818) 457-1742

National Association for Holistic Aromatherapy
2000 Second Avenue, Suite 206
Seattle, WA 98121
Tel: (888) ASK-NAHA or (206) 256-0741
Web site: www.naha.org

Flower Essences

Patricia Kaminski
Flower Essence Society (FES)
P.O. Box 459
Nevada City, CA 95959
Tel: (800) 736-9222 (U.S. & Canada) or (530) 265-9163
Fax: (530) 265-0584
E-mail: pkaminski@flowersociety.org
Web site: www.flowersociety.org

Herbalist, flower essence therapist, codirector of the Flower Essence Society, author of *Flowers That Heal*, and coauthor of *Flower Essence Repertory*.

The Flower Essence Society is an international membership organization of health practitioners, researchers, students, and others interested in deepening knowledge of flower essence therapy. FES is devoted to research and education, and offers training and certification programs, and publications. The Society also provides a free networking service for finding a practitioner in your area.

Richard Katz
Flower Essence Society
P.O. Box 459
Nevada City, CA 95959
Tel: (800) 736-9222 (U.S. & Canada) or (530) 265-9163
Fax: (530) 265-0584
E-mail: mail@flowersociety.org
Web site: www.flowersociety.org

Health educator, naturalist, founder and codirector of Flower Essence Society, coauthor of *Flower Essence Repertory*.

Bach Flower Remedies
Nelson Bach USA Ltd.
100 Research Drive
Wilmington, MA 01887
Tel: (800) 319-9151 or (978) 988-3833
Web site: www.nelsonbach.com

Herbal Medicine

See also Naturopathic Medicine.

Teresa Boardwine
P.O. Box 232
Fairfax Station, VA 22039
Tel: (703) 425-7527
E-mail: grncmfrt@aol.com
Dreamtime Center for Herbal Studies
270 Sunnyside Orchard Road
Washington, VA 22747
Tel: (540) 675-1122
E-mail: drmtime@shentel.net
Web site: www.dreamtimeherbschool.com

Herbalist and cofounder of Dreamtime Center for Herbal Studies, a school dedicated to preserving whole plant medicine and elevating the profession of herbalism.

Chanchal Cabrera, M.N.I.M.H., A.H.G.
Gaia Garden Herbal Dispensary
2672 West Broadway
Vancouver, BC
V6K 2G3 Canada
Tel: (604) 734-4372
Web site: www.gaiagarden.com

Chanchal Cabrera is a medical herbalist. Her company is Canada's largest retail herbal company, with three stores in the Vancouver region, two full-service herbal dispensaries and clinics, and a worldwide mail-order service.

Michael Cottingham
Clinical herbalist/ethnobotanist
Voyage Botanica
P.O. Box 727
Silver City, NM 88062-0727

Tel: (505) 535-2307

E-mail: mikewren@gilanet.com

Web site: www.voyagebotanica.org

Voyage Botanica is a nonprofit ethnobotanical foundation dedicated to educating people about the uses of medicinal plants.

Amanda McQuade Crawford, M.N.I.M.H., Dip.Phyto.

Ojai Center of Phytotherapy

P.O. Box 66

Ojai, CA 93024

Tel: (805) 646-6699

E-mail: amcqc@earthlink.net

North American College of Botanical Medicine

1104 Park Avenue SW

Albuquerque, NM 87102

Tel: (505) 873-8107

E-mail: phyto@swcp.com

Web site: www.mothergaia.com/phyto

Medical herbalist, nutrition counselor, researcher, director of Ojai Center of Phytotherapy, founding member of the American Herbalists Guild, founder of North American College of Botanical Medicine, and author of *Herbal Remedies for Women* and *The Herbal Menopause Book*.

Mindy Green, A.H.G., M.S.

Herbalist

Herb Research Foundation

1007 Pearl Street, #200

Boulder, CO 80302

Tel: (303) 449-2265, Ex. 201

E-mail: mgreen@herbs.org

Web site: www.herbs.org

Sue Reynolds, M.S.W., L.M.T.
Certified herbalist and aromatherapist
Reynolds Office of Health and Nutrition
P.O. Box 591
Goleta, CA 93116
Tel: (805) 692-6912
E-mail: Herbalist@ReynoldsOffice.com
Web site: www.ReynoldsOffice.com

Karen Vaughan, E.M.T., A.H.G.
Clinical herbalist
Creation's Garden
253 Garfield Place
Brooklyn, NY 11215
Tel: (718) 622-6755
E-mail: CreationsGarden@juno.com

David Winston, A.H.G.
Herbalist and Alchemist, Inc.
51 South Wandling Avenue
Washington, NJ 07882
Tel: (908) 689-9020
E-mail: herbalist@nac.net
Web site: www.herbalist-alchemist.com
Clinical herbalist; educator; consultant to physicians, herbalists, and naturopathic physicians; and founder of Herbalist-Alchemist, a company offering a large line of organically grown and consciously wild-crafted herbal tinctures and other products.

Matthew Wood
Herbalist and educator
Sunnyfield Herb Farm
6001 Sunnyfield Road
Minnetrista, MN 55364
Tel: (952) 472-8057

American Botanical Council
P.O. Box 144345
Austin, TX 78714-4345
Tel: (512) 926-4900
Web site: www.herbalgram.org

American Herbalists Guild
1931 Gaddis Road
Canton, GA 30115
Tel: (770) 751-6021
Web site: www.healthy.net/herbalists

Homeopathy

See also Naturopathic Medicine.

Michael G. Carlston, M.D.
987 Airway Court, Suite 19
Santa Rosa, CA 95403
Tel: (707) 545-1554
E-mail: mcarlston@aol.com
Family practice physician who has been using homeopathy for over twenty-five years. "Whenever possible, I prefer the use of homeopathy, diet and lifestyle interventions, and herbs over prescription medication, as they tend to heal more gently and completely." Dr. Carlston teaches medical students, residents, and physicians about homeopathy. In his practice, he sees himself as a teacher and coach, guiding people towards better health choices and helping them to implement those changes.

Roger Morrison, M.D.
Hahnemann Homeopathic Clinic
Hahnemann College of Homeopathy
80 Nichols Avenue
Richmond, CA 94801

Tel (clinic): (510) 412-9040

Tel (college): (510) 232-2079

Physician, homeopath, author of *Desktop Companion to Physical Pathology*, and teacher at the Hahnemann College of Homeopathy.

Dana Ullmann, M.P.H.

Homeopathic Educational Services

2124 Kittredge Street

Berkeley, CA 94704

Tel: (510) 649-0294

E-mail: mail@homeopathic.com

Web site: www.homeopathic.com

Author of *The Consumer's Guide to Homeopathy and Homeopathic Medicine for Children and Infants*, and coauthor of *Everybody's Guide to Homeopathic Medicines*. HES is a resource center offering books, tapes, software, and medicinal products.

National Center for Homeopathy

801 North Fairfax Street, Suite 306

Alexandria, VA 22314

Tel: (877) 624-0613 or (703) 548-7790

Web site: www.homeopathic.org

Naturopathic Medicine

(Essential Oils, Food Therapy, Herbal Medicine, Homeopathy, Nutritional Supplements)

Bradley Bongiovanni, N.D.

Mosaics Integrated Health

6611 Rockside Road, Suite 215

Independence, OH

Tel: (216) 524-7772

E-mail: Dr.Bongiovanni@aol.com

Web site: www.wellspace.com

Dr. Bongiovanni, a graduate of the National College of Naturopathic Medicine in Portland, Oregon, practices natural family health care and is a frequent contributor to print, online, and other publications including *Reader's Digest* "Ask the Experts," *Prevention,* and *Natural Health*.

Nick Buratovich, N.M.D.
2435 East Southern Avenue, #9
Tempe, AZ 85282
Tel: (480) 831-0717
Fax: (480) 345-9336
E-mail: nicknaturo@earthlink.net

Naturopathic physician and department chair of physical medicine at Southwest College of Naturopathic Medicine and Health Sciences in Tempe, Arizona (www.scnm.edu), Dr. Buratovich maintains a general practice in family medicine. His area of expertise is the treatment of musculoskeletal disorders and chronic pain conditions.

Alan Christianson, N.M.D.
Integrative Health Care, PC
8952 East Desert Cove, Suite 209
Scottsdale, AZ 85260
Tel: (480) 657-0003
Fax: (480) 657-8693
E-mail: alannmd@msn.com
Web site: www.integrativehealthcare.com

Naturopathic physician incorporating conventional and progressive diagnostic procedures, nutrition, botanical medicine, homeopathy, acupuncture, spinal manipulation, and IV therapies; commonly treated disorders include chronic pain, cancer, arteriosclerosis, and heavy metal toxicity.

Boyer B. Cole, N.M.D.
851 South Main Street
Cottonwood, AZ 86326
Tel: (520) 649-0269
E-mail: boyer@wildapache.net

Naturopathic physician Dr. Cole employs a wide range of natural therapies in his practice, including nutrition, spinal manipulation, hydrotherapy, physical therapy, homeopathy, and botanical medicine. He is one of a handful of doctors nationwide using NeuroCranial Restructuring (NCR), a technique that has had success with difficult-to-treat conditions such as sleep apnea, chronic nasal difficulties, headaches, TMJ, and spinal problems.

David R. Field, N.D., L.Ac.
46 Doctors Park Drive
Santa Rosa, CA 95405
Tel: (707) 576-7388
E-mail: doctordf@aol.com
Web site: www.doctordavidfield.net

Naturopathic physician and licensed acupuncturist, specializing in therapeutic nutrition, botanical medicine, homeopathy, and acupuncture.

Ann Louise Gittleman, N.D., C.N.S., M.S.
ALG, Inc.
P.O. Box 882
Bozeman, MT 59771
Tel: (406) 585-9837 or (704) 895-9104
E-mail: gittleman@mindspring.com
Web site: www.annlouise.com

Nutritionist and author of numerous books, including *Beyond Pritikin, The 40/30/30 Phenomenon,* and *The Living Beauty Detox Program.*

Kathi Head, N.D.
E-mail: kathi@kathi.net
Web site: www.kathi.net

Naturopathic physician, technical advisor at Thorne Research, which formulates and manufactures nutritional supplements and botanical formulas, senior editor of *Alternative Medicine Review*, and author of *The Natural Pharmacist: Everything You Need to Know about Diabetes* and *The Natural Pharmacist: Natural Treatments for Diabetes*.

Joanne B. Mied, N.D.
Psychogenic Solutions, Inc.
711 Diablo Avenue, #19
Novato, CA 94947
Tel: (415) 898-0067

Herbalist, naturopath, and iridologist who helps people heal minor aches and pains as well as serious ailments; certified in herbology, iridology, and psychogenics.

Jody E. Noé, M.S., N.D.
Brattleboro Naturopathic Clinic
1063 Marlboro Road
Brattleboro, VT 05301
Tel: (802) 254-9332
Fax: (802) 258-2629
E-mail: brattnat@together.net

Naturopathic physician, ethnobotanist, founding member of the Botanical Medicine Academy. Among the therapeutic modalities used at the Brattleboro Naturopathic Clinic are botanical and homeopathic medicine, nutritional supplements, diet and lifestyle counseling, hydrotherapy, and traditional Chinese medicine.

Paul Reilly, N.D., L.Ac.
Seattle Cancer Treatment and Wellness Center
901 Boren Avenue, Suite 901
Seattle, WA 98104
Tel: (206) 292-2277

Naturopathic physician and licensed acupuncturist who specializes in integrated care of cancer and disorders of the blood. Seattle Cancer Treatment and Wellness offers integrated care for patients with cancer or blood disorders, with the services of board-certified oncologists, naturopathic physicians, and Oriental Medical Doctors/acupunturists.

Susan Roberts, N.D.
National College of Naturopathic Medicine
Natural Health Center Corbett
4444 SW Corbett
Portland, OR 97201
Tel: (503) 224-4003
E-mail: WNHC@aol.com
    Naturopathic family practice physician specializing in women's health care, pediatrics, and natural childbirth at home.

American Association of Naturopathic Physicians
8201 Greensboro Drive, Suite 300
McLean, VA 22102
Tel: (703) 610-9037
Fax: (703) 610-9005
Web site: www.naturopathic.org

Reflexology

International Institute of Reflexology
P.O. Box 12642
St. Petersburg, FL 33733-2642
Tel: (727) 343-4811
Web site: www.reflexology-usa.net

Reflexology Association of America
4012 Rainbow, Suite K
PMB #585
Las Vegas, NV 89103-2059
Web site: www.reflexology-usa.org

Stones/Crystal Therapy

Melody
Author of the stone/crystal reference series *Love Is in the Earth*,
published by:
Earth Love Publishing House
3440 Youngfield Street, #353
Wheat Ridge, CO 80033
Tel: (303) 233-9660

Katrina Raphaell
Crystal healing therapist, founder of the Crystal Academy of
Advanced Healing Arts, and author of *The Crystal Trilogy*: *Crystal
Enlightenment, Vol. I*; *Crystal Healing, Vol. II*; and *The Crystalline Transmission,
Vol. III* (all from Aurora Press)
The Crystal Academy of Advanced Healing Arts
P. O. Box 1334
Kapaa, Kauai, HI 96746
Tel: (808) 823-6959
Fax: (808) 821-1165
Web site: www.crystalacademy.cncfamily.com

Daya Sarai Chocron
12 Wilson Avenue
Northampton, MA 01060
Tel: (413) 584-1022
E-mail: dayasarai@worldnet.att.net
Vibrational/spiritual healer, shaman, educator, and author of
Healing with Crystals and Gemstones and *Healing the Heart*; offers appren-
ticeship programs in vibrational healing in addition to seeing individual
clients.

Endnotes

Part II

Abscess

1. Patricia Davis, *Aromatherapy: An A-Z.* Saffron Walden, Essex, England: C.W. Daniel Co., 1988: 11.

Acne

1. L. Juhlin and G. Michaelsson, "Fibrin microclot formation in patients with acne," *Acta Derm Venerol* 63 (1983): 538–40.

2. Maesimund B. Panos, M.D., and Jane Heimlich, *Homeopathic Medicine at Home.* New York: Jeremy P. Tarcher, 1980: 193.

3. A chelated form of a mineral supplement is one in which the mineral is attached to a protein molecule that carries the mineral to the bloodstream. The body chelates minerals naturally, but you can enhance absorption by taking a supplement in this form. Picolinates are one type of chelates.

Allergic Reaction

1. Robert Ullman, N.D., and Judyth Reichenberg-Ullman, N.D., *Homeopathic Self-Care.* Rocklin, Calif.: Prima Publishing, 1997: 62–65.

2. Ibid., 63.

Anxiety

1. Colleen K. Dodt, *The Essential Oils Book.* Pownal, Vt.: Storey Communications, 1996: 31.

2. Kathi Keville with Peter Korn, *Herbs for Health and Healing.* New York: Berkley Books, 1996: 386.

Backache

1. Linda Rector Page, *Healthy Healing.* Healthy Healing Publications (Internet: healthyhealing.com), 1997: B243; Janet Zand, et al., *Smart Medicine for Healthier Living.* Garden City Park, N.Y.: Avery Publishing Group, 1999: 126.

2. Tom Monte and the editors of *Natural Health* Magazine, *The Complete Guide to Natural Healing.* New York: Perigee/Berkley Publishing Group, 1997: 48.

3. Michael Tierra, L.Ac., OMD, *The Way of Herbs.* New York: Pocket Books, 1990: 317–18.

4. James Kusick, *A Treasury of Natural First Aid Remedies From A to Z.* New York: Parker, 1995: 19.

5. James A. Duke, Ph.D., *The Green Pharmacy.* New York: St. Martin's, 1997: 90.

6. Stephen Cummings, M.D., and Dana Ullman, M.P.H., *Everybody's Guide to Homeopathic Medicines.* New York: Jeremy P. Tarcher/Putnam, 1997: 289.

7. H.R. Liberman et al., "Mood, performance and pain sensitivity: Changes induced by food constituents," *Journal of Psychiatric Research* 17 (1983): 135–45.

Bacterial Infection

1. Jane Buckle, R.N., "Ask the physician: Aromatherapy in nursing," *Alternative Medicine* 27 (December 1998/January 1999): 36–37.

2. Kurt Schnaubelt, Ph.D., *Advanced Aromatherapy*. Rochester, Vt.: Healing Arts Press, 1995: 31–36.

3. Ibid., 97.

4. "Ask the physician: Aromatherapy in nursing," *Alternative Medicine* 27 (December 1998/January 1999): 38.

5. Michael T. Murray, N.D., *The Healing Power of Herbs*. Rocklin, CA: Prima Publishing, 1995.

6. Kathi Keville with Peter Korn, *Herbs for Health and Healing*. New York: Berkley Books, 1996: 142.

7. Allan Sachs, D.C., C.C.N., *The Authoritative Guide to Grapefruit Seed Extract*. Mendocino, Calif.: LifeRhythm, 1997: 17.

Bad Breath

1. Karen Sullivan and C. Norman Shealy, M.D., Ph.D., eds., *The Complete Family Guide to Natural Home Remedies*. Rockport, Mass.: Element Books, 1997: 61.

2. Simon Y. Mills, M.A., M.N.I.M.H., *The Dictionary of Modern Herbalism*. Rochester, Vt.: Healing Arts Press, 1988: 37.

3. Dr. Barry Rose, *The Family Health Guide to Homeopathy*. Berkeley, Calif.: Celestial Arts, 1992: 103–04.

Bed-Wetting (Childhood)

1. James F. Balch, M.D., and Phyllis A. Balch, C.N.C., *Prescription for Nutritional Healing*. Garden City Park, N.Y.: Avery Publishing Group, 1990: 104; Michael T. Murray, N.D., and Joseph Pizzorno, N.D., *Encyclopedia of Natural Medicine*. Rocklin, Calif.: Prima Publishing, 1991: 311.

2. Robert B. Tisserand, *The Art of Aromatherapy*. Rochester, Vt.: Healing Arts Press, 1977: 300.

3. Kathi Keville with Peter Korn, *Herbs for Health and Healing*. New York: Berkley Books, 1996: 286–87.

4. Miranda Castro, R.S.Hom., *The Complete Homeopathy Handbook*. New York: St. Martin's, 1990.

5. David Carroll, *The Complete Book of Natural Medicines*. New York: Summit Books, 1980: 109.

6. Tom Monte and the editors of *Natural Health* Magazine, *The Complete Guide to Natural Healing*. New York: Perigee/Berkley Publishing Group, 1997: 164; James F. Balch, M.D., and Phyllis A. Balch, C.N.C., *Prescription for Nutritional Healing*. Garden City Park, N.Y.: Avery Publishing Group, 1990: 104.

7. J.I. Rodale and staff, *The Health Seeker*. Emmaus, Pa.: Rodale Press, 1962: 794.

Black Eye

1. Valerie Ann Worwood, *The Complete Book of Essential Oils and Aromatherapy*. Novato, Calif.: New World Library, 1991: 24.

2. Mark Mayell and the editors of *Natural Health* Magazine, *The Natural Health First-Aid Guide*. New York: Pocket Books, 1994: 250.

3. Janet Zand, L.Ac., O.M.D., et al., *Smart Medicine for Healthier Living*. Garden City Park, N.Y.: Avery Publishing Group, 1999: 152–3; Michael T. Murray, N.D., *Encyclopedia of Nutritional Supplements*. Rocklin, Calif.: Prima Publishing, 1996: 323.

Bladder Infection (Cystitis)

1. Jacqueline Young, *The Natural Way: Cystitis*. Rockport, Mass.: Element Books, 1997: 15.

2. Diane Stein, *The Natural Remedy Book for Women*. Freedom, Calif.: Crossing Press, 1992: 170.

3. A.E. Sobota, "Inhibition of bacterial adherence by cranberry juice: Potential use for the treatment of urinary tract infections," *Journal of Urology* 131 (1984): 1013–16.

Blister

1. Patricia Davis, *Aromatherapy: An A-Z.* Saffron Walden, Essex, England: C.W. Daniel Co., 1988: 55.

2. Maesimund B. Panos, M.D., and Jane Heimlich, *Homeopathic Medicine at Home.* New York: Jeremy P. Tarcher, 1980: 75.

3. James Kusick, *A Treasury of Natural First Aid Remedies From A to Z.* New York: Parker, 1995: 41.

4. Ibid., 41.

Body Odor

1. James A. Duke, Ph.D., *The Green Pharmacy.* New York: St. Martin's, 1997: 104–5.

2. Robert B. Tisserand, *The Art of Aromatherapy.* Rochester, Vt.: Healing Arts Press, 1977: 309.

3. Patricia Davis, *Aromatherapy: An A-Z.* Saffron Walden, Essex, England: C.W. Daniel Co., 1988: 353.

4. Linda Rector Page, N.D., Ph.D., *Healthy Healing.* Carmel Valley, Calif.: Healthy Healing Publications, 1997: 244.

5. James A. Duke, Ph.D., *The Green Pharmacy.* New York: St. Martin's, 1997: 106–07.

6. Allan Sachs, D.C., C.C.N., *The Authoritative Guide to Grapefruit Seed Extract.* Mendocino, Calif.: LifeRhythm, 1997: 76.

7. John Heinerman, *Heinerman's New Encyclopedia of Fruits and Vegetables.* Paramus, N.J.: Prentice Hall, 1995: 5.

Boil

1. James F. Balch, M.D., and Phyllis A. Balch, C.N.C., *Prescription for Nutritional Healing.* Garden City Park, NY: Avery Publishing Group, 1990: 108; Linda Rector Page, N.D., Ph.D., *Healthy Healing.* Carmel Valley, Calif.: Healthy Healing Publications, 1997: A215.

2. Janet Zand, L.Ac., O.M.D., et al., *Smart Medicine for Healthier Living.* Garden City Park, N.Y.: Avery Publishing Group, 1999: 144.

3. Mildred Jackson, N.D., and Terri Teague, N.D., D.C., *The Handbook of Alternatives to Chemical Medicine.* Novato, Calif.: New World Library, 1997: 158.

4. Dr. Andrew Lockie and Dr. Nicola Geddes, *The Complete Guide to Homeopathy.* New York: DK Publishing, 1995: 188–89.

5. Bill Gottlieb, ed., *New Choices in Natural Healing.* Emmaus, Pa.: Rodale Press, 1995: 206.

Bone Spur (Heel Spur)

1. L. Randol Barker, M.D., et al., eds., *Principles of Ambulatory Medicine, 2d ed.* Baltimore, Md: Williams & Wilkins, 1986: 887, 1449–50.

2. James F. Balch, M.D., and Phyllis A. Balch, C.N.C., *Prescription for Nutritional Healing.* Garden City Park, N.Y.: Avery Publishing Group, 1990: 197.

3. Earl Mindell, R.Ph., Ph.D., *Earl Mindell's Food as Medicine.* New York: Fireside/Simon & Schuster, 1994: 65; Linda Rector Page, N.D., Ph.D., *Healthy Healing.* Carmel Valley, Calif.: Healthy Healing Publications, 1997: 305.

4. Dr. Barry Rose, *The Family Health Guide to Homeopathy.* Berkeley, Calif.: Celestial Arts, 1992: 196.

5. "Prescribing—for yourself: Vitamin C for relief from heel spurs," *Alternative Medicine Digest* 22 (February/March 1998): 24.

6. James F. Balch, M.D., and Phyllis A. Balch, C.N.C., *Prescription for Nutritional Healing.* Garden City Park, N.Y.: Avery Publishing Group, 1990: 197.

7. Judithann H. David, Ph.D., and J.P. Van Hulle, *Michael's Gemstone Dictionary.* Orinda, Calif.: Affinity Press, 1990: 107, 114.

Bruise

1. Miranda Castro, R.S.Hom., *The Complete Homeopathy Handbook*. New York: St. Martin's, 1990.

Bunion

1. Valerie Ann Worwood, *The Complete Book of Essential Oils and Aromatherapy*. Novato, Calif.: New World Library, 1991: 24.

2. Penelope Ody, *Herbs for First Aid*. Los Angeles: Keats Publishing, 1999: 61.

3. Dr. Barry Rose, *The Family Health Guide to Homeopathy*. Berkeley, Calif.: Celestial Arts, 1992: 190.

4. Janet Zand, L.Ac., O.M.D., et al., *Smart Medicine for Healthier Living*. Garden City Park, N.Y.: Avery Publishing Group, 1999: 156.

5. Karen Sullivan and C. Norman Shealy, M.D., Ph.D., eds., *The Complete Family Guide to Natural Home Remedies*. Rockport, Mass.: Element Books, 1997: 79.

6. Inge Dougans, *Reflexology: An Introductory Guide to Foot Massage for Total Health*. Boston, Mass.: Element Books, 1999: 89–90.

Burn

1. Janet Zand, L.Ac., O.M.D., et al., *Smart Medicine for Healthier Living*. Garden City Park, N.Y.: Avery Publishing Group, 1999: 159.

Bursitis

1. Anne Woodham and David Peters, M.D., *Encyclopedia of Healing Therapies*. New York: Dorling Kindersley, 1997: 253.

2. K. Folkers and J. Ellis, "Successful therapy with vitamin B6 and vitamin B2 of the carpal tunnel syndrome and need for determination of the RDA's for vitamin B6 and B2 disease states." *Annals of the New York Academy of Science* 585 (1990): 295–301.

Canker Sore

1. Donald J. Brown, N.D., *Herbal Prescriptions for Better Health*. Rocklin, Calif.: Prima Publishing, 1996: 259.

2. Robert Ullman, N.D., and Judyth Reichenberg-Ullman, N.D., *Homeopathic Self-Care*. Rocklin, Calif.: Prima Publishing, 1997: 93–96.

Cold Sore (Fever Blister)

1. Allan Sachs, D.C., C.C.N., *The Authoritative Guide to Grapefruit Seed Extract*. Mendocino, Calif.: LifeRhythm, 1997: 78–79.

2. Roger Morrison, M.D., *Desktop Companion to Physical Pathology*. Nevada City, Calif.: Hahnemann Clinic Publishing, 1998.

3. Michael T. Murray, N.D., and Joseph Pizzorno, N.D., *Encyclopedia of Natural Medicine*. Rocklin, Calif.: Prima Publishing, 1991: 531.

Colic (Infant)

1. Kathi Keville with Peter Korn, *Herbs for Health and Healing*. New York: Berkley Books, 1996: 317.

Common Cold

1. Linda Rector Page, N.D., Ph.D., *Healthy Healing*. Carmel Valley, Calif.: Healthy Healing Publications, 1997: 274.

2. Kurt Schnaubelt, Ph.D., *Advanced Aromatherapy*. Rochester, Vt.: Healing Arts Press, 1995: 109.

3. James Kusick, *A Treasury of Natural First Aid Remedies From A to Z*, New York: Parker, 1995: 75.

4. Maesimund B. Panos, M.D., and Jane Heimlich, *Homeopathic Medicine at Home*. New York: Jeremy P. Tarcher, 1980: 105–07.

5. David Carroll, *The Complete Book of Natural Medicines*. New York: Summit Books, 1980: 159.

Conjunctivitis (Pinkeye)

1. Roger Morrison, M.D., *Desktop Companion to Physical Pathology*. Nevada City, Calif.: Hahnemann Clinic Publishing, 1998.

2. Linda Rector Page, N.D., Ph.D., *Healthy Healing*. Carmel Valley, Calif.: Healthy Healing Publications, 1997: 299.

Constipation

1. James F. Balch, M.D., and Phyllis A. Balch, C.N.C., *Prescription for Nutritional Healing*. Garden City Park, N.Y.: Avery Publishing Group, 1990: 145.

2. D. LeRoith et al., "Insulin or a closely related molecule is native to Escherichia coli," *Journal of Biochemistry* 256 (1981): 6, 533–36; M. Weiss and S.H. Ingbar. "Demonstration of a saturable binding site for thyrotropin in Yersinia enterocolitica," *Science* 219 (1983): 1331–35; J. Ballard and M. Shiner, "Evidence of cytotoxicity in ulcerative colitis from immunofluorescent staining of the rectal mucosa," *Lancet* (1974i): 1014–17.

3. Michael Tierra, L.Ac., OMD, *The Way of Herbs*. New York: Pocket Books, 1990: 298, 324. Dr. Christopher died in 1983. His family and former students are carrying on his work.

4. Dr. Barry Rose, *The Family Health Guide to Homeopathy*. Berkeley: Celestial Arts, 1992: 151.

5. Christopher Hobbs, *Foundations of Health: Healing with Herbs and Food*. Loveland, Colo.: Botanica Press, 1992: 134.

Cough

1. Clayton L. Thomas, M.D., M.P.H., ed., *Taber's Cyclopedic Medical Dictionary*, 17th ed. Philadelphia: F.A. Davis, 1993: 458.

2. James A. Duke, Ph.D., *The Green Pharmacy*. New York: St. Martin's, 1997: 180.

3. Stephen Cummings, M.D., and Dana Ullman, M.P.H., *Everybody's Guide to Homeopathic Medicines*. New York: Jeremy P. Tarcher/Putnam, 1997: 78–82.

Cuts and Scrapes

1. Melvyn R. Werbach, M.D., and Michael T. Murray, N.D., *Botanical Influences on Illness: A Sourcebook of Clinical Research*. New Canaan, Conn.: Keats Publishing, 1988: 211.

2. Allan Sachs, D.C., C.C.N., *The Authoritative Guide to Grapefruit Seed Extract*. Mendocino, Calif.: LifeRhythm, 1997: 79.

3. Maesimund B. Panos, M.D., and Jane Heimlich, *Homeopathic Medicine at Home*. New York: Jeremy P. Tarcher, 1980: 55–58.

Dandruff

1. Linda Rector Page, N.D., Ph.D., *Healthy Healing*. Carmel Valley, Calif.: Healthy Healing Publications, 1997: 283.

2. David L. Hoffman, M.N.I.M.H., *The New Holistic Herbal*. Boston: Element Books, 1990: 186.

3. Karen Sullivan and C. Norman Shealy, M.D., Ph.D., eds., *The Complete Family Guide to Natural Home Remedies*. Rockport, Mass.: Element Books, 1997: 78.

4. Dr. Barry Rose, *The Family Health Guide to Homeopathy*. Berkeley: Celestial Arts, 1992: 72–73.

Dental Abscess

1. Linda Rector Page, N.D., Ph.D., *Healthy Healing.* Carmel Valley, Calif.: Healthy Healing Publications, 1997: 215.

2. Allan Sachs, D.C., C.C.N., *The Authoritative Guide to Grapefruit Seed Extract.* Mendocino, Calif.: LifeRhythm, 1997: 79.

Depression

1. Patricia Davis, *Aromatherapy: An A-Z.* Saffron Walden, Essex, England: C.W. Daniel Co., 1988: 11.

2. Melvyn R. Werbach, M.D., and Michael T. Murray, N.D., *Botanical Influences on Illness: A Sourcebook of Clinical Research.* New Canaan, Conn.: Keats Publishing, 1988: 135–36.

3. Jason Elias, M.A., L.Ac., and Shelagh Ryan Masline, *The A to Z Guide to Healing Herbal Remedies.* New York: Wings Books, 1996: 240.

4. Dr. Andrew Lockie and Dr. Nicola Geddes, *The Complete Guide to Homeopathy.* New York: DK Publishing, 1995: 194–95.

Dermatitis (Eczema)

1. Clayton L. Thomas, M.D., M.P.H., ed., *Taber's Cyclopedic Medical Dictionary*, 17th ed. Philadelphia: F.A. Davis, 1993: 605; *Dorland's Illustrated Medical Dictionary*, 26th ed. Philadelphia: W.B. Saunders, 1985: 420.

2. N. Soter and H. Baden, *Pathophysiology of Dermatologic Disease.* New York: McGraw-Hill, 1984.

3. Kurt Schnaubelt, Ph.D., *Advanced Aromatherapy.* Rochester, Vt.: Healing Arts Press, 1995: 113.

4. Karen Sullivan and C. Norman Shealy, M.D., Ph.D., eds., *The Complete Family Guide to Natural Home Remedies.* Rockport, Mass.: Element Books, 1997: 113.

Diaper Rash

1. Maesimund B. Panos, M.D., and Jane Heimlich, *Homeopathic Medicine at Home.* New York: Jeremy P. Tarcher, 1980: 160–61.

Diarrhea

1. James A. Duke, Ph.D., *The Green Pharmacy.* New York: St. Martin's, 1997: 204–05.

Dizziness (Vertigo)

1. Janet Zand, L.Ac., O.M.D., et al., *Smart Medicine for Healthier Living.* Garden City Park, N.Y.: Avery Publishing Group, 1999: 581.

2. James A. Duke, Ph.D., *The Green Pharmacy.* New York: St. Martin's, 1997: 212.

3. Roger Morrison, M.D., *Desktop Companion to Physical Pathology.* Nevada City, Calif.: Hahnemann Clinic Publishing, 1998.

4. James F. Balch, M.D., and Phyllis A. Balch, C.N.C., *Prescription for Nutritional Healing.* Garden City Park, N.Y.: Avery Publishing Group, 1990: 308.

Ear Infection

1. Robert B. Tisserand, *The Art of Aromatherapy.* Rochester, Vt.: Healing Arts Press, 1977: 199–200, 248.

Edema (Water Retention)

1. James F. Balch, M.D., and Phyllis A. Balch, C.N.C., *Prescription for Nutritional Healing.* Garden City Park, N.Y.: Avery Publishing Group, 1990: 164.

2. Patricia Davis, *Aromatherapy: An A-Z.* Saffron Walden, Essex, England: C.W. Daniel Co., 1988: 235.

3. Ibid., 235.

4. Dr. Barry Rose, *The Family Health Guide to Homeopathy.* Berkeley: Celestial Arts, 1992: 212.

5. Linda Rector Page, N.D., Ph.D., *Healthy Healing.* Carmel Valley, Calif.: Healthy Healing Publications, 1997: 425.

Eye Problems (Eyestrain, Bloodshot, Dry Eyes, Circles)

1. Linda Rector Page, N.D., Ph.D., *Healthy Healing.* Carmel Valley, Calif.: Healthy Healing Publications, 1997: 299.

2. Earl Mindell, R.Ph., Ph.D., *Earl Mindell's Herb Bible.* New York: Fireside/ Simon & Schuster, 1992: 91.

3. Dr. Andrew Lockie and Dr. Nicola Geddes, *The Complete Guide to Homeopathy.* New York: DK Publishing, 1995: 166–67.

4. Bill Gottlieb, ed., *New Choices in Natural Healing.* Emmaus, Pa.: Rodale Press, 1995: 295.

5. James F. Balch, M.D., and Phyllis A. Balch, C.N.C., *Prescription for Nutritional Healing.* Garden City Park, N.Y.: Avery Publishing Group, 1990: 174.

6. Ann Louise Gittleman, M.S., C.N.S., *The Living Beauty Detox Program.* San Francisco: HarperSanFrancisco, 2000: 128.

7. James Kusick, *A Treasury of Natural First Aid Remedies From A to Z.* New York: Parker, 1995: 105.

Fatigue

1. Roberta Wilson, *Aromatherapy for Vibrant Health and Beauty.* Garden City Park, N.Y.: Avery Publishing Group, 1995: 141.

2. Dr. Andrew Lockie and Dr. Nicola Geddes, *The Complete Guide to Homeopathy.* New York: DK Publishing, 1995: 196-97.

3. David Carroll, *The Complete Book of Natural Medicines.* New York: Summit Books, 1980: 227.

Flu

1. Bill Gottlieb, ed., *New Choices in Natural Healing.* Emmaus, Pa.: Rodale Press, 1995: 307–08.

2. Karen Sullivan and C. Norman Shealy, M.D., Ph.D., eds., *The Complete Family Guide to Natural Home Remedies.* Rockport, Mass.: Element Books, 1997: 58.

3. Stephen Cummings, M.D., and Dana Ullman, M.P.H., *Everybody's Guide to Homeopathic Medicines.* New York: Jeremy P. Tarcher/Putnam, 1997: 58–60.

Food Poisoning

1. James Kusick, *A Treasury of Natural First Aid Remedies From A to Z.* New York: Parker, 1995: 115.

2. Mark Mayell and the editors of *Natural Health* Magazine, *The Natural Health First-Aid Guide.* New York: Pocket Books, 1994: 458.

3. Maesimund B. Panos, M.D., and Jane Heimlich, *Homeopathic Medicine at Home.* New York: Jeremy P. Tarcher, 1980: 86.

Fungal Infection (Athlete's Foot, Jock Itch, Nails, Oral Thrush)

1. Kathi Keville with Peter Korn, *Herbs for Health and Healing.* New York: Berkley Books, 1996: 325–26.

Gas (Flatulence)

1. James A. Duke, Ph.D., *The Green Pharmacy.* New York: St. Martin's, 1997: 243.

2. Valerie Ann Worwood, *The Complete Book of Essential Oils and Aromatherapy.* Novato, Calif.: New World Library, 1991: 298–89.

3. Maesimund B. Panos, M.D., and Jane Heimlich, *Homeopathic Medicine at Home.* New York: Jeremy P. Tarcher, 1980: 131.

4. Joy Gardner, *Color and Crystals: A Journey Through the Chakras.* Freedom, Calif.: Crossing Press, 1988: 78-79, 128, 136.

Gingivitis

1. Dr. Barry Rose, *The Family Health Guide to Homeopathy.* Berkeley: Celestial Arts, 1992: 110–11.

Gout

1. Michael T. Murray, N.D., *The Healing Power of Herbs.* Rocklin, Calif.: Prima Publishing, 1995: 364.

2. Robert B. Tisserand, *The Art of Aromatherapy.* Rochester, Vt.: Healing Arts Press, 1977: 186–87, 300.

3. James A. Duke, Ph.D., *The Green Pharmacy.* New York: St. Martin's, 1997: 272–75.

4. Dr. Barry Rose, *The Family Health Guide to Homeopathy.* Berkeley: Celestial Arts, 1992: 193–94.

Hay Fever

1. Janet Zand, L.Ac., O.M.D., et al., *Smart Medicine for Healthier Living.* Garden City Park, N.Y.: Avery Publishing Group, 1999: 316; Linda Rector Page, N.D., Ph.D., *Healthy Healing.* Carmel Valley, Calif.: Healthy Healing Publications, 1997: A230.

2. Anne Woodham and David Peters, M.D., *Encyclopedia of Healing Therapies.* New York: Dorling Kindersley, 1997: 299.

3. Miranda Castro, R.S.Hom., *The Complete Homeopathy Handbook.* New York: St. Martin's Press, 1990.

Headache

1. James A. Duke, Ph.D., *The Green Pharmacy.* New York: St. Martin's, 1997: 283.

2. Diane Stein, *The Natural Remedy Book for Women.* Freedom, Calif.: Crossing Press, 1992: 192.

Heartburn/Indigestion

1. Penelope Ody, *Herbs for First Aid.* Los Angeles: Keats Publishing, 1999: 76.

2. Karen Sullivan and C. Norman Shealy, M.D., Ph.D., eds., *The Complete Family Guide to Natural Home Remedies.* Rockport, Mass.: Element Books, 1997: 65.

3. James F. Balch, M.D., and Phyllis A. Balch, C.N.C., *Prescription for Nutritional Healing.* Garden City Park, N.Y.: Avery Publishing Group, 1990: 196.

4. Ibid., 197.

Hemorrhoids

1. J.F. Johanson and A. Sonnenberg, "Constipation is not a risk factor for hemorrhoids: A case-control study of potential etiological agents," *American Journal of Gastroenterology* 89 (1994): 1981–86; Dr. Andrew Lockie and Dr. Nicola Geddes, *The Complete Guide to Homeopathy.* New York: DK Publishing, 1995: 181.

2. Jeanne Rose, *The Aromatherapy Book.* Berkeley: North Atlantic Books, 1992: 115.

3. Robert Ullman, N.D., and Judyth Reichenberg-Ullman, N.D., *Homeopathic Self-Care.* Rocklin, Calif.: Prima Publishing, 1997: 212–16.

4. Joy Gardner, *Color and Crystals: A Journey Through the Chakras.* Freedom, Calif.: Crossing Press, 1988: 99–100; Judithann H. David, Ph.D., and J.P. Van Hulle, *Michael's Gemstone Dictionary.* Orinda, Calif.: Affinity Press, 1990: 107.

Hiccups

1. Diane Stein, *The Natural Remedy Book for Women.* Freedom, Calif.: Crossing Press, 1992: 211.

2. David Carroll, *The Complete Book of Natural Medicines.* New York: Summit Books, 1980: 279.

3. Mildred Jackson, N.D., and Terri Teague, N.D., D.C., *The Handbook of Alternatives to Chemical Medicine.* Novato, Calif.: New World Library, 1997: 187.

4. Dr. Barry Rose, *The Family Health Guide to Homeopathy*. Berkeley, Calif.: Celestial Arts, 1992: 140, 145, 181.

5. Diane Stein, *The Natural Remedy Book for Women*. Freedom, Calif.: Crossing Press, 1992: 208-09.

6. Ibid., 211.

Hives (Urticaria)

1. Michael T. Murray, N.D., and Joseph Pizzorno, N.D., *Encyclopedia of Natural Medicine*. Rocklin, Calif.: Prima Publishing, 1991: 364–69.

2. Patricia Davis, *Aromatherapy: An A-Z*. Saffron Walden, Essex, England: C.W. Daniel Co., 1988: 11.

3. Michael T. Murray, N.D., *Encyclopedia of Nutritional Supplements*. Rocklin, Calif.: Prima Publishing, 1996: 324.

Hot Flashes (Menopausal)

1. John R. Lee, M.D., *What Your Doctor May Not Tell You About Menopause*. New York: Warner Books, 1996: 117–28.

Inflammation (Natural Anti-Inflammatories)

1. Kurt Schnaubelt, Ph.D., *Advanced Aromatherapy*. Rochester, Vt.: Healing Arts Press, 1995: 116.

2. Chanchal Cabrera, "Healing inflammation: A functional approach," Presentation at Gaia Symposium, 1999. Tape available from Medicines from the Earth; (800) 252-0688.

3. M.L. Ferrandiz and M.J. Alcaraz, "Anti-inflammatory activity and inhibition of arachidonic acid metabolism by flavonoids," *Agents Action* 32 (1991): 283–87.

Insect Bites and Stings

1. Valerie Ann Worwood, *The Complete Book of Essential Oils and Aromatherapy*. Novato, Calif.: New World Library, 1991: 53.

2. Dr. Andrew Lockie and Dr. Nicola Geddes, *The Complete Guide to Homeopathy*. New York: DK Publishing, 1995: 221.

3. Mark Mayell and the editors of *Natural Health* Magazine, *The Natural Health First-Aid Guide*. New York: Pocket Books, 1994: 161.

4. James Kusick, *A Treasury of Natural First Aid Remedies From A to Z*. New York: Parker, 1995: 26.

Insomnia

1. H. Kaplan and B. Sadock, *Modern Synopsis of Comprehensive Textbook of Psychiatry*, vol. IV. Baltimore: Williams & Wilkins, 1985: 558–74.

2. Valerie Ann Worwood, *The Complete Book of Essential Oils and Aromatherapy*. Novato, Calif.: New World Library, 1991: 285.

3. Stephen Cummings, M.D., and Dana Ullman, M.P.H., *Everybody's Guide to Homeopathic Medicines*. New York: Jeremy P. Tarcher/Putnam, 1997: 289.

4. Michael T. Murray, N.D., *Encyclopedia of Nutritional Supplements*. Rocklin, Calif.: Prima Publishing, 1996: 162.

5. Ann Louise Gittleman, M.S., C.N.S., *The Living Beauty Detox Program*. San Francisco: HarperSanFrancisco, 2000: 140.

6. C. Mallo et al., "Effects of a four-day nocturnal melatonin treatment on the 24 h plasma melatonin, cortisol and prolactin profiles in humans," *Acta Endocrnologia* 119 (1988): 474–80.

7. I Haimov et al., "Sleep disorders and melatonin rhythms in elderly people," *British Medical Journal* 309 (1994): 167.

Jet Lag

1. Bill Gottlieb, ed., *New Choices in Natural Healing.* Emmaus, Pa.: Rodale Press, 1995: 399.

2. Mark Mayell and the editors of *Natural Health* Magazine, *The Natural Health First-Aid Guide.* New York: Pocket Books, 1994: 503.

Joint Soreness

1. Penelope Ody, *Herbs for First Aid.* Los Angeles: Keats Publishing, 1999: 79.

2. Jeanne Rose, *Herbs & Things.* New York: Perigee Books, 1972.

3. James Kusick, *A Treasury of Natural First Aid Remedies From A to Z.* New York: Parker, 1995: 18.

4. Miranda Castro, R.S.Hom., *The Complete Homeopathy Handbook.* New York: St. Martin's Press, 1990.

5. H.R. Liberman et al., "Mood, performance and pain sensitivity: Changes induced by food constituents," *Journal of Psychiatric Research* 17 (1983): 135–45.

Kidney Stones

1. Michael T. Murray, N.D., and Joseph Pizzorno, N.D., *Encyclopedia of Natural Medicine.* Rocklin, Calif.: Prima Publishing, 1991: 401.

2. Ibid., 402, 403.

3. G.C. Curhan et al., "A prospective study of dietary calcium and other nutrients and the risk of symptomatic kidney stones," *New England Journal of Medicine* 328:12 (March 25, 1993): 833–8.

4. Michael T. Murray, N.D., and Joseph Pizzorno, N.D., *Encyclopedia of Natural Medicine.* Rocklin, Calif.: Prima Publishing, 1991: 405.

5. R.P. Heavey and R.R. Recker, "Effects of nitrogen, phosphorus, and caffeine on calcium balance in women," *Journal of Laboratory and Clinical Medicine* 99 (1982): 46–55; G.C. Curhan et al., "A prospective study of dietary calcium and other nutrients and the risk of symptomatic kidney stones," *New England Journal of Medicine* 328:12 (March 25, 1993): 833–8; F.P. Muldowney et al., "Importance of dietary sodium in the hypercalciuria syndrome," *Kidney Int* 22 (1982): 292–96; J. Silver et al., "Sodium-dependent idiopathic hypercalciuria in renal-stone formers," *Lancet* ii (1983): 484–86.

6. J. Shuster et al., "Soft drink consumption and urinary stone recurrence: A randomized prevention trial," *Journal of Clinical Epidemiology* 45 (1992): 911–16.

7. Robert B. Tisserand, *The Art of Aromatherapy.* Rochester, Vt.: Healing Arts Press, 1977: 225, 302.

8. Dr. Barry Rose, *The Family Health Guide to Homeopathy.* Berkeley: Celestial Arts, 1992: 158–59.

9. E. Prien and S. Gershoff, "Magnesium oxide-pyridoxine therapy for recurrent calcium oxalate calculi," *Journal of Urology* 112 (1974): 509–12

Laryngitis

1. Kathi Keville with Peter Korn, *Herbs for Health and Healing.* New York: Berkley Books, 1996: 174, 177–79.

2. David L. Hoffman, M.N.I.M.H., *The New Holistic Herbal.* Boston: Element Books, 1990: 47.

3. Dr. Andrew Lockie and Dr. Nicola Geddes, *The Complete Guide to Homeopathy.* New York: DK Publishing, 1995: 188–89.

4. Linda Rector Page, N.D., Ph.D., *Healthy Healing.* Carmel Valley, Calif.: Healthy Healing Publications, 1997: 410.

5. Mildred Jackson, N.D., and Terri Teague, N.D., D.C., *The Handbook of Alternatives to Chemical Medicine.* Novato, Calif.: New World Library, 1997: 53.

Memory Problems

1. Kathi Keville with Peter Korn, *Herbs for Health and Healing.* New York: Berkley Books, 1996: 386.

2. Dr. Barry Rose, *The Family Health Guide to Homeopathy.* Berkeley: Celestial Arts, 1992: 51.

3. Janet Zand, L.Ac., O.M.D., et al., *Smart Medicine for Healthier Living*. Garden City Park, N.Y.: Avery Publishing Group, 1999: 405–6.

4. Michael T. Murray, N.D., *Encyclopedia of Nutritional Supplements*. Rocklin, Calif.: Prima Publishing, 1996: 140.

5. J.M. Candy et al., "Aluminosilicates and senile plaque formation in Alzheimer's disease," *Lancet* I (1986): 354–57.

Menstrual Cramps

1. Clayton L. Thomas, M.D., M.P.H., ed., *Taber's Cyclopedic Medical Dictionary*, 17th ed. Philadelphia: F.A. Davis, 1993: 591.

2. Susan M. Lark, M.D., *Menstrual Cramps: A Self-Help Program*. Los Altos, Calif.: Westchester, 1993: 12.

3. M.C. P. Rees et al., "Prostaglandins in menstrual fluid in menorrhagia and dysmenorrhea," *British Journal of Obstetrics and Gynaecology* 91 (1984): 673.

4. Robert Ullman, N.D., and Judyth Reichenberg-Ullman, N.D., *Homeopathic Self-Care*. Rocklin, Calif.: Prima Publishing, 1997:253–57.

5. Janet Zand, L.Ac., O.M.D., et al., *Smart Medicine for Healthier Living*. Garden City Park, N.Y.: Avery Publishing Group, 1999: 417.

Migraine

1. Lauran Neergaard, "Findings spell relief for victims of migraines," *San Francisco Chronicle* (June 13, 2000): A2.

2. Michael T. Murray, N.D., and Joseph Pizzorno, N.D., *Encyclopedia of Natural Medicine*. Rocklin, Calif.: Prima Publishing, 1991: 413–14, 420.

3. Jeanne Rose, *The Aromatherapy Book*. Berkeley: North Atlantic Books, 1992: 88, 114, 164.

4. E.S. Johnson et al., "Efficacy of feverfew as prophylactic treatment of migraine," *British Medical Journal*, 291 (1985): 569–73.

5. J. Schoenen et al., "High-dose riboflavin as a prophylactic treatment of migraine: Results of an open pilot study," *Cephalgia* 14 (1994): 328–29.

Motion Sickness

1. Bill Gottlieb, ed., *New Choices in Natural Healing*. Emmaus, Pa.: Rodale Press, 1995: 432.

2. James F. Balch, M.D., and Phyllis A. Balch, C.N.C., *Prescription for Nutritional Healing*. Garden City Park, N.Y.: Avery Publishing Group, 1990: 245.

Muscle Aches and Pains

1. Colleen K. Dodt, *The Essential Oils Book*. Pownal, Vt.: Storey Communications, 1996: 35, 65.

2. Earl Mindell, R.Ph., Ph.D., *Earl Mindell's Herb Bible*. New York: Fireside/Simon & Schuster, 1992: 243–44.

3. Maesimund B. Panos, M.D., and Jane Heimlich, *Homeopathic Medicine at Home*. New York: Jeremy P. Tarcher, 1980: 131.

Muscle Cramp/Spasm

1. Penelope Ody, *Herbs for First Aid*. Los Angeles: Keats Publishing, 1999: 67.

2. Karen Sullivan and C. Norman Shealy, M.D., Ph.D., eds., *The Complete Family Guide to Natural Home Remedies*. Rockport, Mass.: Element Books, 1997: 80.

Nail Problems (Brittle, Ingrown)

1. Valerie Ann Worwood, *The Complete Book of Essential Oils and Aromatherapy*. Novato, Calif.: New World Library, 1991: 99.

2. Bill Gottlieb, ed., *New Choices in Natural Healing*. Emmaus, Pa.: Rodale Press, 1995: 211.

3. Dr. Barry Rose, *The Family Health Guide to Homeopathy.* Berkeley: Celestial Arts, 1992: 198–89.

4. Ann Louise Gittleman, M.S., C.N.S., *The Living Beauty Detox Program.* San Francisco: HarperSanFrancisco, 2000: 135–36.

5. Jean Valnet, M.D., *The Practice of Aromatherapy.* Rochester, Vt.: Healing Arts Press, 1990: 153.

Nausea and Vomiting

1. Robert B. Tisserand, *The Art of Aromatherapy.* Rochester, Vt.: Healing Arts Press, 1977: 206, 247, 269.

2. Patricia Davis, *Aromatherapy: An A-Z.* Saffron Walden, Essex, England: C.W. Daniel Co., 1988: 11.

3. Roger Morrison, M.D., *Desktop Companion to Physical Pathology.* Nevada City, Calif.: Hahnemann Clinic Publishing, 1998.

4. Linda Rector Page, N.D., Ph.D., *Healthy Healing.* Carmel Valley, Calif.: Healthy Healing Publications, 1997: 373.

5. James Kusick, *A Treasury of Natural First Aid Remedies From A to Z.* New York: Parker, 1995: 184.

Nosebleed

1. Janet Zand, L.Ac., O.M.D., et al., *Smart Medicine for Healthier Living.* Garden City Park, N.Y.: Avery Publishing Group, 1999: 445.

2. Karen Sullivan and C. Norman Shealy, M.D., Ph.D., eds., *The Complete Family Guide to Natural Home Remedies.* Rockport, Mass.: Element Books, 1997: 231.

3. James F. Balch, M.D., and Phyllis A. Balch, C.N.C., *Prescription for Nutritional Healing.* Garden City Park, N.Y.: Avery Publishing Group, 1990: 253.

4. Jean Valnet, M.D., *The Practice of Aromatherapy.* Rochester, Vt.: Healing Arts Press, 1990: 153.

Pain (Natural Pain Relievers)

1. S. Bhathena et al., "Decreased plasma enkephalins in copper deficiency in man," *American Journal of Clinical Nutrition* 43 (1986): 42–46.

2. Melvyn R. Werbach, M.D., and Michael T. Murray, N.D., *Nutritional Influences on Illness: A Sourcebook of Clinical Research.* Tarzana, Calif.: Third Line Press, 1994: 342.

3. Kurt Schnaubelt, Ph.D., *Advanced Aromatherapy.* Rochester, Vt.: Healing Arts Press, 1995: 69, 75, 94.

4. G.A. Cordell and O.E. Araujo, "Capsaicin: Identification, nomenclature, and pharmacotherapy," *Annals of Pharmacotherapy* 27 (1993): 330–36; R. Patacchini et al., "Capsaicin-like activity of some natural pungent substances on peripheral ending of visceral primary afferents," *Arch Pharmacology* 342 (1990): 72–77.

5. Chanchal Cabrera, "Healing inflammation: A functional approach," Presentation at Gaia Symposium, 1999. Tape available from Medicines from the Earth; (800) 252-0688.

6. Miranda Castro, R.S.Hom., *The Complete Homeopathy Handbook.* New York: St. Martin's, 1990.

7. H.R. Liberman et al., "Mood, performance and pain sensitivity: Changes induced by food constituents," *Journal of Psychiatric Research* 17 (1983): 135–45.

Poison Ivy/Oak Rash

1. Tom Monte and the editors of *Natural Health* Magazine, *The Complete Guide to Natural Healing.* New York: Perigee/Berkley Publishing Group, 1997: 325.

2. Michael Tierra, L.Ac., OMD, *The Way of Herbs.* New York: Pocket Books, 1990: 336.

3. Roger Morrison, M.D., *Desktop Companion to Physical Pathology.* Nevada City, Calif.: Hahnemann Clinic Publishing, 1998.

Psoriasis

1. J. Voorhees and E. Duell, "Imbalanced cyclic AMP-cyclic GMP levels in psoriasis," *Advances in Cyclic Nucleotide Research* 5 (1975): 755–57.

2. Michael T. Murray, N.D., and Joseph Pizzorno, N.D., *Encyclopedia of Natural Medicine*. Rocklin, Calif.: Prima Publishing, 1991: 487-88; Janet Zand, L.Ac., O.M.D., et al., *Smart Medicine for Healthier Living*. Garden City Park, N.Y.: Avery Publishing Group, 1999: 493.

3. Jean Valnet, M.D., *The Practice of Aromatherapy*. Rochester, Vt.: Healing Arts Press, 1990: 101–2.

4. Valerie Ann Worwood, *The Complete Book of Essential Oils and Aromatherapy*. Novato, Calif.: New World Library, 1991: 96.

5. James A. Duke, Ph.D., *The Green Pharmacy*. New York: St. Martin's, 1997: 452–54.

6. C.N. Ellis et al., "A double-blind evaluation of topical capsaicin in pruritic psoriasis," *Journal of the American Academy of Dermatology* 29:3 (1993): 438–42.

7. Michael T. Murray, N.D., *The Healing Power of Herbs*. Rocklin, Calif.: Prima Publishing, 1995: 75.

8. Roger Morrison, M.D., *Desktop Companion to Physical Pathology*. Nevada City, Calif.: Hahnemann Clinic Publishing, 1998.

Puncture Wound

1. Mark Mayell and the editors of *Natural Health* magazine, *The Natural Health First-Aid Guide*. New York: Pocket Books, 1994: 121.

2. Maesimund B. Panos, M.D., and Jane Heimlich, *Homeopathic Medicine at Home*. New York: Jeremy P. Tarcher, 1980: 59.

3. Mark Mayell and the editors of *Natural Health* Magazine, *The Natural Health First-Aid Guide*. New York: Pocket Books, 1994: 492.

Rash

1. Penelope Ody, *Herbs for First Aid*. Los Angeles: Keats Publishing, 1999: 78.

2. James Kusick, *A Treasury of Natural First Aid Remedies From A to Z*. New York: Parker, 1995: 198.

3. Dr. Barry Rose, *The Family Health Guide to Homeopathy*. Berkeley: Celestial Arts, 1992: 206.

4. Bill Gottlieb, ed., *New Choices in Natural Healing*. Emmaus, Pa.: Rodale Press, 1995: 483–84.

5. James Kusick, *A Treasury of Natural First Aid Remedies From A to Z*. New York: Parker, 1995: 199.

Sciatica

1. Roger Morrison, M.D., *Desktop Companion to Physical Pathology*. Nevada City, Calif.: Hahnemann Clinic Publishing, 1998.

2. H.R. Liberman et al., "Mood, performance and pain sensitivity: Changes induced by food constituents," *Journal of Psychiatric Research* 17 (1983): 135–45.

Shingles (Herpes Zoster)

1. Patricia Davis, *Aromatherapy: An A-Z*. Saffron Walden, Essex, England: C.W. Daniel Co., 1988: 346–47.

2. Stephen Cummings, M.D., and Dana Ullman, M.P.H., *Everybody's Guide to Homeopathic Medicines*. New York: Jeremy P. Tarcher/Putnam, 1997: 263–65.

Shock

1. Patricia Davis, *Aromatherapy: An A-Z*. Saffron Walden, Essex, England: C.W. Daniel Co., 1988: 292.

2. Janet Zand, L.Ac., O.M.D., et al., *Smart Medicine for Healthier Living*. Garden City Park, N.Y.: Avery Publishing Group, 1999: 521.

Sinus Congestion/Infection

1. James F. Balch, M.D., and Phyllis A. Balch, C.N.C., *Prescription for Nutritional Healing.* Garden City Park, N.Y.: Avery Publishing Group, 1990: 286.

2. Roger Morrison, M.D., *Desktop Companion to Physical Pathology.* Nevada City, Calif.: Hahnemann Clinic Publishing, 1998.

Sore Throat

1. Bill Gottlieb, ed., *New Choices in Natural Healing.* Emmaus, Pa.: Rodale Press, 1995: 509–10.

2. Michael T. Murray, N.D., and Joseph Pizzorno, N.D., *Encyclopedia of Natural Medicine.* Rocklin, Calif.: Prima Publishing, 1991: 512.

Sprain/Pulled Ligament

1. Robert Ullman, N.D., and Judyth Reichenberg-Ullman, N.D., *Homeopathic Self-Care.* Rocklin, Calif.: Prima Publishing, 1997: 312.

2. Stephen Cummings, M.D., and Dana Ullman, M.P.H., *Everybody's Guide to Homeopathic Medicines.* New York: Jeremy P. Tarcher/Putnam, 1997: 285.

3. Robert Ullman, N.D., and Judyth Reichenberg-Ullman, N.D., *Homeopathic Self-Care.* Rocklin, Calif.: Prima Publishing, 1997: 311–13.

4. H.R. Liberman et al., "Mood, performance and pain sensitivity: Changes induced by food constituents," *Journal of Psychiatric Research* 17 (1983): 135–45.

Stomachache

1. Bill Gottlieb, ed., *New Choices in Natural Healing.* Emmaus, Pa.: Rodale Press, 1995: 515.

Strep Throat

1. Stephen Cummings, M.D., and Dana Ullman, M.P.H., *Everybody's Guide to Homeopathic Medicines.* New York: Jeremy P. Tarcher/Putnam, 1997: 135.

2. Jeanne Rose, *The Aromatherapy Book.* Berkeley: North Atlantic Books, 1992: 116.

3. Robert B. Tisserand, *The Art of Aromatherapy.* Rochester, Vt.: Healing Arts Press, 1977: 305.

Ibid., 320; Patricia Davis, *Aromatherapy: An A-Z.* Saffron Walden, Essex, England: C.W. Daniel Co., 1988: 208.

5. David Carroll, *The Complete Book of Natural Medicines.* New York: Summit Books, 1980: 390.

Stye

1. David L. Hoffman, M.N.I.M.H., *The New Holistic Herbal.* Boston: Element Books, 1990: 47.

2. Linda Rector Page, N.D., Ph.D., *Healthy Healing.* Carmel Valley, Calif.: Healthy Healing Publications, 1997: 300.

3. Ibid.

Sunburn

1. David L. Hoffman, M.N.I.M.H., *The New Holistic Herbal.* Boston: Element Books, 1990: 82, 164.

2. Penelope Ody, *Herbs for First Aid.* Los Angeles: Keats Publishing, 1999: 95.

3. Bill Gottlieb, ed., *New Choices in Natural Healing.* Emmaus, Pa.: Rodale Press, 1995: 526–27.

4. Editors of *Prevention* Health Books. *Prevention's Healing with Vitamins.* Emmaus, Pa.: Rodale Press, 1996: 522–25.

Surgery (Pre-op and Post-op Support)

1. Web site: www.gaiagarden.com. "Surgical Care" in Health Information Notes. Personal interview with Chanchal Cabrera.

2. Maesimund B. Panos, M.D., and Jane Heimlich, *Homeopathic Medicine at Home.* New York: Jeremy P. Tarcher, 1980: 93.

3. H.R. Liberman et al., "Mood, performance and pain sensitivity: Changes induced by food constituents," *Journal of Psychiatric Research* 17 (1983): 135–45.

Swollen Glands

1. Kurt Schnaubelt, Ph.D., *Advanced Aromatherapy.* Rochester, Vt.: Healing Arts Press, 1995: 74–75, 102.

2. James Kusick, *A Treasury of Natural First Aid Remedies From A to Z.* New York: Parker, 1995: 224.

3. Robert Ullman, N.D., and Judyth Reichenberg-Ullman, N.D., *Homeopathic Self-Care.* Rocklin, Calif.: Prima Publishing, 1997: 334–38.

4. James Kusick, A Treasury of Natural First Aid Remedies From A to Z. New York: Parker, 1995: 225.

Tendonitis

1. Valerie Ann Worwood, *The Complete Book of Essential Oils and Aromatherapy.* Novato, Calif.: New World Library, 1991: 75.

2. James A. Duke, Ph.D., *The Green Pharmacy.* New York: St. Martin's, 1997: 132–33.

3. Ibid., 132.

4. Maesimund B. Panos, M.D., and Jane Heimlich, *Homeopathic Medicine at Home.* New York: Jeremy P. Tarcher, 1980: 78.

5. H.R. Liberman et al., "Mood, performance and pain sensitivity: Changes induced by food constituents," *Journal of Psychiatric Research* 17 (1983): 135–45.

Tinnitus (Ringing in the Ears)

1. Janet Zand, L.Ac., O.M.D., et al., *Smart Medicine for Healthier Living.* Garden City Park, N.Y.: Avery Publishing Group, 1999: 557.

2. P. Yanick, "Solving problematic tinnitus: A clinical scientific approach," *Townsend Letter for Doctors* (February/March 1985): 31; P. Yanick, "Nutritional aspects of tinnitus and hearing disorders," in *Tinnitus and Its Management*, P. Yanick, Jr., and J.G. Clark, eds., Springfield, Ill.: Charles C. Thomas, 1984.

3. Dr. Barry Rose, *The Family Health Guide to Homeopathy.* Berkeley: Celestial Arts, 1992: 90.

4. Jean Valnet, M.D., *The Practice of Aromatherapy.* Rochester, Vt.: Healing Arts Press, 1990: 166.

Tonsillitis

1. Dr. Andrew Lockie and Dr. Nicola Geddes, *The Complete Guide to Homeopathy.* New York: DK Publishing, 1995: 178–79.

2. James F. Balch, M.D., and Phyllis A. Balch, C.N.C., *Prescription for Nutritional Healing.* Garden City Park, N.Y.: Avery Publishing Group, 1990: 301, 318.

Tooth Extraction (Pre-op and Post-op Support)

1. Web site: www.gaiagarden.com. "Surgical Care" in Health Information Notes. Personal interview with Chanchal Cabrera.

2. Dr. Andrew Lockie and Dr. Nicola Geddes, *The Complete Guide to Homeopathy.* New York: DK Publishing, 1995: 164–65.

3. "Prescribing for yourself: Natural remedies for healing after tooth extraction," *Alternative Medicine* 26 (October/November 1998): 16.

4. Stephen Cummings, M.D., and Dana Ullman, M.P.H., *Everybody's Guide to Homeopathic Medicines.* New York: Jeremy P. Tarcher/Putnam, 1997: 289.

5. Maesimund B. Panos, M.D., and Jane Heimlich, *Homeopathic Medicine at Home*. New York: Jeremy P. Tarcher, 1980: 93.

Toothache

1. Miranda Castro, R.S.Hom., *The Complete Homeopathy Handbook*. New York: St. Martin's Press, 1990.

Ulcer (Stomach)

1. R. Petersdorf, *Harrison's Principles of Internal Medicine*, 10th ed. New York: McGraw-Hill, 1983.

2. J. Siegel, "Gastrointestinal ulcer: Arthus reaction," *Annals of Allergy* 32 (1974): 127–30.

3. M. Guslandi, "Importance of defensive factors in the prevention of peptic ulcer recurrence," *Acta Gastro-Enterologica Belgica* 46 (1983): 411–18.

4. Robert B. Tisserand, *The Art of Aromatherapy*. Rochester, Vt.: Healing Arts Press, 1977: 198, 232.

5. W. Shive et al., "Glutamine in treatment of peptic ulcer," *Texas State Journal of Medicine* (November 1957): 840–43.

6. A.G. Turpie et al., "Clinical trial of deglycrrhizinate liquorice in gastric ulcer," *Gut* 10 (1969): 299–303.

7. Dr. Barry Rose, *The Family Health Guide to Homeopathy*. Berkeley: Celestial Arts, 1992: 146–47.

Vaginal Yeast Infection

1. F. Heidrich et al., "Clothing factors and vaginitis," *Journal of Family Practice* 19 (1984): 491–94.

2. Colleen K. Dodt, *The Essential Oils Book*. Pownal, Vt.: Storey Communications, 1996: 42–43.

3. Karen Sullivan and C. Norman Shealy, M.D., Ph.D., eds., *The Complete Family Guide to Natural Home Remedies*. Rockport, Mass.: Element Books, 1997: 84; Stephen Cummings, M.D., and Dana Ullman, M.P.H., *Everybody's Guide to Homeopathic Medicines*, New York: Jeremy P. Tarcher/Putnam, 1997: 181–83.

4. Joy Gardner, *Color and Crystals: A Journey Through the Chakras*. Freedom, Calif.: Crossing Press, 1988: 99–100, 128; Judithann H. David, Ph.D., and J.P. Van Hulle, *Michael's Gemstone Dictionary*, Orinda, Calif.: Affinity Press, 1990: 107.

Vaginitis

1. Diane Stein, *The Natural Remedy Book for Women*. Freedom, Calif.: Crossing Press, 1992: 318.

2. Robert Ullman, N.D., and Judyth Reichenberg-Ullman, N.D., *Homeopathic Self-Care*. Rocklin, Calif.: Prima Publishing, 1997: 352–56.

3. Joy Gardner, *Color and Crystals: A Journey Through the Chakras*. Freedom, Calif.: Crossing Press, 1988: 99-100, 128; Judithann H. David, Ph.D., and J.P. Van Hulle, *Michael's Gemstone Dictionary*. Orinda, Calif.: Affinity Press, 1990: 107.

Viral Infection

1. Kurt Schnaubelt, Ph.D., *Advanced Aromatherapy*. Rochester, Vt.: Healing Arts Press, 1995: 37–39.

2. Patricia Davis, *Aromatherapy: An A-Z*. Saffron Walden, Essex, England: C.W. Daniel Co., 1988: 331.

3. Michael T. Murray, N.D., and Joseph Pizzorno, N.D., *Encyclopedia of Natural Medicine*. Rocklin, Calif.: Prima Publishing, 1991: 60; Michael T. Murray, N.D., *Encyclopedia of Nutritional Supplements*. Rocklin, Calif.: Prima Publishing, 1996: 224.

4. Allan Sachs, D.C., C.C.N., *The Authoritative Guide to Grapefruit Seed Extract*. Mendocino, Calif.: LifeRhythm, 1997: 17.

Wart

1. Dr. Andrew Lockie and Dr. Nicola Geddes, *The Complete Guide to Homeopathy*. New York: DK Publishing, 1995: 188–89.

2. Allan Sachs, D.C., C.C.N., *The Authoritative Guide to Grapefruit Seed Extract*. Mendocino, Calif.: LifeRhythm, 1997: 99–100.

Part III

About the Therapies

1. Kurt Schnaubelt, Ph.D., *Advanced Aromatherapy*. Rochester, Vt.: Healing Arts Press, 1995.

2. Patricia Kaminski and Richard Katz, *Flower Essence Repertory*. Nevada City, Calif.: Flower Essence Society, 1996: 3.

3. Edward Bach and F. J. Wheeler, *The Bach Flower Remedies*. New Canaan, Conn.: Keats Publishing, 1977.

4. Patricia Kaminski and Richard Katz, *Flower Essence Repertory*. Nevada City, Calif.: Flower Essence Society, 1996: 5; Patricia Kaminski and Richard Katz, "Using Flower Essences: A Practical Overview," Nevada City, Calif.: Flower Essence Society, 1994.

5. The information on how to use flower essences is from personal correspondence with Patricia Kaminski and a Flower Essence Society publication: Patricia Kaminski and Richard Katz, "Using Flower Essences: A Practical Overview," Nevada City, Calif.: Flower Essence Society, 1994.

6. Melvyn R. Werbach, M.D., and Michael T. Murray, N.D., *Nutritional Influences on Illness: A Sourcebook of Clinical Research*. Tarzana, Calif.: Third Line Press, 1994: 243; Michael T. Murray, N.D., and Joseph Pizzorno, N.D., *Encyclopedia of Natural Medicine*. Rocklin, Calif.: Prima Publishing, 1991: 459; Linda Rector Page, N.D., Ph.D., *Healthy Healing*. Carmel Valley, Calif.: Healthy Healing Publications, 1997: 196.

7. Linda Rector Page, N.D., Ph.D., *Healthy Healing*. Carmel Valley, Calif.: Healthy Healing Publications, 1997: 202.

8. A. Bu-Abbas et al., "Marked Antimutagenic potential of aqueous green tea extracts: Mechanism of action," *Mutagenesis* 9 (1994): 325–31; J. Wilner, "Green Tea," in *The Cancer Solution*, Boca Raton, FL: Peltec, 1994: 75; H. Mukhtar et al., "Green tea and skin: Anticarcinogenic effects," *Journal of Investigative Dermatology* 102 (1994): 3-7.

9. N.R. Farnsworth et al., "Medicinal plants in therapy," *Bulletin of the World Health Organization* 63:6 (1985): 965–81.

10. Miranda Castro, R.S.Hom., *The Complete Homeopathy Handbook*. New York: St. Martin's Press, 1990: 3–5; Anne Woodham and David Peters, M.D., *Encyclopedia of Healing Therapies*. New York: Dorling Kindersley, 1997: 126.

11. Dr. Barry Rose, *The Family Health Guide to Homeopathy*. Berkeley: Celestial Arts, 1992: 11.

12. Michael T. Murray, N.D., *Encyclopedia of Nutritional Supplements*. Rocklin, Calif.: Prima Publishing, 1996: 8–9.

13. Linda Rector Page, N.D., Ph.D., *Healthy Healing*. Carmel Valley, Calif.: Healthy Healing Publications, 1997: 74.

14. Melvyn R. Werbach, M.D., and Michael T. Murray, N.D., *Botanical Influences on Illness: A Sourcebook of Clinical Research*. New Canaan, Conn.: Keats Publishing, 1988: 256.

15. James F. Balch, M.D., and Phyllis A. Balch, C.N.C., *Prescription for Nutritional Healing*. Garden City Park, N.Y.: Avery Publishing Group, 1990: 33.

16. Linda Rector Page, N.D., Ph.D., *Healthy Healing*. Carmel Valley, Calif.: Healthy Healing Publications, 1997: 103.

17. James F. Balch, M.D., and Phyllis A. Balch, C.N.C., *Prescription for Nutritional Healing*. Garden City Park, N.Y.: Avery Publishing Group, 1990: 7.

18. Inge Dougans, *Reflexology: An Introductory Guide to Foot Massage for Total Health*. Boston, Mass.: Element Books, 1999: 10.

19. Ibid., 14–15.

20. Linda Rector Page, N.D., Ph.D., *Healthy Healing*. Carmel Valley, Calif.: Healthy Healing Publications, 1997: 20.

21. Kevin and Barbara Kunz, *The Complete Guide to Foot Reflexology.* Englewood Cliffs, N.J.: Prentice-Hall, 1980: 19.

22. Ibid., 36.

23. Ann Gillanders, *The Family Guide to Reflexology.* New York: Little, Brown and Co., 1998: 84.

24. Melody, *Love Is in the Earth: A Kaleidoscope of Crystals.* Wheat Ridge, Colo.: Earth-Love Publishing House, 1995: 9–10.

25. Judithann H. David, Ph.D., and J.P. Van Hulle, *Michael's Gemstone Dictionary.* Orinda, Calif.: Affinity Press, 1990: 9.

26. Katrina Raphaell, *Crystal Enlightenment: The Transforming Properties of Crystals and Healing Stones, vol. 1.* Santa Fe, N.M.: Aurora Press, 1985: 10.

27. Daya Sarai Chocron, *Healing with Crystals and Gemstones.* York Beach, Maine: Samuel Weiser, 1986: 104.

28. Judithann H. David, Ph.D., and J.P. Van Hulle, *Michael's Gemstone Dictionary.* Orinda, Calif.: Affinity Press, 1990: 13–15.

29. Daya Sarai Chocron, *Healing with Crystals and Gemstones.* York Beach, Maine: Samuel Weiser, 1986: 30; Melody, *Love Is in the Earth: A Kaleidoscope of Crystals.* Wheat Ridge, Colo.: Earth-Love Publishing House, 1995: 54–55; Katrina Raphaell, *Crystal Enlightenment: The Transforming Properties of Crystals and Healing Stones, vol. 1.* Santa Fe, N.M.: Aurora Press, 1985: 30.

30. Diane Stein, *The Natural Remedy Book for Women.* Freedom, Calif.: Crossing Press, 1992: 84.

31. Joy Gardner, *Color and Crystals: A Journey Through the Chakras.* Freedom, Calif.: Crossing Press, 1988: 78–79.

32. Melody, *Love Is in the Earth: A Kaleidoscope of Crystals.* Wheat Ridge, Colo.: Earth-Love Publishing House, 1995: 62; Katrina Raphaell, *Crystal Enlightenment: The Transforming Properties of Crystals and Healing Stones, vol. 1.* Santa Fe, N.M.: Aurora Press, 1985: 18–19.

Index

The entries in SMALL CAPITAL LETTERS refer to the 102 common conditions addressed in this book.

About the Author

Stephanie Marohn has over fifteen years of experience as a writer and editor. She has coauthored four books on alternative health, published articles in newspapers and magazines, served as senior editor for both *Alternative Medicine* magazine and Future Medicine Publishing, and edited numerous books for Prima Publishing, a leader in the alternative medicine field. Since 1993, Marohn has operated Angel Editing Services, an editing and writing consulting business specializing in nonfiction books, with a particular focus on psychospirituality, metaphysics, and other alternative thought. She lives in Sebastopol, California, north of San Francisco.

Hampton Roads Publishing Company

...for the evolving human spirit

Hampton Roads Publishing Company
publishes books on a variety of subjects,
including metaphysics, health, integrative medicine,
visionary fiction, and other related topics.

For a copy of our latest catalog, call toll-free
(800) 766-8009, or send your name and address to:

Hampton Roads Publishing Company, Inc.
1125 Stoney Ridge Road
Charlottesville, VA 22902

e-mail: hrpc@hrpub.com
www.hrpub.com